T0263465

Melanoma and Pigmented Lesions

Guest Editors

JULIE E. RUSSAK, MD
DARRELL S. RIGEL, MD

DERMATOLOGIC CLINICS

www.derm.theclinics.com

Consulting Editor
BRUCE H. THIERS, MD

July 2012 • Volume 30 • Number 3

SAUNDERS an imprint of ELSEVIER, Inc.

W.B. SAUNDERS COMPANY
A Division of Elsevier Inc.

1600 John F. Kennedy Boulevard • Suite 1800 • Philadelphia, PA 19103-2899

http://www.theclinics.com

DERMATOLOGIC CLINICS Volume 30, Number 3
July 2012 ISSN 0733-8635, ISBN-13: 978-1-4557-3853-3

Editor: Stephanie Donley

Dermatologic Clinics (ISSN 0733-8635) is published quarterly by Elsevier Inc., 360 Park Avenue South, New York, NY 10010-1710. Months of publication are January, April, July, and October. Business and editorial offices: 1600 John F. Kennedy Blvd., Suite 1800, Philadelphia, PA 19103-2899. Customer service office: 11830 Westline Drive, St. Louis, MO 63146. Periodicals postage paid at New York, NY, and additional mailing offices. Subscription prices are USD 346.00 per year for US individuals, USD 512.00 per year for US institutions, USD 404.00 per year for Canadian individuals, USD 613.00 per year for Canadian institutions, USD 473.00 per year for international individuals, USD 613.00 per year for international institutions, USD 161.00 per year for US students/residents, and USD 233.00 per year for Canadian and international students/residents. International air speed delivery is included in all *Clinics* subscription prices. All prices are subject to change without notice. **POSTMASTER:** Send address changes to *Dermatologic Clinics*, Elsevier Health Sciences Division, Subscription Customer Service, 3251 Riverport Lane, Maryland Heights, MO 63043. **Customer Service: 1-800-654-2452 (U.S. and Canada); 314-447-8871 (outside U.S. and Canada). Fax: 314-447-8029. E-mail: journalscustomerservice-usa@elsevier.com (for print support); journalsonlinesupport-usa@elsevier.com (for online support).**

Reprints. For copies of 100 or more, of articles in this publication, please contact the Commercial Reprints Department, Elsevier Inc., 360 Park Avenue South, New York, New York 10010-1710. Tel.: (212) 633-3813; Fax: (212) 462-1935; Email: reprints@elsevier.com.

The *Dermatologic Clinics* is covered in *MEDLINE/PubMed (Index Medicus), Current Contents/Clinical Medicine, Excerpta Medica, Chemical Abstracts,* and *ISI/BIOMED.*

Printed and bound by CPI Group (UK) Ltd, Croydon, CR0 4YY

Transferred to Digital Print 2012

Contributors

CONSULTING EDITOR

BRUCE H. THIERS, MD
Professor and Chairman, Department of
Dermatology and Dermatologic Surgery,
Medical University of South Carolina,
Charleston, South Carolina

GUEST EDITORS

JULIE E. RUSSAK, MD
Clinical Instructor, Department of
Dermatology, Mt. Sinai School of Medicine,
New York, New York

DARRELL S. RIGEL, MD
Clinical Professor, Department of
Dermatology, New York University School
of Medicine, New York, New York

AUTHORS

CHRISTINE S. AHN, BA
Department of Dermatology, Wake Forest
School of Medicine, Winston Salem,
North Carolina

MARY KATE BAKER, MPH
Doctoral Candidate, Department of
Community & Behavioral Health, East
Tennessee State University College of
Public Health, Johnson City, Tennessee

CHRISTOPHER A. BARKER, MD
Department of Radiation Oncology, Memorial
Sloan-Kettering Cancer Center, New York,
New York

NORMAN A. BROOKS, MD
Skin Cancer Medical Center, Encino,
California

SUNANDANA CHANDRA, MD
NYU Medical Oncology Fellow, NYU School of
Medicine, New York, New York

CLAY J. COCKERELL, MD
Clinical Professor, Departments of
Dermatology and Pathology, UT Southwestern
Medical Center, Dallas, Texas

MELODY J. EIDE, MD, MPH
Departments of Dermatology and Public
Health Sciences, Henry Ford Hospital,
Detroit, Michigan

MICHELE J. FARBER, MD
Jefferson Medical College, Thomas Jefferson
University, Philadelphia, Pennsylvania

LAURA KORB FERRIS, MD, PhD
Assistant Professor of Dermatology,
Department of Dermatology, University
of Pittsburgh Medical Center, Pittsburgh,
Pennsylvania

ROBERT J. FRIEDMAN, MD, MSc (Med)
Department of Dermatology, Clinical
Professor, NYU School of Medicine, New York,
New York

RYAN J. HARRIS, MD
Dermatology Research Fellow, Department of
Dermatology, University of Pittsburgh Medical
Center, Pittsburgh, Pennsylvania

EDWARD R. HEILMAN, MD
Clinical Associate Professor, Departments of
Dermatology and Pathology, State University
of New York Downstate Medical Center,
Brooklyn, New York

JOEL J. HILLHOUSE, PhD
Professor, Department of Community &
Behavioral Health, East Tennessee State
University College of Public Health, Johnson
City, Tennessee

ANDREA M. HUI, MD
Department of Dermatology, State University
of New York Downstate Medical Center,
Brooklyn, New York

MICHAEL JACOBSON, MD
Department of Dermatology, State University
of New York Downstate Medical Center,
Brooklyn, New York

SVEN KRENGEL, MD
Department of Dermatology, University of
Lübeck; Dermatological Group Practice,
Lübeck, Germany

NANCY Y. LEE, MD
Department of Radiation Oncology, Memorial
Sloan-Kettering Cancer Center, New York,
New York

STEVEN M. LEVINE, MD
Institute of Reconstructive Plastic Surgery,
Department of Plastic Surgery, New York
University Langone Medical Center, New York,
New York

EMILY G. LITTLE, MD
University of Michigan Medical School,
Ann Arbor, Michigan; Section of Dermatology,
East Carolina University School of Medicine,
Greenville, North Carolina

ASHFAQ A. MARGHOOB, MD
Memorial Sloan-Kettering Skin Cancer Center
at Hauppauge, Hauppauge, New York

KAVITA MARIWALLA, MD
Assistant Clinical Professor, Columbia
University, New York; Assistant Clinical
Professor of Dermatology, State University of
New York at Stony Brook, East Setauket,
New York

ORIT MARKOWITZ, MD
Department of Dermatology, State University
of New York Downstate Medical Center,
Brooklyn; Department of Dermatology, Mount
Sinai School of Medicine, New York, New York

JENNIFER S. MULLIKEN, MA, BA
New York University School of Medicine,
New York, New York

ANNA C. PAVLICK, BSN, MS, DO
Associate Professor of Medicine and
Dermatology, Director, NYU Melanoma
Program, NYU Cancer Institute, New York,
New York

BABAR K. RAO, MD
Clinical Associate Professor of Dermatology
and Pathology, Department of Dermatology,
Robert Wood Johnson Medical School,
University of Medicine and Dentistry of
New Jersey, Somerset, New Jersey

DARRELL S. RIGEL, MD
Clinical Professor, Department of
Dermatology, New York University School
of Medicine, New York, New York

JUNE K. ROBINSON, MD
Research Professor of Dermatology, Department
of Dermatology, Northwestern University
Feinberg School of Medicine, Chicago, Illinois

JULIE E. RUSSAK, MD
Clinical Instructor, Department of
Dermatology, Mt. Sinai School of Medicine,
New York, New York

RICHARD L. SHAPIRO, MD, FACS
Associate Professor of Surgery, Division of
Surgical Oncology, Department of Surgery, NYU
Clinical Cancer Center, New York University
Langone Medical Center, New York, New York

DANIEL M. SIEGEL, MD
Department of Dermatology, State University
of New York Downstate Medical Center,
Brooklyn, New York

DAVID SILVERSTEIN, MD
State University of New York at Stony Brook,
East Setauket, New York

ARTHUR J. SOBER, MD, FAAD
Medical Director, Medical Dermatology,
Department of Dermatology, Massachusetts
General Hospital; Professor of Dermatology,
Harvard Medical School, Boston, Massachusetts

OLIVER J. WISCO, DO, FAAD
Director of Mohs Surgery, Dermatology Clinic,
81st Medical Group, Keesler AFB, Mississippi;
Visiting Melanoma Research Fellow,
Massachusetts General Hospital's Wellman
Center for Photobiology Research, Boston,
Massachusetts

Contents

The incidence of melanoma is rising worldwide, and in the United States has increased by approximately 2.8% annually since 1981. Melanoma is more common in whites, and is generally more prevalent in men. However, there is a 6.1% annual increase in US incidence of melanomas in white women younger than age 44, with growing concern that increases in skin cancer in younger women may reflect recent trends in indoor tanning. Melanoma incidence is also greater in higher economic groups. Globally, melanoma incidence is highest in Australia, followed by the United States and parts of Europe.

Melanoma is an important public health problem in the United States and worldwide. The incidence of melanoma continues to increase at a high rate and deaths from melanoma are also increasing. The endogenous risk factors that are currently recognized are in many cases surrogates for genetic markers yet to be determined. Exogenous risk factors need to be better defined and understood to help develop better public education programs that can change risk behaviors and subsequently lower future incidence and mortality from melanoma.

Total cumulative sun exposure is associated with the development of squamous cell and basal cell cancers, whereas intense intermittent sun exposure is associated with the development of melanoma. Exposure to UV radiation is the only known modifiable cause of melanoma, but the role of sunscreen in melanoma prevention remains somewhat controversial. This article discusses how UV radiation contributes to the pathogenesis of melanoma, how sunscreen modulates the action of UV radiation on the skin, and the effect of sunscreen on the risk of developing melanoma. A review of available sunscreen agents and their sun-protective properties is also included.

Lack of information and misinformation abounds regarding the potential risks of malignancy, management approaches, benefits of surgical intervention, follow-up strategies, and overall prognosis for individuals with congenital melanocytic nevi (CMN). This review is intended to provide answers to questions that frequently arise shortly after the birth of individuals with CMN, especially of larger types.

Dysplastic nevi have been a subject of much debate since their original description in 1978. Although some question the biological potential of dysplastic nevi themselves, several studies have shown that their presence confers substantial risk for melanoma. In addition to predisposing patients to melanoma, dysplastic nevi have been shown to harbor genetic mutations, indicating their position on a continuum between banal nevi and melanomas. Dysplastic nevi are also clinically relevant as mimickers of melanoma, and can be challenging diagnostically. This article reviews the history, epidemiology, biology and genetics, clinical features, histopathologic features, and management guidelines for patients with these lesions.

Skin cancer is a major public health concern, and tanning remains a modifiable risk factor. Multidimensional influences, including psychosocial, individual, environmental, and policy-related factors, create the milieu for individuals to engage in tanning. Parents and physicians can modify the behavior of teens and young adults using strategies based on harm reduction. Environmental and policy-related factors similar to those used to limit smoking by restricting access of minors to cigarettes in the United States in the 20th century need to be created. Federal regulations can restrict direct advertising and the excise tax can be increased to a prohibitive amount. Social networking may assist with affect regulation.

This article presents an overview of the history and development of dermatoscopy over the last 2 decades. The common dermatoscopic diagnostic algorithms are discussed, including classic pattern analysis, the ABCD rule (asymmetry, border, color, and dermatoscopic structures), 7-point checklist, and Menzies method, as well as a new method by the authors (ASAP: a simple and practical approach). In addition, evidence on the clinical impact and challenges of dermatoscopy for the diagnosis and management of pigmented lesions and the importance of training are reviewed.

Although new technologies are becoming available to aid in diagnosis, the skin biopsy continues to be the fundamental tool of the dermatologist to evaluate the nature of a pigmented lesion. There are 3 major techniques for the biopsy of a pigmented lesion: shave biopsy, punch/incisional biopsy, and excisional biopsy. This article discusses when to biopsy a pigmented lesion and reviews the different biopsy techniques, with reference to specific clinical scenarios.

Although melanoma represents only 10% of all skin cancer diagnoses, it accounts for at least 65% of all skin cancer–related deaths. The number of new cutaneous melanoma cases projected during 2010 was 68,000—a 23% increase from the 2004 prediction of 55,100 cases. In 2015, the lifetime risk of developing melanoma is estimated to increase to 1 in 50. As the incidence of melanoma continues to rise, now more than ever, clinicians and histopathologists must have familiarity with the various clinical and pathologic features of cutaneous melanoma.

Radiation therapy is used infrequently for cutaneous melanoma, despite research suggesting benefit in certain clinical scenarios. This review presents data forming the highest level of evidence supporting the use of radiation therapy. Retrospective and prospective studies demonstrate radiation therapy for primary tumors is associated with high control rates. Two randomized trials have found improvements in regional control with adjuvant radiotherapy to regional lymphatics. Retrospective and prospective studies demonstrate radiation therapy is associated with palliative response and metastatic tumor control. Optimal care of melanoma patients involves radiation therapy; awareness of this is incumbent of clinicians caring for patients with this disease.

Detection of melanoma at an early stage is crucial to improving survival rates in melanoma. Accurate diagnosis by current techniques including dermatoscopy remains difficult, and new tools are needed to improve our diagnostic abilities. This article discusses recent advances in diagnostic techniques including confocal scanning laser microscopy, MelaFind, SIAscopy, and noninvasive genomic detection, as well as other future possibilities to aid in diagnosing melanoma. Advantages and barriers to implementation of the various technologies are also discussed.

DERMATOLOGIC CLINICS

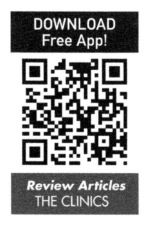

Preface

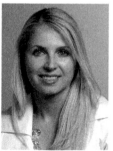 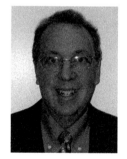

Julie E. Russak, MD   Darrell S. Rigel, MD
Guest Editors

Skin cancer rates are rising dramatically. Melanoma particularly is an increasingly important public health problem in the United States and worldwide. The incidence of melanoma has been increasing faster than that of any other cancer in the United States. Overall, melanoma incidence increased 2.9% annually from 1981 to 2006. Statistically significant increases are occurring for tumors of all histologic subtypes and thicknesses, including those greater than 4 mm. Invasive melanoma currently is the fifth most frequently diagnosed cancer in men and the sixth most frequently diagnosed cancer in women in the United States. In 2012, 76,250 newly diagnosed cases of invasive melanoma and 55,560 cases of in situ melanoma are expected. At current rates, the lifetime risk of an American developing invasive melanoma is 1 in 52 overall and 1 in 38 for Caucasian men and 1 in 56 in Caucasian women. This contrasts dramatically with a lifetime risk of 1 in 1500 for Americans born in 1935. Approximately 9180 people are expected to die from melanoma in the United States during 2012, accounting for 66% of all skin cancer deaths.

The public health ramifications of these facts and the importance of early detection are profound. Melanoma, once viewed as a relatively uncommon disease limited in recognition to dermatologists and surgeons alone, is now being seen on a daily basis by primary care physicians, oncologists, and other health care professionals. The resulting need to educate all of these groups on early recognition and managing patients with melanoma is also increasing.

Primary prevention efforts are also becoming increasingly important. Melanoma is one of the few cancers where we can identify and modify the risk factors. Excess ultraviolet exposure whether from the sun or artificial exposure has been proven to increase the risk of the developing melanoma. Simple behavioral changes can lead to a significant decrease in a person's chance of developing skin cancer. An understanding of the mechanisms and risk factors is critical in counseling patients to facilitate prevention. Melanoma is the one of the most clear-cut cases of the disease where early detection and treatment are critical. Therefore, the need for medical practitioners to be able to recognize and treat melanoma in its earliest stages cannot be overemphasized.

Approaches to melanoma diagnosis have dynamically evolved during the past twenty years. In the 1990s, dermoscopy enabled the recognition of new subsurface features to differentiate between malignant and benign pigmented lesions. During the last decade, new computer-based technologies, confocal microscopy, digital photographic documentation, topical immune response modulators,

Dermatol Clin 30 (2012) xi–xii
doi:10.1016/j.det.2012.05.003
0733-8635/12/$ – see front matter © 2012 Published by Elsevier Inc.

and advances in immunotherapy, lymph node biopsies, photoprotection agents, and our understanding of the biologic basis of this cancer and the deleterious effects of tanning salons also emphasize our need to understand this cancer within a broader context. All of these topics are covered in depth in this issue to facilitate a wide-range understanding of this cancer.

We hope that you will find this issue of *Dermatologic Clinics* useful in navigating current and developing techniques to diagnose melanoma and it will enhance the goal that we all strive for—lowering the morbidity and mortality from this disease.

Julie E. Russak, MD
Department of Dermatology
Mt. Sinai School of Medicine
One Gustave L. Levy Place
New York, NY 10029-6574, USA

Darrell S. Rigel, MD
Department of Dermatology
New York University School of Medicine
550 First Avenue
New York, NY 10016, USA

E-mail addresses:
julierussak@gmail.com (J.E. Russak)
Darrell.rigel@gmail.com (D.S. Rigel)

Update on the Current State of Melanoma Incidence

Emily G. Little, MD[a,b], Melody J. Eide, MD, MPH[c,d],*

KEYWORDS

• Melanoma • Incidence • Epidemiology • SEER registry

KEY POINTS

• Melanoma incidence has been increasing since data collection began in the United States in the 1970s.
• There is an increase in melanoma incidence in young women, and there is concern that this may reflect recent trends in indoor tanning.
• Melanoma incidence is highest in higher socioeconomic groups, but when it occurs in lower socioeconomic groups it is usually diagnosed at a later stage.

Although advances have been made in the war on cancer, melanoma incidence and mortality have continued to increase over the past three decades. The American Cancer Society anticipates more than 70,000 cases of melanoma in 2011,[1] and based on rates from 2005 to 2007, it is estimated that almost 2% of Americans will be diagnosed with melanoma during their lifetime.[2] This correlates with 1 in 52 Americans receiving a melanoma diagnosis during their lifetime.[2] This article discusses the current state of melanoma incidence, including time trends and sociodemographic patterns, and discusses plausible explanations for these findings.

US TRENDS IN MELANOMA INCIDENCE OVER TIME

Melanoma incidence has been on the rise in the United States for several decades as tracked by the US Surveillance, Epidemiology, and End Results (SEER) program (**Fig. 1**). The SEER program, which is supported through the National Cancer Institute, provides cancer surveillance in the United States through registries representative of the US population.[3] Data collection began in 1973 and it has grown from the original nine locations to include more than 17 registries and 28% of the US population. Melanoma age-adjusted incidence in 2008 (the most recent SEER data available) in the United States has reached 22.5 per 100,000 (2000 US population).[4] Melanoma incidence has been increasing steadily by roughly 2.8% annually from 1981 to 2008.[4] According to a recently published study, which includes SEER and National Program of Cancer Registries data, the national rate of melanoma was 19.2 per 100,000 from 2004 to 2006.[5] Combining the two databases during that time period covers 77.6% of the US population.[5]

Gender

The incidence and the mortality of melanoma are generally greater in men than women. In 2008,

No relationships to disclose.

[a] University of Michigan Medical School, 3225 Chamberlain Circle, Ann Arbor, MI 48103, USA; [b] Section of Dermatology, East Carolina University School of Medicine, 517 Moye Boulevard, Greenville, NC 27834-2847, USA; [c] Department of Dermatology, Henry Ford Hospital, 3031 West Grand Boulevard, Suite 800, Detroit, MI 48202, USA; [d] Department of Public Health Sciences, Henry Ford Hospital, One Ford Place, Detroit, MI 48202, USA

* Corresponding author. Department of Dermatology, Henry Ford Hospital, 3031 West Grand Boulevard, Suite 800, Detroit, MI 48202.

E-mail address: Meide1@hfhs.org

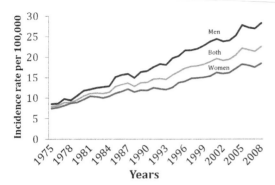

Fig. 1. Age-adjusted melanoma incidence rates, SEER, 1973 to 2008.

the incidence of melanoma in all males was 29.1 per 100,000 compared with 19 per 100,000 in women.[4] In 2008, age-adjusted incidence for men remains higher than for women at 28.3 and 18.5 cases per 100,000, respectively.[4] The percent increase from 1986 to 2008 in men is 3% (delay-adjusted), and is 2.4% annually for women between 1980 and 2008.[4]

Similarly, the annual percent increase in melanoma for all ages is greater in men than women, 6.1% compared with 2.8%.[4] However, there is growing concern about a shift toward higher incidence in young women. Younger than age 44 the incidence for women is 8.2 per 100,000, whereas for men it is 5.3 per 100,000.[4] This higher incidence of melanoma in young women compared with young men is generally an increase in thin lesions.[6] There is growing concern that increases in skin cancer in younger women may reflect recent trends in indoor tanning.

The most common location for melanoma in men is on the trunk, followed by the upper extremities.[5] In women, the lower extremities are the most common location for melanoma.[5]

Race and Ethnicity

Melanoma most commonly affects whites, but it also occurs in other races. From 2004 to 2008 the age-adjusted rates in Hispanic, black, Asian/Pacific Islander (API), and American Indian/Alaska Native (AI/AN) were 3.9, 1, 1.4, and 3.7 per 100,000, respectively (**Fig. 2**).[4] This is in comparison with non-Hispanic whites, in whom the incidence is 28.7 per 100,000.[4] The lower incidence of melanoma in darker-skinned individuals is attributed to the protective effects of higher melanin densities.[7]

In Hispanics, AI/AN, and APIs, a greater percentage of melanomas occurred in younger age groups (24.4%, 22.9%, and 20.8% less than 40 years old, respectfully) compared with blacks and whites (15.8% and 14.3% younger than 40 years old).[7] Most cases in blacks, API, and Hispanics were female, compared with whites, in which men were more likely to develop melanoma.[7] In blacks, acral lentiginous was the most common subtype, whereas superficial spreading was the most common in all other racial groups.[7] The rates of melanoma rise with increasing age in all groups.[7] Nonwhite groups were more likely to be diagnosed with distant melanomas. Only 4% of melanomas in whites are distant at diagnosis, whereas anywhere between 7% and 13% of other ethnic groups have advanced melanomas at diagnosis.[7]

Tumor Characteristics

In the United States from 1992 to 2004, in non-Hispanic whites 37.5% were superficial spreading melanoma, 7.4% were nodular melanoma, 7.3%

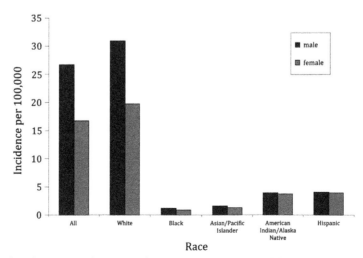

Fig. 2. Age-adjusted melanoma incidence rates by race, SEER-17, 2004 to 2008.

were lentigo maligna, 0.9% were acral lentiginous melanoma, and 4.4% were other subtypes.[8] There were no significant differences in the proportions of the histologic subtypes over the time interval.[8] Similar proportions are reported from 2004 to 2006 as 28.8% superficial spreading, 6.9% nodular, 6% lentigo maligna, and 1% acral lentiginous, although 57.2% were reported as melanoma not-otherwise-specified.[5] Of the subcategories of melanoma not-otherwise-specified, 1.2% were desmoplastic melanoma and 0.4% were amelanotic melanoma.[5]

In non-Hispanic whites aged 0 to 85 and older from 1992 to 2004, there were increases in all groups of tumor thickness.[8] For tumors less than or equal to 1 mm there was a 4.8% increase for men and 4.7% for women, and for tumors greater than or equal to 4.01 mm a 4.1% increase for men and 3.3% increase for women.[8] The annual percent change in incidence rates for tumor thickness were even greater in the subgroup older than age 65.[8] In a similar analysis of SEER data from 1992 to 2006, there were increases in melanoma incidence in men of all tumor thickness for those aged 65 and older.[6] In younger men, only thin tumors increased in incidence.[6] Similarly, among women, tumors of all depth increased in incidence over the time interval, except tumors greater than 2 mm in women aged 40 to 64 and tumors 2.01 to 4 mm deep in women younger than 40 years old.[6] In men and women older than 65 years, there was almost a twofold increase in the rates of thick tumors compared with thin tumors.[6]

International

Melanoma incidence is significant outside of the United States. Australia has the largest incidence of melanoma, with incidence rates roughly twice that of the United States. The Australian Institute of Health and Welfare has been collecting statistics about melanoma incidence in Australia since 1982, and these are available through 2007.[9] In 2007, there were 10,342 melanomas, an incidence of 46.7 per 100,000 people (age-standardized to 2001 Australian population).[9] For Australians, there is a 1 in 28 risk of developing melanoma by the age of 75.[9] The average annual change in incidence rates for melanoma of the skin in Australia from 1982 to 2007 is 2.3%, comparable with US changes.[9]

In Europe, incidence has not reached the same magnitude as the United States and Australia.[10] In the United Kingdom the incidence from 1998 to 2002 for men ranges from 6.9 to 10.7 age-standardized rate per 100,000 and 7.1 to 12.6 per 100,000 for females.[10] In males, the incidence is

the greatest in Germany, Norway, and Switzerland, with age-standardized rates of 12.7, 14.2, and 18.6 per 100,000, respectively.[10] In females, Denmark, Norway, Iceland, and Switzerland have the highest age-standardized rates at 14.1, 14.6, 19, and 19.6 per 100,000, respectively.[10] In general, melanoma incidence rates in whites decrease with distance from the equator.[11] However, in Western Europe, the inverse pattern is observed, with greatest incidence in the North.[11] This has been postulated to be because lighter-skinned northern Europeans travel to southern Europe where they receive intense, intermittent sun exposure.[11]

Risk Factors

Established risk factors for melanoma are genetic and phenotypic traits, risk behaviors, and environmental factors.[12] Genetic and phenotypic predisposition can be further specified as increasing age, fair skin and hair color, greater than 20 nevi, freckling, greater than or equal to three atypical nevi, greater likelihood of burning with sun exposure, immunosuppression, previous psoralen UV-A treatment, solar keratoses, squamous cell carcinoma, xeroderma pigmentosum, and family history of dysplastic nevi or melanoma.[12] Environmental exposure is important in melanoma with attention being given to history of greater or equal to three episodes of sunburn; periodic excessive sunlight exposure (vacations with intense exposure); possibly long-term continuous sunlight exposure; and UV exposure at tanning salons.[12] Other environmental factors, such as ozone depletion and latitudes closer to the equator, may also relate.[12]

SOCIODEMOGRAPHIC FACTORS IN MELANOMA INCIDENCE
Income

Over the past several years it has come to light that melanoma is generally more common in those of higher economic class. Reyes-Ortiz and colleagues[12] performed a review of 25 studies in the United States and other countries examining socioeconomic status (SES) and melanoma incidence. In all except two, there was a positive association between higher SES and increased melanoma incidence.[12] This effect was greatest in men of higher SES.[12] The authors proposed several possible explanations. The first is biologic susceptibility.[12] Patients that have melanomas and increased SES are likely to have phenotypic risk factors, including fair skin and hair color, increased likelihood to burn instead of tan, increased freckling, and a large number of atypical melanocytic nevi.[12]

The second is increased UV exposure.[12] High SES groups have greater leisure time and more opportunity for periodic excessive sunlight exposure.[11,12] In the Norwegian Women and Cancer Study, the average number of sunburns yearly increased by level of education, which likely represents greater travel to southern climates, common in middle and high SES in Norway.[13] Similarly, people living in larger towns in Sweden (higher incidence of melanoma) have increased frequency of foreign travel, detected by increased passport use.[14]

Although melanoma incidence parallels SES, a recent US study suggested that all SES groups may actually have increasing incidences of melanoma. According to Linos and colleagues,[8] California patients living in areas of highest SES were at higher absolute risk of all melanomas. However, patients living in low SES areas experienced the greatest increases in incidence, and the greatest increases in incidence were among the thickest tumors (2.01–4 and $\geq$4 mm).[8] Similarly, Greenlee and Howe[15] demonstrated that living at higher poverty levels increased the odds of late-stage melanoma by twofold.

A similar relationship between SES and melanoma incidence has been reported in Europe.[16] In Denmark, Birch-Johansen and colleagues[16] evaluated all 3.22 million Danish residents born between 1925 and 1973 without a previous history of cancer. Socioeconomic, demographic, and health-related indicators were obtained from Danish registers.[16] Melanomas diagnosed from 1994 to 2003 were associated with the highest disposable income, an incidence rate ratio (IRR) of 1.4 (confidence interval [CI], 1.3–1.5); higher education, with an IRR of 1.7 (CI, 1.6–1.9); and unemployment was negatively associated, with an IRR of 0.8 (CI, 0.7–0.9).[16]

Similar results have been found in England, where the most deprived had a relative risk of 0.5.[17] Shack and colleagues[17] assigned a socioeconomic group based on their address at the time of diagnosis, using the income domain of the Index of Multiple Deprivation.

Similar findings have been reported by Goodman and colleagues,[18] who showed there is a lower incidence of melanoma in outdoor workers. Among indoor occupations, funeral director/embalmers and dentists had the highest incidence (odds ratio, 5.3 [CI, 2.1–13.6] and 3.1 [CI, 1.9–5.1], respectively).[18]

Education

In 1999, the National Cancer Institute initiated the SEER-National Longitudinal Mortality Study, which connects the SEER registry to self-reported, detailed demographic and socioeconomic data from the Census Bureau's Current Population Survey.[19] Of the categories of education, family income, poverty status, and place of residence, only education and income were significant for differences in incidence of melanoma.[19] Those with less than a high school education had a relative risk of 0.55 (CI, 0.37–0.82), signifying a lower risk of melanoma in the less-educated population.[19] Similarly, those with a family income less than $12,500 had a relative risk of 0.59 (CI, 0.36–0.95).[19]

In Iceland, the population is small and ethnically similar and has been postulated to have high social equity.[20] However, there are still differences in SES, and education has been found to be the most reliable measure of social status in Iceland.[20] Vidarsdottir and colleagues[20] conducted a study linking the Icelandic Cancer Registry and information on education from the 1981 census. Higher educational level was associated with an increased risk of melanoma. The least educated had a standardized incidence ratio of 0.60 (CI, 0.36–0.85), and the standardized incidence ratio was 147% higher in the highest-educated group.[20]

The effect of education on melanoma incidence was also reported in the United States.[21] Harrison and colleagues[21] compared SEER melanoma incidence statistics from 1973 to 1993 with SES information from the 1950, 1960, 1970, 1980, and 1990 census data. The percentage of high school graduates over time was significantly associated with an increase in melanoma incidence, which was not mediated by income, age, or gender.[21]

ENVIRONMENTAL IMPACT ON MELANOMA
Indoor UV

Solar radiation is divided into UV-A and UV-B, which represent 95% and 5% of the UV radiation, respectively.[22] Sunburn is most often caused by UV-B; however, high doses of UV-A have also been implicated.[23] Tanning beds contain a similar ratio of UV-A/UV-B to natural sunlight, but they can have much higher UV amounts, 10 to 15 times greater than the noonday sun.[23] Since their first inception in the 1970s, tanning beds have gained enormous popularity, with 60% of women and 50% of men in Northern Europe aged 18 to 50 years old stating ever-use of tanning beds by the late 1990s.[23] This time course correlates with an increase in melanoma incidence, particularly among young women,[24] who are most likely to use tanning beds.[23] Purdue and colleagues[24] evaluated SEER data by year of birth and incidence by 5-year age groups and time periods. The age-adjusted annual incidence increased from 5.5 per

100,000 (4.5–6.6) in 1973 to 13.9 per 100,000 (12.7–15.2) in 2004.[24]

There have been individual studies that report a positive association between tanning beds and melanoma, and others that report a negative association. A meta-analysis published in 2005 sought to gather the information from smaller case-controlled studies.[25] The summary odds ratio has an elevated risk of 1.25 (1.05–1.49)[25] of having a melanoma if ever exposed to a tanning bed. A greater risk was reported if the first exposure to tanning beds was as a young adult (odds ratio, 1.69 [CI, 1.32–2.18]).[25] Similar results were found in a more comprehensive meta-analysis performed by the International Agency for Research on Cancer Working Group on artificial UV light and skin cancer,[23] where ever use of tanning beds was associated with a relative risk of 1.15 (1.00–1.31) for developing melanoma. Also, first exposure before the age of 35 years increased the relative risk to 1.75 (1.35–2.26).[23] Recently, the International Agency for Research on Cancer has determined that there is sufficient evidence that UV-emitting tanning devices are carcinogenic to humans.[22] California has become the first state to ban tanning bed use for those younger than 18.[26]

Health Care Use

Melanoma prognosis is dependent on thickness. Aitken and colleagues[27] performed a case-control study to assess if whole-body skin examination is associated with a reduced incidence of thick melanoma. They determined that a whole-body clinical skin examination in the 3 years before the diagnosis of melanoma was associated with a 14% lower risk of having a greater than 0.75-mm melanoma.[27]

More skin examination screening data are necessary, as evidenced by differing screening recommendation guidelines. The American Cancer Society recommends skin cancer screening every 3 years for adults until age 40, and annually thereafter. The US Preventive Services Task Force has not believed evidence was sufficient to support the use of full skin examination as a recommended cancer screening.[28]

Receipt of full-body skin examination varies based on several factors. Individuals with lower SES are also less likely to report having a skin examination.[28] Older (≥50 years), white non-Hispanic, educated (high school diploma or greater) adults who have a usual place of care and have health insurance are more likely to have a recent skin examination.[28] According to the National Health Interview Surveys, the

percentage of the US adult population who had ever had a skin examination conducted by a doctor was 20.6% in 1992, 20.9% in 1998, and 14.5% in 2000.[28]

Overdiagnosis

The substantial increase in the reported incidence of melanoma has caused some to argue that there is not an actual increase; rather, it is an effect of over biopsying. Welch and colleagues[29] used Medicare claims to obtain annual population-based rates of skin biopsy in patients aged 65 and older and correlated them with the rates of melanoma incidence in the SEER program from 1986 to 2001. During the time period there was a 2.5-fold increase in the average biopsy rate, and a 2.4-fold increase in average melanoma incidence.[29] Most of the increase in melanomas were in situ and local disease, and there was no increase in mortality during this time period.[29] From this, the authors concluded that the growth in rate of skin biopsies correlates with an increased rate of melanoma detection, and suggested that increases in incidence might be attributable to healthcare overuse.[29]

However, Linos and colleagues[8] state that persistent increases among thicker tumors contest the argument that increases in incidence are caused by increased surveillance and detection. In their study, which also analyzed SEER data, there was an increase of 3.86% of thick (>4 mm) melanomas. Hollestein and coworkers[30] also conclude that because the incidence of melanomas of all Breslow thickness categories has increased, as have the mortality rates, the melanoma epidemic in The Netherlands (and likewise around the world) is real, and not just an artifact of overdiagnosis. In a recent analysis of SEER data, Jemal and colleagues[6] reported that thin lesions can be fatal, accounting for approximately 30% of the total melanoma deaths. Regardless of the mortality rate, if thin melanomas represent a substantial part of melanoma mortality, then thin tumors are not biologically insignificant.[6]

Access to Care

An increased incidence of melanoma is associated with a higher SES; however, a low SES is related to a more-advanced stage at diagnosis.[12] A population-based study in California compared Medicaid enrollment with melanoma stage at diagnosis.[31] Late-stage disease was diagnosed in 27% of Medicaid and 9% of non-Medicaid patients with melanoma.[31] Those with intermittent or enrolled in Medicaid within 1 month of diagnosis were more likely to have their melanoma diagnosed at a later stage.[31] Those who had been enrolled in Medicaid for the year before the study were not at increased risk for late-stage melanoma.[31] This suggests that continuous healthcare coverage may be protective.

Similarly, a 2008 study examined the effect of insurance status and race on cancer diagnosis, using the US National Cancer Database.[32] Compared with privately insured patients, uninsured patients had a 2.3 (2.1–2.5) greater chance of having advanced-stage melanoma, and Medicaid patients had a 3.3 (3–3.6) increased risk.[32]

The management of melanoma has changed throughout the past several decades. Bilimoria and colleagues[33] investigated how standardized melanoma treatment is across the nation. They identified 26 quality indicators, and 10 are easily assessed through cancer registry data. There was wide variation in adherence from the patient level (11.8%–96.5%) and the hospital level (3.7%–83%).[33]

Physician density also plays a role in detection of earlier, thinner melanomas. Increased density of dermatologists is highly correlated with decreased Breslow depth at diagnosis and better melanoma prognosis.[34] This association was present even after controlling for other SES measures.[34]

Skin examinations are more commonly reported among those with higher education, a standard place of care, and health insurance. Of college graduates, 14.5% reported having a recent skin examination, compared with 3.4% of patients with less than a high school education.[28] Nine percent of patients with a usual place of health care report a recent skin examination, compared with 2.7% of those without a usual place of health care.[28] Of those with health insurance, 9.1% of patients report a recent skin examination, compared with 3.5% of those who did not.[28]

SUMMARY

The incidence of melanoma has increased significantly over the past several decades. Although incidence remains significantly higher among men, recent analyses suggest melanoma is rising among young women perhaps because of indoor UV exposure trends. Although race, age, gender, and phenotypic factors remain important risk factors, other associations are emerging as relevant to the melanoma epidemic, including those related to SES and healthcare use. Melanoma remains an easily screenable, life-threatening cancer. More attention to understanding the scope and relationship of melanoma with its associated risks is necessary to impact disease outcomes.

REFERENCES

1. American Cancer Society. Cancer facts and figures 2011. Atlanta (GA): American Cancer Society; 2011.
2. Available at: http://seer.cancer.gov/statfacts/html/melan.html. Accessed November 1, 2011.
3. Surveillance Epidemiology and End Results (SEER) Program (www.seer.cancer.gov) SEER*Stat Database: Incidence - SEER 17 Regs Research Data + Hurricane Katrina Impacted Louisiana Cases, Nov 2010 Sub (1973-2008 varying) - Linked To County Attributes - Total U.S., 1969-2009 Counties, National Cancer Institute, DCCPS, Surveillance Research Program, Cancer Statistics Branch, released April 2011, based on the November 2010 submission.
4. Howlader N, Noone AM, Krapcho M, et al. SEER cancer statistics review, 1975-2008. Bethesda (MD): National Cancer Institute; 2011. Available at: http://seercancergov/csr/1975_2008/. based on November 2010 SEER data submission, posted to the SEER web site. Accessed August 6, 2011.
5. Watson M, Johnson CJ, Chen VW, et al. Melanoma surveillance in the United States: overview of methods. J Am Acad Dermatol 2011;65(5):S6–16.
6. Jemal A, Saraiya M, Patel P, et al. Recent trends in cutaneous melanoma incidence and death rates in the United States, 1992-2006. J Am Acad Dermatol 2011;65(5):S17–25.e3.
7. Wu X-C, Eide MJ, King J, et al. Racial and ethnic variations in incidence and survival of cutaneous melanoma in the United States, 1999-2006. J Am Acad Dermatol 2011;65(5):S26–37.
8. Linos E, Swetter SM, Cockburn MG, et al. Increasing burden of melanoma in the United States. J Invest Dermatol 2009;129(7):1666–74.
9. Australian cancer incidence and mortality books. Canberra (Australia): AIHW; 2010.
10. Cancer incidence in five continents, volumes I to IX: IARC cancer base no. 9 [database on the internet]. Lyon (France): International Agency for Research on Cancer; 2010. Available at: http://ci5.iarc.fr. Accessed August 6, 2011.
11. de Vries E, Willem Coebergh J. Cutaneous malignant melanoma in Europe. Eur J Cancer 2004;40(16):2355–66.
12. Reyes-Ortiz CA, Goodwin JS, Freeman JL. The effect of socioeconomic factors on incidence, stage at diagnosis and survival of cutaneous melanoma. Med Sci Monit 2005;11(5):RA163–72.
13. Braaten T, Weiderpass E, Kumle M, et al. Explaining the socioeconomic variation in cancer risk in the Norwegian Women and Cancer Study. Cancer Epidemiol Biomarkers Prev 2005;14(11):2591–7.

14. Perez-Gomez B, Aragones N, Gustavsson P, et al. Socio-economic class, rurality and risk of cutaneous melanoma by site and gender in Sweden. BMC Public Health 2008;8(33):1471–2458.

15. Greenlee R, Howe H. County-level poverty and distant stage cancer in the United States. Cancer Causes Control 2009;20(6):989–1000.

16. Birch-Johansen F, Hvilsom G, Kjaer T, et al. Social inequality and incidence of and survival from malignant melanoma in a population-based study in Denmark, 1994-2003. Eur J Cancer 2008;44(14): 2043–9.

17. Shack L, Jordan C, Thomson C, et al. Variation in incidence of breast, lung and cervical cancer and malignant melanoma of skin by socioeconomic group in England. BMC Cancer 2008;8(1):271.

18. Goodman KJ, Bible ML, London S, et al. Proportional melanoma incidence and occupation among white males in Los Angeles County (California, United States). Cancer Causes Control 1995;6(5):451–9.

19. Clegg L, Reichman M, Miller B, et al. Impact of socioeconomic status on cancer incidence and stage at diagnosis: selected findings from the Surveillance, Epidemiology, and End Results: National Longitudinal Mortality Study. Cancer Causes Control 2009;20(4):417–35.

20. Vidarsdottir H, Gunnarsdottir HK, Olafsdottir EJ, et al. Cancer risk by education in Iceland; a census-based cohort study. Acta Oncol 2008;47(3):385–90.

21. Harrison RA, Haque AU, Roseman JM, et al. Socio-economic characteristics and melanoma incidence. Ann Epidemiol 1998;8(5):327–33.

22. El Ghissassi F, Baan R, Straif K, et al. A review of human carcinogens–part D: radiation. Lancet Oncol 2009; 10(8):751–2. DOI:10.1016/S1470-2045(09)70213-X.

23. The International Agency for Research on Cancer Working Group on Artificial Ultraviolet I, Skin Cancer. The association of use of sunbeds with cutaneous malignant melanoma and other skin cancers: a systematic review. Int J Cancer 2006;120(5):1116–22.

24. Purdue MP, Freeman LE, Anderson WF, et al. Recent trends in incidence of cutaneous melanoma among US caucasian young adults. J Invest Dermatol 2008; 128(12):2905–8.

25. Gallagher RP, Spinelli JJ, Lee TK. Tanning beds, sunlamps, and risk of cutaneous malignant melanoma. Cancer Epidemiol Biomarkers Prev 2005; 14(3):562–6.

26. O'Connor A. California bans indoor tanning for minors. The New York Times. October 10, 2011. Available at: http://well.blogs.nytimes.com/2011/10/10/california-bans-indoor-tanning-for-minors/. Accessed October 17, 2011.

27. Aitken JF, Elwood M, Baade PD, et al. Clinical whole-body skin examination reduces the incidence of thick melanomas. Int J Cancer 2010;126(2):450–8.

28. Saraiya M, Hall HI, Thompson T, et al. Skin cancer screening among U.S. adults from 1992, 1998, and 2000 National Health Interview surveys. Prev Med 2004;39(2):308–14.

29. Welch HG, Woloshin S, Schwartz LM. Skin biopsy rates and incidence of melanoma: population based ecological study. BMJ 2005;331(7515):481.

30. Hollestein LM, van den Akker SA, Nijsten T, et al. Trends of cutaneous melanoma in The Netherlands: increasing incidence rates among all Breslow thickness categories and rising mortality rates since 1989. Ann Oncol 2012;23(2):524–30.

31. Pollitt RA, Clarke CA, Shema SJ, et al. California Medicaid enrollment and melanoma stage at diagnosis: a population-based Study. Am J Prev Med 2008;35(1):7–13.

32. Halpern MT, Ward EM, Pavluck AL, et al. Association of insurance status and ethnicity with cancer stage at diagnosis for 12 cancer sites: a retrospective analysis. Lancet Oncol 2008;9(3):222–31.

33. Bilimoria KY, Raval MV, Bentrem DJ, et al. National assessment of melanoma care using formally developed quality indicators. J Clin Oncol 2009;27(32): 5445–51.

34. Eide MJ, Weinstock MA, Clark MA. The association of physician-specialty density and melanoma prognosis in the United States, 1988 to 1993. J Am Acad Dermatol 2009;60(1):51–8.

Risk Factors for the Development of Primary Cutaneous Melanoma

Julie E. Russak, MD[a],*, Darrell S. Rigel, MD[b]

KEYWORDS

- Melanoma • UV radiation • UV tanning • Nevi

KEY POINTS

- Melanoma is an important public health problem in the United States and worldwide.
- Factors that increase the risk of developing melanoma are:
  - History of blistering sunburns as a teenager
  - Red or blonde hair
  - Marked freckling of upper back - sign of excessive sun exposure and that a person is susceptible to it
  - Family history of melanoma
  - History of actinic keratoses (AKs) - considered the earliest stage in the development of skin cancer
  - Intermittent high intensity sun exposure.
- Exogenous risk factors need to be better defined and understood to help develop better public education programs.

INTRODUCTION

Melanoma is an important public health problem in the United States and worldwide. The incidence of melanoma has been increasing faster than that of any other cancer in the United States.[1] Overall, melanoma incidence increased 2.9% annually from 1981 to 2006.[2] Statistically significant increases are occurring for tumors of all histologic subtypes and thicknesses, including those greater than 4 mm. Invasive melanoma currently is the fifth most frequently diagnosed cancer in men and the sixth most frequently diagnosed cancer in women in the United States. In 2012, 76,250 newly diagnosed cases of invasive melanoma and 55,560 cases of in situ melanoma were expected.[3] At current rates, the lifetime risk of an American developing invasive melanoma is 1 in 52 (**Fig. 1**) overall, 1 in 38 for Caucasian men, and 1 in 56 in Caucasian women. This rate contrasts dramatically with a lifetime risk of 1 in 1500 for Americans born in 1935.[4] Approximately 9180 people are expected to die from melanoma in the United States during 2012, accounting for 66% of all deaths caused by skin cancer.[5]

The importance of diagnosing melanoma early in its evolution cannot be understated.[6] Because the primary treatment modality of cutaneous melanoma, surgical excision, has not changed substantially over the past several decades, the improved 5-year survival rate can be primarily attributed to earlier detection. There has been

[a] Department of Dermatology, Mt. Sinai School of Medicine, One Gustave L. Levy Place, New York, NY 10029-6574, USA; [b] Department of Dermatology, New York University School of Medicine, 550 First Avenue, New York, NY 10016, USA
* Corresponding author.
E-mail address: julierussak@gmail.com

Dermatol Clin 30 (2012) 363–368
doi:10.1016/j.det.2012.05.002
0733-8635/12/$ – see front matter © 2012 Published by Elsevier Inc.

derm.theclinics.com

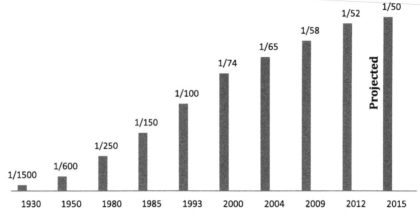

Fig. 1. The lifetime risk of an American developing invasive melanoma by year is depicted. (*Data from* Rigel DS, Robinson JK, Ross MI, et al. In: Kirkwood JM, editor. Cancer of the skin. 2nd edition. Saunders; 2011.)

steady improvement in survival from melanoma over decades with the 5-year survival for invasive melanoma increasing from 82% in 1979 to 92% in 2002.[7] Early detection depends on recognition and identification of patients at high risk for the development of melanoma.

The factors that significantly influence a person's risk of developing melanoma are discussed subsequently.

NATURAL UV LIGHT EXPOSURE (SUNLIGHT)

Exposure to UV radiation from the sun is the most important environmental risk factor for the development of melanoma. Melanoma risk strongly correlates with UV exposure and sunburns; the face and neck are common anatomic sites for skin cancer. Exposure to UV radiation on the skin results in clearly demonstrable mutagenic effects. The p53 suppressor gene, which is often mutated in melanoma, is directly affected by UV exposure.[8] The primary wavelengths influencing melanoma risk are most likely in the UV-B (290–320 nm) range. However, animal studies have also demonstrated a small effect on melanoma development due to exposure to UV-A wavelengths.[9,10] Individuals with type I and II skin types who are more sensitive to the effects of exposure at these wavelengths are at higher risk for the development of skin cancer.[11]

The amount of average annual UV radiation correlates with the incidence of melanoma.[12] The closer an individual is to the equator, the greater the intensity of UV exposure that occurs. The US Surveillance, Epidemiology and End Results (SEER) incidence of melanoma shows a direct relationship between the incidence of melanoma and latitude. The correlation of melanoma incidence to UV radiation exposure is greater when

ambient UV-A (320–400 nm) radiation is also included.[13] High-altitude regions have a higher melanoma rate that may be related to the higher UV fluences (J/cm^2) noted at these sites.[14] Melanoma risk is directly related to the annual UV exposure. When lifetime residential history was coupled with levels of midrange UV radiation (UV-B flux) to provide a measure of individual exposure to sunlight, a 10% increase in annual UV-B flux was associated with a 19% increased risk for melanoma.[15]

Solar radiation UV photons have direct damaging effects on molecules and cells, including DNA, proteins, and lipids, which cause immunosuppression, photoaging, and photocarcinogenesis. Intermittent recreational exposure to UV has been directly correlated to the increased risk for the development of melanoma.

ARTIFICIAL UV TANNING

Approximately 30 million people tan indoors in the United States annually, including 2.3 million adolescents. Despite increased evidence on the dangers of artificial UV radiation, the popularity of indoor tanning is growing.[16] The relationship between UV exposure from tanning beds and subsequent development of melanoma has now been well documented.

More than 20 case-control studies have investigated a possible link between indoor tanning and melanoma.[17] The more recent and more rigorously designed studies have found a positive correlation with an increased risk of melanoma. A study of 571 first time patients with melanoma compared with 913 healthy controls found a significantly higher odds ratio (OR) of 1.8 between indoor tanning and melanoma.[18] In another study of 1518 patients with dermatologic diseases surveyed for skin cancer history and tanning bed use, a significant increased risk of malignant melanoma was noted for every use of indoor tanning (OR 1.64), and a very strong correlation was noted for women aged 45 years or younger who used indoor tanning equipment (OR 3.2).[19] Persons with a history of tanning bed usage and that of melanoma are at increased risk for additional subsequent primaries.

A meta-analysis of 19 studies of indoor tanning and melanoma risk suggested that every use of indoor tanning was associated with the development of melanoma with a relative risk of 1.15, whereas the first use before the age of 35 showed a significantly increased risk of melanoma, with a summary relative risk of 1.75.[20] Based on this study and other studies, the International Agency for Research on Cancer classified UV exposure from tanning beds at its highest carcinogenic risk category (carcinogenic to humans).[20] The National Institutes of Health has also concluded that "Exposure to sunbeds and sunlamps is known to be a human carcinogen based on sufficient evidence of carcinogenicity from studies in human, which indicate a causal relationship between exposure to sunbeds and sunlamps and cancer." Indoor tanning has also been calculated to be directly associated with deaths due to melanoma.[21]

NEVI

Acquired melanocytic nevi are important markers for the risk of melanoma development. The total number of melanocytic nevi on the whole body is the most important independent risk factor for melanoma, and the risk for melanoma development increases almost linearly with increased numbers of melanocytic nevi.[22] Presence of dysplastic nevi is an additional independent risk factor for the development of melanoma. Studies have demonstrated that dysplastic nevi are reported in up to 34% to 56% of patients with melanoma,[23] and their presence may confer up to a 10-fold increase in the risk of melanoma.[24]

The development of potential precursors to melanoma, such as dysplastic nevi, is inhibited by the regular use of sunscreen.[25–27] Lower nevus counts were found in children who regularly used sunscreens than those who did not, suggesting that sun protection at an early age might lower the subsequent risk of melanoma.[28]

PERSONAL AND FAMILY HISTORY OF MELANOMA

Approximately 10% of melanomas present in familial clusters.[29] To date, the exact genes that increase melanoma risk have not been fully described. Yet, there is a clear relationship between a prior personal or family history and melanoma risk.

Patients with histories of a previous primary melanoma are at higher risk for developing a second primary melanoma (2.8–25.6).[30–32] A recent case series calculated the 5- and 10-year risks for developing a second primary melanoma among patients to be 2.8% and 3.6%, respectively.[33]

In 1820, Norris[34] reported the first case of what is now recognized as familial melanoma syndrome, but it was not until 1978, when Clark and Lynch[35,36] first described families with the familial, atypical multiple mole melanoma (FAMMM) syndrome, which is characterized by the presence of melanoma in first-degree relatives, large numbers of melanocytic nevi (>50–100), and melanocytic nevi demonstrating architectural disorder and atypia. Genetic analysis of FAMMM pedigrees resulted in the identification of 2 high-penetrance susceptibility genes, the cyclin-dependent kinase inhibitor 2A (CDKN2A) on chromosome 19p21 and cyclin-dependent kinase 4 (CDK4) on chromosome 12q14.[37] Mutations in CDKN2A account for approximately 20% to 40% of hereditary melanoma, and 0.2% to 1% of all melanomas.[38] Mutations in CDK4 are rare and have been reported in less than 15 families worldwide, leaving CDKN2A as the most significant melanoma predisposition gene identified thus far.

In a more recent meta-analysis study MC1R gene, which encodes the melanocyte-stimulating hormone receptor, has been identified as a low penetrance melanoma susceptibility gene.[39] Polymorphic variants at this locus behave as the key determinant of red hair and freckling[40] and are established as low-risk melanoma susceptibility genes. Coinheritance of variants in MC1R also increases the penetrance of CDKN2A in families with familial melanoma.[41]

SKIN PHENOTYPE

Inability to tan is also associated with an increased risk of melanoma. The MC1R gene is consistently a major determinant of pigment development in vertebrates. The human MC1R coding region is highly polymorphic with at least 30 allelic variants, most of which are associated with red hair. The red-head phenotype is defined by not only hair color but also fair skin, inability to tan, a propensity to freckle, and high levels of pheomelanin.[42]

GENDER

Gender differences that affect the risk are noted in melanoma incidence. In the United States, melanoma is more common in men than in women. In 1973, the incidence rates were 7.3 per 100,000 in men and 6.4 per 100,000 in women, whereas in the 2003 to 2007 period, the incidence rate increased in men to 25.6 per 100,000 and 16.2 per 100,000 in women.[43] Melanoma incidence is greater in women than men until the age of 40 years. However, by the age of 75 years, the incidence is almost 3 times as high in men compared with women (145.6 vs 47.3 per 100,000).[44] In the United States, more recent generations of men have similar incidence rates compared with prior generations, even though incidence rates are still increasing in older generations of men.[45] However, incidence seems to be increasing in more recent generations of women possibly because of an increased usage of tanning beds by this group.

RACE AND ETHNICITY

Melanoma risk is significantly lower in non–white populations. A recent study comparing Hispanic and non-Hispanic men in California showed that the incidence rates were increasing more rapidly and more advanced tumors were diagnosed in the Hispanic population.[46] In 2007, the SEER data showed an incidence rate of 27.5 and 1.1 per 100,000, respectively, in whites and blacks of the United States.[47]

SOCIOECONOMIC FACTORS

Several studies have reported that melanomas are more prevalent in the wealthier socioeconomic levels. Studies have shown that the incidence of melanoma in age-matched sections of the population is higher in those with a larger income and other measures of affluence.[48] This relationship may be because of the greater opportunity of the

more affluent for recreational sun exposure and sunny holidays in the winter months. However, the mortality rate from melanoma is lower in the more affluent groups,[49] which may be related to better access to care. Certain occupations are associated with an increased risk of melanoma. Firefighters,[50] pilots, and finance professionals[51] are consistently found to be at the highest risk for melanoma in studies.

RISK FACTORS LEADING TO AN INCREASED CHANCE OF MELANOMA DETECTION

Factors that are related to the risk of detecting melanoma during mass skin cancer screenings have been identified. The National Melanoma/Skin Cancer Screening Program was designed by the American Academy of Dermatology to enhance early detection of cutaneous malignant melanoma by providing nationwide education campaigns on skin cancer in combination with free skin cancer screenings. Goldberg and colleagues[52] analyzed data generated from the program from 2001 to 2005. The study was designed to identify factors associated with melanoma detection and derive a model of increased likelihood for melanoma detection through visual skin examinations at screenings.

Five factors, which were described with the acronym HARMM, were shown to independently increase the likelihood of suspected melanoma (**Table 1**): History of previous melanoma (OR = 3.5, 95% confidence interval (CI) 2.9–3.8); Age over 50 (OR = 1.2, CI 1.1–1.3); Regular dermatologist absent (OR = 1.40, CI 1.3–1.5); Mole Changing (OR = 2.0, CI 1.9–2.2); and Male gender (OR = 1.4, CI 1.3–1.5). Individuals at highest risk (4 or 5 factors) comprised only 5.8% of the total population screened; however, they accounted

Table 1
HARMM melanoma risk model

Melanoma Risk	Melanoma Univariate Analyses, OR (95% CI)[a]	Melanoma Multivariate Analysis, Adjusted OR (95% CI)[a]
History of previous melanoma	3.5 (3.1–4.0)	3.3 (2.9–3.8)
Age older than 50 y	1.2 (1.1–1.3)	1.2 (1.1–1.3)
Regular dermatologist absent	1.3 (1.2–1.5)	1.4 (1.3–1.5)
Mole changing	2.0 (1.9–2.2)	2.0 (1.9–2.2)
Male gender	1.4 (1.3–1.5)	1.4 (1.3–1.5)

Abbreviation: CI, confidence interval.
   Total Valid Cases = 334,422; Total Valid Melanoma = 3053.
   [a] All *P* values <.001.
   Adapted from Risk Factors For Presumptive Melanoma In Skin Cancer Screening: American Academy of Dermatology National Melanoma/Skin Cancer Screening Program Experience 2001-2005.

for 13.6% melanoma findings and were 4.4 times (CI 3.8–5.1) more likely to be diagnosed with suspected melanoma than individuals at lowest risk (zero or one factor).

SUMMARY

Melanoma is a significant public health problem in the United States. The incidence of melanoma continues to increase at a high rate and deaths from melanoma are also increasing. The endogenous risk factors that are currently recognized are in many cases surrogates for genetic markers yet to be determined. Exogenous risk factors need to be better defined and understood to help develop better public education programs that can change risk behaviors and subsequently lower future incidence and mortality from melanoma.

REFERENCES

1. Linos E, Swetter SM, Cockburn MG, et al. Increasing burden of melanoma in the United States. J Invest Dermatol 2009;129:1666–74.
2. Available at: http://seer.cancer.gov/csr/1975_2006/. Accessed April 30, 2012.
3. Jemal A, Siegel R, Ward E, et al. Cancer Statistics, 2009. CA Cancer J Clin 2009;59:225–49.
4. Kopf AW, Rigel DS, Friedman RJ. The rising incidence and mortality rate of malignant melanoma. J Dermatol Surg Oncol 1982;8:760–1.
5. Albert MR, Weinstock MA. Keratinocyte carcinoma. CA Cancer J Clin 2003;53:292–302.
6. Jemal A, Siegel R, Ward E, et al. Cancer statistics, 2007. CA Cancer J Clin 2007;57(1):43–66.
7. Siegel R, Naihadsham MA, Jemal A. Cancer statistics, 2012. CA Cancer J Clin 2012;62(1):43–66.
8. Ouhtit A, Nakazawa H, Armstrong BK, et al. UV-Radiation-Specific p53 mutation frequency in normal skin as a predictor of risk of basal cell carcinoma. J Natl Cancer Inst 1998;90:523–31.
9. Setlow RB, Grist E, Thompson K, et al. Wavelengths effective in induction of malignant melanoma. Proc Natl Acad Sci U S A 1993;90:6666–70.
10. Ley RD. Dose response for ultraviolet radiation A-induced focal melanocytic hyperplasia and non-melanoma skin tumors in Monodelphis domestica. Photochem Photobiol 2001;73:20–3.
11. Markovic SN, Erickson LA, Rao RD, et al. Malignant melanoma in the 21st century, part 1: epidemiology, risk factors, screening, prevention, and diagnosis. Mayo Clin Proc 2007;82(3):364–80.
12. Armstrong BK, Kricker A. Epidemiology of skin cancer. Photochem Photobiol 2001;63:8–18.
13. Moan J, Dahlback A, Setlow AB. Epidemiological support for an hypothesis for melanoma induction indicating a role for UVA radiation. Photochem Photobiol 1999;70:243–7.
14. Rigel DS, Rigel EG, Rigel AC. Effects of altitude and latitude on ambient UVB radiation. J Am Acad Dermatol 1999;40(1):114–6.
15. Fears TR, Bird CC, Guerry D 4th, et al. Average mid-range ultraviolet radiation flux and time outdoors predict melanoma risk. Cancer Res 2002;62(14): 3992–6.
16. Levine JA, Sorace M, Spencer J, et al. The indoor UV tanning industry: a review of skin cancer risk, health benefit claims, and regulation. J Am Acad Dermatol 2005;53(6):1038–44.
17. Swerdlow AJ, Weinstock MA. Do tanning lamps cause melanoma? An epidemiologic assessment. J Am Acad Dermatol 1998;38(1):89–98.
18. Westerdahl J, Ingvar C, Masback A, et al. Risk of cutaneous melanoma in relation to use of sunbeds: further evidence for UV-A carcinogenicity. Br J Cancer 2000;82(9):1593–9.
19. Ting W, Schultz K, Cac NN, et al. Tanning bed exposure increases the risk of malignant melanoma. Int J Dermatol 2007;46(12):1253–7.
20. International Agency for Research on Cancer Working Group on artificial ultraviolet (UV) light and skin cancer. The association of use of sunbeds with cutaneous malignant melanoma and other skin cancers: a systematic review. Int J Cancer 2007; 120(5):1116–22.
21. Diffey BL. A quantitative estimate of melanoma mortality from ultraviolet A sunbed use in the U.K. Br J Dermatol 2003;149(3):578–81.
22. Snels DG, Hille ET, Gruis NA, et al. Risk of cutaneous malignant melanoma in patients with nonfamilial atypical nevi from a pigmented lesions clinic. J Am Acad Dermatol 1999;40(5 Pt 1):686–93.
23. Tucker MA. Melanoma epidemiology. Hematol Oncol Clin North Am 2009;23(3):383–95, vii.
24. Gandini S, Sera F, Cattaruzza MS, et al. Meta-analysis of risk factors for cutaneous melanoma: I. Common and atypical naevi. Eur J Cancer 2005; 41(1):28–44.
25. Marks R. Epidemiology of melanoma. Clin Exp Dermatol 2000;25(6):459–63.
26. Green A, Williams G, Neale R, et al. Daily sunscreen application and betacarotene supplementation in prevention of basal-cell and squamous-cell carcinomas of the skin: a randomised controlled trial. Lancet 1999;354:723–9.
27. Naylor MF, Boyd A, Smith DW, et al. High sun protection factor sunscreens in the suppression of actinic neoplasia. Arch Dermatol 1995;131:170–5.
28. MacLennan R, Kelly JW, Rivers JK, et al. The Eastern Australian Childhood Nevus Study: site differences in density and size of melanocytic nevi in relation to latitude and phenotype. J Am Acad Dermatol 2003;48(3):367–75.

29. Florell SR, Boucher KM, Garibotti G, et al. Population-based analysis of prognostic factors and survival in familial melanoma. J Clin Oncol 2005; 23:7168–77.

30. Tucker MA, Boice JD Jr, Hoffman DA. Second cancer following cutaneous melanoma and cancers of the brain, thyroid, connective tissue, bone, and eye in Connecticut, 1935–82. Natl Cancer Inst Monogr 1985;68:161–89.

31. Kang S, Barnhill RL, Mihm MC, et al. Multiple primary cutaneous melanomas. Cancer 1992;70:1911–6.

32. DiFronzo LA, Wanek LA, Elashoff R, et al. Increased incidence of second primary melanoma in patients with a previous cutaneous melanoma. Ann Surg Oncol 1999;6:705–11.

33. Goggins WB, Tsao H. A population-based analysis of risk factors for a second primary cutaneous melanoma among melanoma survivors. Cancer 2003; 97(3):639–43.

34. Norris W. Case of fungoid disease. Edinb Med Surg J 1820;16:562–5.

35. Lynch HT, Krush AJ. Hereditary and malignant melanoma: implications for early cancer detection. Can Med Assoc J 1968;99:789–92.

36. Clark WH Jr, Reimer RR, Greene M, et al. Origin of familial malignant melanomas from heritable melanocytic lesions: the B-K mole syndrome. Arch Dermatol 1978;114(5):732–8.

37. Meyer K, Guldberg P. Genetic risk factors for melanoma. Hum Genet 2009;120:499–510.

38. Begg CB, Orlow I, Hummer AJ, et al. Lifetime risk of melanoma in CDKN2A mutation carriers in a population-based sample. J Natl Cancer Inst 2005;97: 1507–15.

39. Suzuki I, Cone RD, Im S, et al. Binding of melanotropic hormones to the melanocortin receptor MC1R on human melanocytes stimulates proliferation and melanogenesis. Endocrinology 1996;137:1627–33.

40. Valverde P, Healy E, Jackson I, et al. Variants of the melanocyte stimulating hormone receptor gene are associated with red hair and fair skin in humans. Nat Genet 1995;11:328–30.

41. Box NF, Duff y DL, Chen W, et al. MC1R genotype modifies risk of melanoma in families segregating CDKN2A mutations. Am J Hum Genet 2001;69:765–73.

42. Lin JY, Fisher DE. Melanocyte biology and skin pigmentation. Nature 2007;445:843–50.

43. Available at: http://seer.cancer.gov/statfacts/html/melan.html#incidence-mortality. Accessed September 1, 2010.

44. Fast Stats: an interactive tool for access to SEER cancer statistics. Surveillance Research Program, National Cancer Institute. Available at: http://seer.cancer.gov/faststats. Accessed September 3, 2010.

45. Eide MJ, Weinstock MA. Epidemiology of skin cancer. In: Rigel DS, editor. Cancer of the skin. Philadelphia: Elevier; 2011.

46. Pollitt RA, Clarke CA, Swetter SM, et al. The expanding melanoma burden in California hispanics: importance of socioeconomic distribution, histologic subtype, and anatomic location. Cancer 2011;117(1):152–61.

47. Available at: http://seer.cancer.gov/faststats/selections.php?#Output. Accessed September 01, 2010.

48. MacKie RM, Hole DJ. Incidence and thickness of primary tumours and survival of patients with cutaneous malignant melanoma in relation to socioeconomic status. BMJ 1996;312(7039):1125–8.

49. Eide MJ, Weinstock MA, Clark MA. Demographic and socioeconomic predictors of melanoma prognosis in the United States. J Health Care Poor Underserved 2009;20(1):227–45.

50. Bates MN. Registry-based case-control study of cancer in California firefighters. Am J Ind Med 2007;50(5):339–44.

51. Vågerö D, Swerdlow AJ, Beral V. Occupation and malignant melanoma: a study based on cancer registration data in England and Wales and in Sweden. Br J Ind Med 1990;47(5):317–24.

52. Goldberg MS, Doucette JT, Lim HW, et al. Risk factors for presumptive melanoma in skin cancer screening: American Academy of Dermatology National Melanoma/Skin Cancer Screening Program experience 2001-2005. J Am Acad Dermatol 2007; 57(1):60–6.

The Effect of Sunscreen on Melanoma Risk

Jennifer S. Mulliken, MA, BA[a], Julie E. Russak, MD[b],*,
Darrell S. Rigel, MD[c]

KEYWORDS

- Cutaneous melanoma • Melanoma risk reduction • Sunscreen • UV protection • SPF

KEY POINTS

- While the etiology of melanoma is multifactorial, individuals who are exposed to intense sunlight intermittently are at highest risk for developing melanoma.
- Intermittent exposure to ultraviolet radiation is the only known modifiable cause of melanoma, but the role of sunscreen in preventing melanoma remains somewhat controversial.
- Evidence suggesting a positive association between sunscreen application and melanoma risk reduction is growing.
- Recent studies suggest that the regular use of sunscreen can prevent the development of melanoma by up to 10 years.

INTRODUCTION

Exposure to UV radiation is a known risk factor for the development of melanoma and nonmelanoma skin cancers.[1] Over time, sun exposure is known to cause DNA damage and systemic immunosuppression, which are factors for carcinogenesis.[2–4] Total cumulative sun exposure is associated with the development of squamous cell and basal cell cancers, whereas intense intermittent sun exposure has been associated with the development of melanoma.[5,6]

A history of sunburn in particular seems to be an important risk factor for the development of melanoma.[7] The results of a meta-analysis conducted by Dennis and colleagues[8] showed that sunburn carries a lifetime relative risk for melanoma of up to 1.6 across all age groups. In addition, the relationship between UV exposure and melanoma risk was found to be dose dependent. An increasing number of lifetime sunburns was associated with a linear increase in the risk of melanoma. It should be noted, however, that a history of sunburns might simply be a proxy for a strong history of recreational sun exposure because individuals who are infrequently exposed to UV radiation are more likely to burn when exposed to sunlight intermittently.

The cause of melanoma is multifactorial. In addition to genetic predisposition, phenotypic characteristics, such as fair skin, red hair, freckling, and proclivity to sunburn, all contribute to melanoma risk as does living in sunny locations or at high altitudes. Although exposure to UV radiation is the only known modifiable cause of melanoma, the role of sunscreen in melanoma prevention remains somewhat controversial.

Conflicts of interest: Dr Russak has received honoraria from Medicis and Warner Chilcott. Dr Rigel has received honoraria from Neutrogena Corporation, Aveeno, and Beiersdorf. Ms Mulliken has no conflicts of interest to declare.
[a] New York University School of Medicine, 550 First Avenue, New York, NY 10016, USA; [b] Department of Dermatology, Mt. Sinai School of Medicine, One Gustave L. Levy Place, New York, NY 10029-6574, USA; [c] Department of Dermatology, New York University School of Medicine, 550 First Avenue, New York, NY 10016, USA
* Corresponding author.
E-mail address: julierussak@gmail.com

derm.theclinics.com

UV RADIATION AND THE PATHOGENESIS OF MELANOMA

UV light is classified according to its physical properties, namely wavelength. UV-A light occurs in the 320- to 400-nm wavelengths, UV-B light in 290- to 320-nm wavelengths, and UV-C light in 100- to 290-nm wavelengths. UV-C radiation is filtered by the ozone layer, whereas UV-A and UV-B radiation reach the earth's surface and have been strongly implicated in the development of cutaneous melanomas.[9,10]

UV-A radiation is far more abundant in natural sunlight than UV-B radiation. The primary mechanism through which UV-A radiation injures cells is through the formation of free radical species. By causing oxidative DNA damage, UV-A light acts as a potential mutagen.[11] UV-A radiation is also thought to have substantial immunosuppressive effects. Exposure to UV-A radiation in mice has been shown to prevent the local immunologic rejection of certain skin cancers.[12] In other studies, UV-A radiation has been shown to induce the development of melanomas in opossums and in certain fish.[13,14]

Although only 5% to 10% of the UV radiation that reaches the earth's surface falls in the UV-B spectrum, UV-B radiation is the major contributor to sunburn and is responsible for causing DNA damage. UV-B penetrates to the basal layer of the epidermis where it leads to the formation of pyrimidine (thymine) dimers in DNA.[15–18] The incorrect repair of these DNA lesions can lead to mutations that alter cell function.[11,16,18] The role of UV-B in the development of cutaneous melanoma has been demonstrated in melanoma-susceptible transgenic mice.[19]

Individuals who are exposed to intense sunlight intermittently are at the highest risk for developing melanoma. Melanoma is most common in persons with indoor occupations whose primary exposure to UV radiation is recreational, such as on weekends and vacations. This pattern of sun exposure in melanoma is further evidenced by the fact that melanoma tends to develop in areas of the body that are primarily subject to intermittent UV radiation. For example, men are typically affected on the back, whereas women are typically affected on the lower legs. In contrast to squamous cell and basal cell cancers, melanoma typically spares the face, hands, and forearms.

SUNSCREENS
Mechanism

UV light is a known carcinogen and, therefore, it is important to protect against the harmful effects of UV-A and UV-B radiation. Sunscreens are agents that temporarily block UV radiation absorption by the skin. Lotions, creams, protective clothing, umbrellas, sunglasses, and hats all qualify as sunscreen agents. Topically applied sunscreen agents are categorized as either organic or inorganic UV filters. Organic filters absorb UV radiation, whereas inorganic filters scatter and reflect UV radiation. There are advantages and disadvantages to both types of formulations. Most commercially available sunscreens contain a combination of organic and inorganic filters.

Inorganic UV filters, such as zinc oxide and titanium dioxide, were previously known as physical sunscreens. When photons of UV radiation contact submicroscopic sunscreen particles, they are dispersed in various directions. These agents do not break down over time and are generally well tolerated. Their major drawback is cosmetic; inorganic filters do not blend into the skin as easily as organic preparations and can result in a whitish discoloration of the skin.

Organic UV filters, previously known as chemical sunscreens, function by absorbing photons of UV radiation. These agents are highly effective and are typically more easily applied than inorganic agents because they are in the form of creams and lotions. Unlike inorganic agents, they tend to degrade with sun exposure and require frequent reapplication. In addition, organic sunscreens have the potential to penetrate the skin, resulting in systemic exposure.[20,21] Finally, organic agents may cause a variety of adverse skin reactions, including allergic contact dermatitis, photoallergic dermatitis, irritant dermatitis, acne, and other aesthetic issues.[22] These reactions occur infrequently, but the prominence of organic UV filters as allergens is increasing because of the increased use of soluble UV filters in daily face moisturizers.

The Sun Protection Factor System

The efficacy of a sunscreen should ideally be measured by the extent to which the sunscreen protects from skin cancer, but because these studies are difficult to perform, surrogate endpoints are used. The sun protection factor (SPF) system measures the ratio of time it takes to sunburn with sunscreen protection divided by the time it takes to burn without protection.[23] When determining the SPF, a sunscreen application thickness of 2 mg/cm^2 is used. Because UV-B radiation causes sunburn, the SPF of a sunscreen measures protection from UV-B radiation only. For example, an SPF of 15 filters 94% of UV-B and an SPF of 30 filters 97% of UV-B. As SPF increases to more than

30, there are only marginal increases in the protection offered.[24]

UV-A protection is more challenging to measure because UV-A radiation is 1000 times less erythemogenic than UV-B radiation.[25] The American Academy of Dermatology recommends that UV-A protection be determined by measuring the dose of UV-A needed to produce minimal persistent pigment darkening (PPD) at 2 to 24 hours.[26,27] The UV-A protection factor of a sunscreen should reflect a 10-fold increase in the UV-A dose needed to induce a PPD. In addition, the ratio of UV-A/UV-B protection should be 1:3 at minimum, and only sunscreens that offer both UV-A and UV-B protection may claim broad-spectrum coverage. Generally speaking, an ideal sunscreen should protect against both UV-B and UV-A radiation and have an SPF of 30 or greater.[26]

There are several problems with the SPF system. For example, SPF is measured under ideal and controlled conditions. On average, 1 oz of sunscreen is required to cover the body, and it takes approximately 15 to 20 minutes from the time of application until a sunscreen becomes optimally effective.[22] However, most people tend to underapply sunscreens, and the resulting SPF may attain only 20% to 50% of the labeled SPF.[28] In addition, SPF tends to degrade 8 hours after application by about 55% with activity and by about 25% with indoor rest.[29]

There has been some question as to whether the maximum SPF on sunscreen labels should be limited to 50+ because products with SPF values more than 50 may not provide superior protection to products with SPF values less than 50. A 2010 study sought to compare the sun-protective effects of an SPF 50 sunscreen with an SPF 85 sunscreen by measuring the grade of erythema after an average of 5 hours of skiing or snowboarding.[30] The results of this study demonstrated that sunscreens with an SPF higher than 50 (SPF 85) provided significantly better sun protection than SPF 50 sunscreens. Because people typically underapply sunscreens, higher SPF sunscreens may also offer a margin of safety over lower SPF sunscreens by maximizing the effective SPF.

UV Filters in Sunscreens

Organic sunscreens can be classified by whether they filter UV-B radiation, UV-A radiation, or both. Organic UV-B filters have been used since the 1970s when the first true sunscreen, para-aminobenzoic acid (PABA), became available.[22] Since then, many other UV-B filters have become available; their properties are summarized in **Table 1.**

PABA derivatives
Although PABA is an effective UV-B absorber, it is rarely used in sunscreens because of its potential to cause allergic contact dermatitis and photoallergic dermatitis.[27] It is also known to stain clothing. PABA derivatives, such as padimate O, are less effective than PABA at filtering UV radiation, but they are also less likely to cause hypersensitivity reactions or stain clothing.[31]

Cinnamates
As their name implies, cinnamates are derivatives of cinnamon. They are chemically related to balsam of Peru and cocoa leaves, and individuals who are sensitized to these items may cross-react to sunscreens that contain cinnamates.[22] Because cinnamates are comprised of polar oils, sunscreens that contain cinnamates may leave a greasy sensation on the skin when applied.[32] Octinoxate, a cinnamate, is currently the most commonly used UV-B filter in the United States.[27] A weak absorber of UV-B radiation, octinoxate is frequently combined with other UV filters in sunscreens to achieve adequate sun protection. Cinoxate is another cinnamate derivative that is rarely used in modern sunscreen formulations.

Salicylates
Salicylates are photostable agents with high substantivity; as a result, they are frequently incorporated into water-resistant products and combined with photolabile UV-A filters, such as avobenzone.[24,31] Octisalate, homosalate, and trolamine salicylate are commonly found in sunscreens. Trolamine salicylate is also often used in hair products as a UV filter.[33]

Octocrylene
Octocrylene lacks substantivity, but it is frequently used with the UV-A filter, avobenzone, as a photostabilizer.[34]

Ensulizole
As a water-soluble agent, ensulizole is commonly used as a component in cosmetic moisturizers.[31]

Protection from UV-B has historically been the focus of sunscreen development. However, as the role of UV-A radiation in photocarcinogenesis, photoimmunosuppression, and photoaging has been better understood, UV-A filters have increasingly been incorporated into commercial sunscreens. UV-A is classified as either UV-A-2 (320–340 nm) or UV-A-1 (340–400 nm) depending on wavelength, and these filters vary in their absorptive properties along the UV-A spectrum. The UV-A filter agents are summarized in **Table 1.**

Table 1
Available sunscreen agents

Sunscreen	UV Spectrum	US Availability	Peak Absorption (nm)
Organic Filters			
PABA	UV-B	Yes	283
Padimate O	UV-B	Yes	311
Octinoxate	UV-B	Yes	311
Cinoxate	UV-B	Yes	289
Octisalate	UV-B	Yes	307
Homosalate	UV-B	Yes	306
Trolamine salicylate	UV-B	Yes	260–355
Octocrylene	UV-B	Yes	303
Ensulizole	UV-B	Yes	310
Parsol SLX	UV-B	No	312
Uvasorb HEB	UV-B	No	312
Univil T150	UV-B	No	314
Meradimate	UV-A	Yes	340
Avobenzone	UV-A	Yes	357
Ecamsule	UV-A	Yes	345
Univil A Plus	UV-A	No	354
Neo Helioplan AT	UV-A	No	334
Oxybenzone	UV-A/UV-B	Yes	288 and 325
Sulisobenzone	UV-A/UV-B	Yes	366
Dioxybenzone	UV-A/UV-B	Yes	352
Silatriazole	UV-A/UV-B	No	303 and 344
Bisoctrizole	UV-A/UV-B	No	303 and 344
Bemotrizinol	UV-A/UV-B	No	305 and 360
Inorganic Filters			
Zinc oxide	UV-A/UV-B	Yes	
Titanium dioxide	UV-A/UV-B	Yes	

Modified from Burnett CT, Rigel D, Lim HW. Current concepts in photoprotection. In: Rigel DS, Robinson JK, Ross M, et al, editors. Cancer of the skin. Philadelphia: Saunders; 2011. p. 80–8.

Benzophenones

Oxybenzone, sulisobenzone, and dioxybenzone are UV-A filters that are commonly incorporated into sunscreens. Of these, oxybenzone is the most commonly used.[31] Although these agents primarily offer protection in the UV-A-2 range, a second protective band is found in the UV-B range.[22] Oxybenzone is the most common cause of contact photoallergy among sunscreens, however, and its use in sunscreens is limited by its allergic properties and by its photolability.[35]

Avobenzone

Avobenzone is currently the only filter approved by the Food and Drug Administration (FDA) and has a peak absorbance in the UV-A-1 spectrum.[27] Although avobenzone has a broad absorbance spectrum, its use has historically been limited by its photolability. Today, avobenzone is frequently incorporated into sunscreens with more photostable agents, such as octocrylene, salicylates, and oxybenzone. The results of recent studies have suggested that combining avobenzone with octocrylene provides the most effective UV-A protection available in the United States.[36]

Meradimate

Meradimate's absorption spectrum lies within the UV-A-2 range. Overall, it is a weak UV-A filter and is rarely used.[24]

Ecamsule

Ecamsule is a recently approved sunscreen agent in the United States. Compared with other agents, ecamsule is a photostable and efficient UV-A filter.[37]

Inorganic sunscreens, such as zinc oxide and titanium dioxide, provide protection in the UV-A and UV-B ranges, but overall they tend to be less efficient at filtering UV radiation than the newer organic agents.[31] Inorganic sunscreens have historically tended to be cosmetically unappealing; they may leave a whitish discoloration on the skin, stain clothing, and be comedogenic.[25,31] Micronized formulations are now more commonly used; because particle size has decreased, these newer formulations are able to protect against shorter UV wavelengths.[37]

The agents discussed previously differ in their UV protective wavelengths, and a combination of several filters is often required to achieve the desired level of protection. In addition, there are several broad-spectrum UV-A and UV-B filters available outside of the United States. Bisoctrizole (absorption peaks: 303 nm and 344 nm) and bemotrizinol (absorption peaks: 305 nm and 360 nm) are examples of 2 broad-spectrum agents available in Europe that are currently undergoing approval in the United States.[38]

SUNSCREEN AND MELANOMA RISK REDUCTION

A variety of factors are known to increase an individual's risk of developing skin cancer, including exposure to UV radiation, decreased skin pigmentation, positive family history, and geographic location. As awareness of the sun's potentially harmful effects has grown, skin-protection efforts have also become more widespread. Sunscreens, protective clothing, and sun avoidance have all been used to modify individual skin cancer risk.

The role of sunscreens in the prolonged prevention of actinic keratoses and squamous cell carcinomas has been well established.[39,40] However, although exposure to UV radiation is a known and modifiable cause of melanoma,[2,41] the ability of sunscreens to reduce the risk of developing melanoma remains controversial. In recent decades, many studies have attempted to establish a link between sunscreen application and the incidence of melanoma, but no consensus has been reached.

The results of 15 case-control studies conducted by the International Agency for Research on Cancer were indecisive regarding the effect of sunscreen on the development of melanoma.[42] Of these studies, 4 showed no association between melanoma and sunscreen use, 3 suggested a lower risk of melanoma with sunscreen use, and 8 suggested a higher risk of melanoma with sunscreen use. Other studies have postulated that because sunscreen prevents symptoms of sunburn, it also permits more time sunbathing; therefore, sunscreen users could be at an increased risk of developing melanoma.[43,44] An increased risk of melanoma with sunscreen use has also been suggested at high altitudes where sunscreens may allow overexposure to UV-A radiation.[45]

As others have previously noted, the studies that found a positive association between sunscreen use and melanoma failed to control adequately for confounding factors.[46] For example, individuals with fair skin who burn easily are the most likely to use sunscreen, but these individuals are also the most likely to develop melanoma in the first place. In addition, those studies that found a lower risk of melanoma with sunscreen use may have overlooked the fact that sunscreen users may be more likely to use other methods of sun protection, including clothing, umbrellas, and tree cover.

Meta-analyses of case-control studies have shown no association between sunscreen use and the development of melanoma,[47,48] although the conclusions that can be drawn from these data are also limited. For example, some of these studies used data collected before 1990 when the median SPF of sunscreen products was less than 10.[49] In more recent years, median SPF trends have been increasing.[50–53] As a result, the outcomes of many earlier studies may no longer be applicable.

The SPF of a sunscreen is assessed at an application thickness of 2 mg/cm^2. Most consumers, however, only apply sunscreen at a thickness of 0.5 to 1.0 mg/cm^2.[54] A sunscreen of SPF 8 applied at a thickness of 0.5 to 1.0 mg/cm^2 will result in an effective SPF of 2 to 3. Given how minimally earlier-generation sunscreens modified UV exposure of the skin, it is not surprising that some case-control studies failed to find any association between sunscreen use and melanoma risk.[46] More broad-spectrum modern sunscreens, on the other hand, provide an effective SPF of around 8 to 10 when applied at an average thickness of 1.0 mg/cm^2. Total UV-A and UV-B exposure to the skin with these sunscreens is about one-third of that with earlier-generation sunscreens.[55]

Overall, epidemiologic studies of melanoma prevention have been limited by insufficient statistical power, recall bias, and the fact that people tend to be poor historians when reporting prior sunscreen usage. The main determinants of sunscreen use are the same as those of melanoma: susceptibility to sunburn, high sun exposure, and a positive family history.[56] There is also a 10- to 50-year latency period between the initial period of sun exposure and the development of melanoma. As a result, it has been difficult to ascertain whether any association exists between sunscreen use and the incidence of melanoma.

Although melanoma incidence reduction through sunscreen use has not been proven, evidence suggesting a positive association between sunscreen application and melanoma risk reduction is growing. For example, the total number of nevi is an important risk factor for the development of melanoma,[57] and the use of sunscreens has been found to attenuate the formation of nevi in light-skinned children.[58] In addition, hepatocyte growth factor/scatter factor transgenic mice treated with sunscreen demonstrated significantly less UV-induced DNA damage (as measured by thymine-thymine dimmer concentration) and fewer UV-induced melanomas than control mice.[59]

Most recently, the first randomized controlled trial to evaluate the association between sunscreen use and melanoma risk has suggested that regular application of sunscreen may, in fact, prevent the development of melanoma for up to 10 years.[60] This trial provides the strongest evidence to date that the regular use of sunscreen can prevent the development of primary cutaneous melanomas. Long-term follow-up showed that, among adults aged 25 to 75 years, daily application of SPF 15+ sunscreen to the head and arms for 5 years was associated with a reduced incidence of new primary melanomas over a 10-year period. After 15 years of follow-up, a 73% reduction in invasive melanomas was also seen with daily sunscreen application. The results of this study have led others to comment on the positive long-term effects of reminding patients to use sunscreen regularly.[61]

NEW DEVELOPMENTS

UV exposure undeniably causes skin damage, and the use of sunscreen or sun-protective clothing is critical in protecting from cutaneous cancers and premature aging. To help consumers select and use sunscreens appropriately, the FDA released a series of sunscreen labeling guidelines in June 2011.[62] Under these guidelines, which will become effective in June 2012, all over-the-counter sunscreen products will be subject to a standard test that will determine which products provide protection against both UV-B and UV-A radiation. Products that pass the test will be labeled as broad spectrum. In addition, only those broad-spectrum sunscreens that have an SPF value of 15 or higher can claim to reduce the risk of skin cancer and premature skin aging if used as directed with other sun-protection measures. Manufacturers will no longer be able to claim that a sunscreen is waterproof or sweat proof because these claims overstate a sunscreen's effectiveness. Unless manufacturers submit data to the FDA for approval, sunscreens will also not be able to claim immediate protection after application or for more than 2 hours after application. Finally, water-resistance claims on sunscreen labels must indicate whether the sunscreen's SPF remains effective for 40 minutes or 80 minutes after swimming or sweating, based on standard testing.

SUMMARY

A strong history of intermittent sun exposure is a well-known risk factor for melanoma. In addition, persons with a fair complexion, red hair, freckles, and inherited gene mutations are also at an increased risk of developing melanoma. As a result, sun protection is extremely relevant in these individuals. Although the role of sunscreen in melanoma prevention remains somewhat controversial, the 2011 study by Green and colleagues[60] provides the strongest evidence to date that the regular use of sunscreen can prevent the development of melanoma for up to 10 years. The daily application of sunscreen to exposed skin can be expensive and time intensive, so counseling about sun-protection efforts should start early to encourage good habits. Given the known role of UV radiation in the pathogenesis of melanoma, it seems foolish not to encourage the regular use of sunscreen in all individuals and especially in those individuals already at increased risk.

REFERENCES

1. American Cancer Society. Cancer facts and figures 2011. Atlanta (GA): American Cancer Society; 2011.
2. Gilchrest BA, Eller MS, Geller AC, et al. The pathogenesis of melanoma induced by ultraviolet radiation. N Engl J Med 1999;340(17):1341–8.
3. Kelly DA, Young AR, McGregor JM, et al. Sensitivity to sunburn is associated with susceptibility to ultraviolet radiation-induced suppression of cutaneous cell-mediated immunity. J Exp Med 2000;191:561–6.
4. Fisher MS, Kripke ML. Systemic alteration induced in mice by ultraviolet light irradiation and its relationship to ultraviolet carcinogenesis. 1977. Bull World Health Organ 2002;80:908–12.
5. Nelemans PJ, Groenendal H, Kiemeney LA, et al. Effect of intermittent exposure to sunlight on melanoma risk among indoor workers and sun-sensitive individuals. Environ Health Perspect 1993;101(3):252–5.
6. Armstrong BK, Kricker A. The epidemiology of UV induced skin cancer. J Photochem Photobiol B 2001;63(1–3):8–18.
7. Gandini S, Sera F, Cattaruzza MS, et al. Meta-analysis of risk factors for cutaneous melanoma: II. Sun exposure. Eur J Cancer 2005;41(1):45–60.

8. Dennis LK, Vanbeek MJ, Beane Freeman LE, et al. Sunburns and risk of cutaneous melanoma: does age matter? A comprehensive meta-analysis. Ann Epidemiol 2008;18:614–27.

9. Ley RD, Applegate LA, Padilla RS, et al. Ultraviolet radiation-induced malignant melanoma in Monodelphis domestica. Photochem Photobiol 1989;50(1): 1–5.

10. Romerdahl CA, Stephens LC, Bucana C, et al. The role of ultraviolet radiation in the induction of melanocytic skin tumors in inbred mice. Cancer Commun 1989;1(4):209–16.

11. Kochevar IE, Pathak MA, Parrish JA. Photophysics, photochemistry, and photobiology. In: Fitzpatrick TB, Eisen AZ, Wolff K, et al, editors. Dermatology in general medicine, vol. 1, 4th edition. NewYork: McGraw-Hill; 1993. p. 1627–38.

12. Bestak R, Halliday GM. Chronic low-dose UVA irradiation induces local suppression of contact hypersensitivity, Langerhans cell depletion and suppressor cell activation in C3H/HeJ mice. Photochem Photobiol 1996;64(6):969–74.

13. Kusewitt DF, Applegate LA, Ley RD. Ultraviolet radiation-induced skin tumors in a South American opossum (Monodelphis domestica). Vet Pathol 1991;28:55–65.

14. Setlow RB, Woodhead AD, Grist E. Animal model for ultraviolet radiation-induced melanoma: platyfish-swordtail hybrid. Proc Natl Acad Sci U S A 1989; 86:8922–6.

15. Freeman SE, Hacham H, Gange RW, et al. Wavelength dependence of pyrimidine dimer formation in DNA of human skin irradiated in situ with ultraviolet light. Proc Natl Acad Sci U S A 1989;86:5605–9.

16. Mitchell DL, Nairn RS. The biology of the (6-4) photoproduct. Photochem Photobiol 1989;49:805–19.

17. Mitchell DL, Jen J, Cleaver JE. Relative induction of cyclobutane dimers and cytosine photohydrates in DNA irradiated in vitro and in vivo with ultraviolet-C and ultraviolet-B light. Photochem Photobiol 1991; 54:741–6.

18. Moriwaki S, Ray S, Tarone RE, et al. The effect of donor age on the processing of UV-damaged DNA by cultured human cells: reduced DNA repair capacity and increased DNA mutability. Mutat Res 1996;364:117–23.

19. Klein-Szanto AJ, Silvers WK, Mintz B. Ultraviolet radiation-induced malignant skin melanoma in melanoma-susceptible transgenic mice. Cancer Res 1994;54:4569–72.

20. Gonzalez H, Farbot A, Larko O, et al. Percutaneous absorption of the sunscreen benzophenone-3 after repeated whole body applications, with and without ultraviolet irradiation. Br J Dermatol 2006;154:337–40.

21. Gonzalez H. Percutaneous absorption with emphasis on sunscreens. Photochem Photobiol Sci 2010;9:482–8.

22. Rigel DS. The effect of sunscreen on melanoma risk. Dermatol Clin 2002;20(4):601–6.

23. Sayre RM, Desrochers DL, Marlowe E, et al. The correlation of indoor solar simulator and natural sunlight: testing of a sunscreen preparation. Arch Dermatol 1978;114(11):1649–51.

24. Kallavanijaya P, Lim HW. Photoprotection. J Am Acad Dermatol 2005;52(6):937–58.

25. Antoniou C, Kosmadaki M, Stratigos A, et al. Sunscreens – what's important to know. J Eur Acad Dermatol Venereol 2008;22(9):1110–8.

26. American Academy of Dermatology. Position statement on broad spectrum protection of sunscreen products. 2009. (Amended by the board of directors November 14, 2009). Available at: http://web1.netonline.com/forms/policies/Uploads/PS/PS-BroadSpectrum%20Protection%20of%20Sunscreen%20Products%2011-16-09.pdf. Accessed February 5, 2012.

27. Burnett CT, Rigel D, Lim HW. Current concepts in photoprotection. In: Rigel DS, et al, editors. Cancer of the skin. Philadelphia: Saunders; 2011. p. 80–8.

28. Eide MJ, Weinstock MA. Public health challenges in sun protection. Dermatol Clin 2006;24(1):119–24.

29. Beyer DM, Faurschou A, Philipsen PA, et al. Sun protection factor persistence on human skin during a day without physical activity or ultraviolet exposure. Photodermatol Photoimmunol Photomed 2010;26(1):22–7.

30. Russak JE, Chen T, Appa Y, et al. A comparison of sunburn protection of high-sun protection factor (SPF) sunscreens: SPF 85 sunscreen is significantly more protective than SPF 50. J Am Acad Dermatol 2010;62(2):348–9.

31. Palm MD, O'Donoghue MN. Update on photoprotection. Dermatol Ther 2007;20(5):360–76.

32. Tanner PR. Sunscreen product formulation. Dermatol Clin 2006;24(1):53–62.

33. González S, Fernández-Lorente M, Gilaberte-Calzada Y. The latest on skin photoprotection. Clin Dermatol 2008;26(6):614–26.

34. Nash J. Human safety and efficacy of ultraviolet filters and sunscreen products. Dermatol Clin 2006;24(1):35–51.

35. Lautenschlager S, Wulf HC, Pittelkow MR. Photoprotection. Lancet 2007;370(9586):528–37.

36. Wang SQ, Stanfield JW, Osterwalder U, et al. Novel emerging sunscreen technologies. Dermatol Clin 2006;24(1):105–17.

37. Lim HW, Rigel DS. UVA: grasping a better understanding of this formidable opponent. Skin Aging 2007;15(7):62.

38. Hexsel CL, Bangert SD, Hebert AA, et al. Current sunscreen issues: 2007 Food and Drug Administration sunscreen labeling recommendations and combination sunscreen/insect repellent products. J Am Acad Dermatol 2008;59(2):316–23.

39. Green A, Williams G, Neale R, et al. Daily sunscreen application and betacarotene supplementation in prevention of basal-cell and squamous-cell carcinomas of the skin: a randomised controlled trial. Lancet 1999;354(9180):723–9.

40. Dummer R, Maier T. UV protection and skin cancer. Recent Results Cancer Res 2002;160:7–12.

41. International Agency for Research on Cancer (IARC). Solar and ultraviolet radiation. IARC monographs on the evaluation of carcinogenic risks to humans, vol. 55. Lyon (France): International Agency for Research on Cancer; 1992.

42. International Agency for Research on Cancer. Sunscreens. Handbooks of cancer prevention, vol. 5. Lyon (France): International Agency for Research on Cancer; 2001.

43. Garland CF, Garland FC, Gorham ED. Could sunscreens increase melanoma risk? Am J Public Health 1992;82(4):614–5.

44. Westerdahl J, Ingvar C, Mâsbäck A, et al. Sunscreen use and malignant melanoma. Int J Cancer 2000;87(1):145–50.

45. Gorham ED, Mohr SB, Garland CF, et al. Do sunscreens increase risk of melanoma in populations residing at higher latitudes? Ann Epidemiol 2007;17(12):956–63.

46. Diffey BL. Sunscreens and melanoma: the future looks bright. Br J Dermatol 2005;153:378–81.

47. Huncharek M, Kupelnick B. Use of topical sunscreens and the risk of malignant melanoma: a meta-analysis of 9067 patients from 11 case-control studies. Am J Public Health 2002;92(7):1173–7.

48. Dennis LK, Beane Freeman LE, VanBeek MJ. Sunscreen use and the risk for melanoma: a quantitative review. Ann Intern Med 2003;139(12):966–78.

49. Rebut D. The sunscreen industry in Europe: past, present, and future. In: Lowe NJ, Shaath N, editors. Sunscreens: development, evaluation and regulatory aspects. New York: Marcel Dekker; 1990. p. 161–71.

50. Gavin A, Boyle R, Donnelly D, et al. Trends in skin cancer knowledge, sun protection practices and behaviours in the Northern Ireland population. Eur J Public Health 2012;22(3):408–12.

51. Buller DB, Andersen PA, Walkosz BJ, et al. Compliance with sunscreen advice in a survey of adults engaged in outdoor winter recreation at high-elevation ski areas. J Am Acad Dermatol 2012;66(1):63–70.

52. Anonymous. Suncare customers reach for new heights. Chemist Druggist 2002;8 June:28.

53. Thieden E, Philipsen PA, Sandby-Møller J, et al. Sunscreen use related to UV exposure, age, sex, and occupation based on personal dosimeter readings and sun-exposure behavior diaries. Arch Dermatol 2005;141(8):967–73.

54. Diffey BL. Sunscreens: use and misuse. In: Giacomoni PU, editor. Sun protection in man. Amsterdam: Elsevier Science BV; 2001. p. 521–34.

55. Diffey BL. Sunscreens as a preventive measure in melanoma: an evidence-based approach or the precautionary principle? Br J Dermatol 2009;161:25–7.

56. Green AC, Williams GM. Point: sunscreen use is a safe and effective approach to skin cancer prevention. Cancer Epidemiol Biomarkers Prev 2007;16(10):1921–2.

57. Gandini S, Sera F, Cattaruzza MS, et al. Meta-analysis of risk factors for cutaneous melanoma: I. Common and atypical naevi. Eur J Cancer 2005;41(1):28–44.

58. Lee TK, Rivers JK, Gallagher RP. Site-specific protective effect of broad-spectrum sunscreen on nevus development among white schoolchildren in a randomized trial. J Am Acad Dermatol 2005; 52(5):786–92.

59. Klug HL, Tooze JA, Graff-Cherry C, et al. Sunscreen prevention of melanoma in man and mouse. Pigment Cell Melanoma Res 2010;23:835–7.

60. Green AC, Williams GM, Logan V, et al. Reduced melanoma after regular sunscreen use: randomized trial follow-up. J Clin Oncol 2011;29(3):257–63.

61. Bigby M, Kim CC. A prospective randomized controlled trial indicates that sunscreen use reduced the risk of developing melanoma. Arch Dermatol 2011;147(7):853–4.

62. Printz C. Dermatology community applauds new FDA sunscreen regulations: labeling requirements aim to make it easier for consumers to select a sunscreen. Cancer 2012;118(1):1–3.

Current Management Approaches for Congenital Melanocytic Nevi

Sven Krengel, MD[a,b], Ashfaq A. Marghoob, MD[c],*

KEYWORDS

- Congenital melanocytic nevi • Neurocutaneous melanocytosis • Multiple medium CMN
- Nevus spilus–like CMN

KEY POINTS

- Congenital melanocytic nevi (CMN) are classified by their projected adult diameter. They display a spectrum of clinical presentations, including nodular variants, multiple medium CMN and nevus spilus-like CMN.
- Leptomeningeal melanocytosis affects 5–15% of patients with CMN >20 cm. Of these, two thirds develop mild to severe neurological symptoms within five years.
- The lifetime risk of melanoma (cutaneous and extracutaneous) in patients with CMN >20 cm is probably less than 5%. Melanomas developing within CMN >40 cm usually arise deep to the dermoepidermal junction and tend to develop in childhood.
- Staged excision after previous tissue expansion is a reasonable therapeutic option for large CMN of the trunk, scalp, and forehead.
- CMN support groups have been founded in several countries, and the parents of a newborn child with a CMN should be encouraged to join these groups.

INTRODUCTION

This article is intended to provide a practice-oriented update on the management of congenital melanocytic nevi (CMN). It is clear that the complexity of the management issues increases with larger CMN, and it is for this reason that this article focuses on these larger CMN. However, many of the management principles outlined in this article may also be relevant for smaller CMN. The scaffold for the article is based on 5 key questions, which are raised in almost every case. The answer to these questions permits the clinician to create a structured management approach for any newborn child with a CMN.

QUESTION 1: WHAT TYPE OF CMN IS PRESENT AND WHAT IS ITS MORPHOLOGY?

The diagnosis of a CMN is usually straightforward. The assessment of the nevus should take into account both its primary and secondary features. The primary features include the location and largest diameter of the nevus. In addition, the presence and number of accompanying smaller (satellite) nevi should be recorded. Traditionally, CMN larger than 20 cm projected adult size (PAS) are designated as large CMN (LCMN) (all metrical data in this article refer to the largest diameter the CMN is expected to attain in adulthood).[1] From birth to adulthood, the area of the head

[a] Department of Dermatology, University of Lübeck, Ratzeburger Allee 160, 23538 Lübeck, Germany; [b] Dermatological Group Practice, Moislinger Allee 95, 23558 Lübeck, Germany; [c] Memorial Sloan-Kettering Skin Cancer Center at Hauppauge, 800 Veterans Memorial Highway, 2nd Floor, Hauppauge, NY 11788, USA
* Corresponding author.
E-mail address: marghooa@mskcc.org

Dermatol Clin 30 (2012) 377–387
doi:10.1016/j.det.2012.04.003
0733-8635/12/$ – see front matter © 2012 Elsevier Inc. All rights reserved.

enlarges by a factor of 2.8, trunk and arms by a factor of 8, and legs by a factor of 12. Consequently, a CMN in a newborn can be expected to reach 20 cm PAS if its largest diameter is around 6 cm on the legs, 7 cm on the trunk and arms, or 12 cm on the face and scalp.[2] The secondary features include the morphologic spectrum of CMN, which can be quite diverse, and comprise variations in color, hairiness, surface topography (ie, rugosity, including mammillated and verrucous changes), and nodularity (ie, palpable dermal or subcutaneous nodules). It is becoming increasingly apparent that these secondary features affect management and thus should be recorded and also included in epidemiologic studies so as to determine any association with complications such as malignancy. In fact, a revised CMN classification system is currently under development, which takes both primary and secondary features into account and classifies nevi on the basis of size and morphology.[3]

On rare occasions, newborns may exhibit unusual CMN variants. The following CMN features may raise difficulties for the clinician:

1. CMN with extensive dermal and/or subcutaneous nodules: Characteristic examples with this morphology are depicted in **Fig. 1**. They

mostly affect CMN larger than 40 cm PAS and are often situated on the back, buttocks, genitalia, or, more rarely, the head/face. Histologically, these tumors consist of monomorphous, often epithelioid nevomelanocytes of variable density, which, at least in older lesions, are embedded in a myxoid stroma. The cells may show variable degrees of peripheral nerve sheath differentiation, neurotization, and mesenchymal or lipomatous changes.[4,5] Larger lesions are sometimes confused for plexiform neurofibroma.[6] A characteristic variant in the genital area has been described as bulky naevocytoma of the perineum.[7] Although most of the dermal or subcutaneous nodules in CMN are present at birth and remain relatively stable, others may develop during infancy or early childhood and enlarge rapidly or even ulcerate. It is quite probable that the former (stable) and the latter (proliferative) nodules represent a congenital and a tardive variant of the same histogenetic process. In enlarging nodules, excision is often necessary to exclude the possible diagnosis of melanoma. The histologic spectrum of proliferative nodules in CMN ranges from benign to atypical variants, the latter exhibiting a certain degree of atypicality of the dermal melanocytes, a blurred demarcation

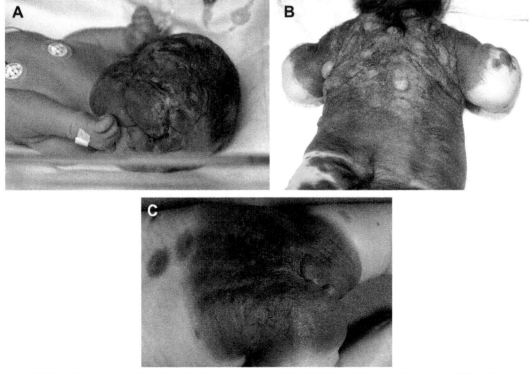

Fig. 1. CMN with extensive dermal and subcutaneous nodules: (A) face, (B) upper back, and (C) genitogluteal area.

of the underlying nevus, and infrequent mitoses.[4] In cases of doubt, molecular differentiation from melanoma may be supported by comparative genomic hybridization from paraffin-embedded tissue.[8]

2. Multiple medium CMN (**Fig. 2**): This variant usually looks much less outstanding than a giant CMN but often carries with it a worse prognosis. These patients manifest only a few (between 3 and 10) medium-sized CMN on the skin (1.5–20 cm PAS). However, multiple foci of abnormal/excessive deposits of melanocytes are often present on the leptomeninges of these patients. These central nervous system (CNS) melanocytic deposits can lead to symptomatic neurologic involvement. The presence of CMN in the skin and CNS is known as neurocutaneous melanocytosis (NCM). The literature review by Kadonaga and Frieden[9] reports that approximately two-thirds of patients with NCM had a giant CMN on the trunk with multiple satellites, and one-third had the variant manifesting multiple medium CMN.

3. Nevus spilus–like variants: Rarely, large or giant CMN may show features reminiscent of speckled lentiginous nevi (SLN, also known as nevus spilus) (**Fig. 3**). Some investigators regard nevus spilus–like variants of CMN as true (large) SLN.[10] However, even if congenital, typical SLN represents a characteristic entity that can in most cases be easily separated from conventional CMN. SLN are defined by the presence of grouped macular or papular melanocytic nevi on a light brown (café au lait macule like) background. The morphologic spectrum of SLN does not include hypertrichosis. In larger SLN, the background café au lait–like lesion sometimes exhibits a sharp midline demarcation and a "checkerboard pattern" distribution.[11] Twin spotting has been discussed as a reason for hybrid forms of large

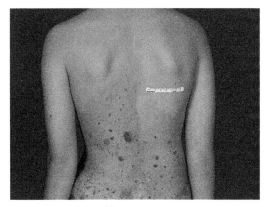

Fig. 3. Nevus spilus–like CMN.

SLN and conventional CMN with hypertrichotic plaques.[12] As yet, there are no indications that nevus spilus–like variants of CMN differ from other forms of CMN in terms of risk of malignancy[13]; death from melanoma has been reported.[14] To the authors' knowledge, no cases of leptomeningeal melanocytosis have been observed in patients with nevus spilus–like variants of CMN.

4. Congenital blue nevi: Congenital dermal melanocytoses, including blue nevi of the epithelioid and spindle cell type, nevus of Ota, and Mongolian spot, represent a distinct group of melanocytic neoplasms (**Fig. 4**). In almost all instances, a clear-cut distinction from a conventional CMN is possible. On the level of pathogenesis, blue nevi (as well as uveal melanoma) frequently exhibit GNAQ mutations, in contrast to NRAS mutations, which is the prevailing finding in CMN.[15,16]

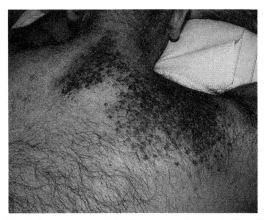

Fig. 4. Large congenital blue nevus of the spindle cell type. The patient underwent operation at age 40 years to alleviate symptoms arising from leptomeningeal involvement. However, he succumbed to CNS melanoma shortly thereafter.

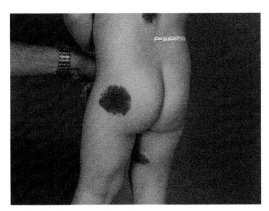

Fig. 2. Multiple medium CMN.

5. Regressive CMN variants is a preliminary term to describe CMN with spontaneous regression. The regression is more often partial than complete. Observations of regression may be made in CMN of all types and sizes, and complete regression is most often seen in scalp nevi.[17] Regression may present as gradual fading of the nevus color or with a halo phenomenon (**Fig. 5**A). In some instances, the reaction involves inflammation and fibrosis.[18] Subtle regressive changes may be indistinguishable from the frequent finding of lightening of the nevus color that commonly occurs during childhood and adolescence (see **Fig. 5**B, C).[19] CMN in fair-skinned children, especially with the Celtic complexion (red hair, freckles), almost always lighten (Krengel, unpublished results, 2012).

QUESTION 2: WHAT IS THE RISK OF CNS INVOLVEMENT?

The hallmark of NCM is the presence of an abnormal deposition of nevomelanocytes along the leptomeninges. This is almost always associated with large (or multiple smaller) CMN on the skin.[9] By logistic regression analysis, the number of satellite nevi has been determined as the predominant significant risk factor for NCM. The statistical risk of a given newborn with a CMN larger than 20 cm PAS was 5 times higher for children with more than 20 satellites than that in children with less than 20 satellites (12.5% vs 2.5%).[20] The presence of melanin deposits in the pia mater of the brain or spine is demonstrable by magnetic resonance imaging (MRI) in approximately 5% to 15% of children with CMN larger than 20 cm PAS ([26/379],[21] [49/1008],[22] [18/120][14]). The presence of melanocytes in the CNS may not result in any neurologic squeal; however, it is not uncommon to develop neurologic symptoms ranging from mild to severe. The numerical ratio between asymptomatic and symptomatic NCM is in the order of 1/3 (asymptomatic) to 2/3 (symptomatic NCM).[21,22] In one study, the rate of progressing from asymptomatic NCM to symptomatic NCM was 7% during a mean follow-up of 5 years.[23] The reported ratios between asymptomatic and symptomatic NCMs are influenced by the clinical threshold criteria used to delineate symptomatic disease and the meticulousness of the neuropsychological examinations.

Symptoms of NCM are usually induced by CNS melanocyte hyperplasia or due to the development of melanoma within the CNS. They include seizures as well as symptoms arising from raised intracranial pressure. Symptoms manifested themselves in 72% within the first 2 years of life[14] (including mild developmental delay) and in 89%

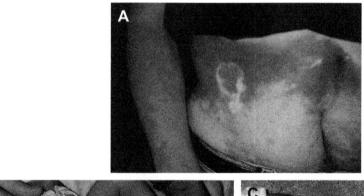

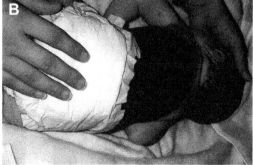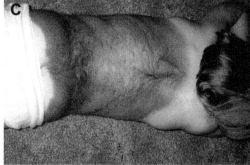

Fig. 5. Regressive CMN. (*A*) Spontaneous partial regression of a CMN, similar to the halo phenomenon occurring in acquired melanocytic nevi. (*B*, *C*) Significant spontaneous lightening of a CMN in the course of 4 years.

within 5 years of life.[22] The long-term prognosis of NCM remains to be determined. Although many symptoms can currently be pharmacologically or surgically controlled, death resulting from progressive neurologic complications or due to CNS melanoma is quite common. Kinsler and colleagues[14] reported that 39% of MRI-positive patients required neurosurgical interventions in the course of their disease and that approximately 8% of symptomatic patients with NCM died of neurologic complications during a mean follow-up of 8.35 years. In another study by Bett,[22] 20.7% of symptomatic patients with NCM died of neurologic complications and 13.8% died of CNS melanoma during a mean follow-up of 5.6 years.

An MRI scan should be obtained for any patient manifesting concerning neurologic symptoms. In addition, an MRI should be considered in asymptomatic patients with CMN larger than 40 cm PAS, especially if they also have more than 20 satellites and in patients with multiple medium CMN or in patients with multiple satellites only. Because myelinization of the brain may obscure the ability to detect subtle NCM deposits, it may be ideal to obtain screening MRI scans between the fourth and eighth month of life. With that said, in most cases, MRI scans appear to be equally sensitive at a later age. MRI scan for NCM-positive patients is valuable in that it can help guide management, including deciding on the feasibility of neurosurgical interventions aimed at alleviating symptoms. In asymptomatic patients at increased risk for NCM, a negative MRI result can help reassure both parents and physicians. On the other hand, if the screening MRI scan in an asymptomatic patient proves positive, it may result in heightened anxiety and may appropriately delay elective excision of cutaneous CMN until after it is confirmed that the NCM is stable and nonprogressive.

QUESTION 3: WHAT IS THE RISK FOR MALIGNANCY?

Numerous malignancies have been associated with CMN, including rhabdomyosarcoma and melanoma. With that said, the association between CMN and melanoma is most clearly established; however, the exact magnitude of the risk for developing melanoma remains to be determined. When discussing the risk for developing melanoma, it is essential to differentiate between cutaneous and extracutaneous melanoma. Some cutaneous CMN can penetrate quite deeply into the subcutaneous tissue, and thus, by convention, any melanoma arising within a CMN, even if located in the adipose tissue, fascia, or muscle, is regarded to have a cutaneous origin. Extracutaneous

melanoma, by and large, refers to primary melanomas arising within the CNS. Studies[24,25] performed in the last 15 years, some prospective by design, have demonstrated that the risk of cutaneous melanoma is in fact lower than that of NCM, which also encompasses CNS melanoma (for a review see[26]).

Regarding melanoma risk, the following 3 points can be made with relative certainty:

1. The risk of melanoma (cutaneous and extracutaneous) correlates with the size of the CMN.

In a comprehensive literature review, Krengel and colleagues[27] determined that the overall melanoma risk was 0.7% for CMN of any size but increased to 2.5% in CMN larger than 20 cm PAS and to 3.1% in CMN larger than 40 cm PAS. They also reported that 73% of all melanomas (and 95% of fatal cases) arose in CMN larger than 40 cm that were situated on the trunk (garment nevi). Similarly, Kinsler and colleagues[28] in a survey of 349 patients reported that 5 out of 6 melanomas were found in patients with giant nevi larger than 60 cm PAS, and 1 melanoma was found in a patient with the multiple medium CMN variant. In this study, 2 of the melanomas were cutaneous, 2 were in the CNS, and the site of the primary melanoma remained unknown in one case. It is currently not known whether, independent of CMN size, truncal localization represents a risk factor for melanoma (note that most CMN larger than 40 cm PAS and almost all CMN larger than 60 cm PAS are situated on the trunk). Bett[29] demonstrated that the absolute melanoma risk of truncal LCMN was 2.9% (15/525) in comparison with 0.3% (1/336) for LCMN of the head and limbs. In their meticulous review, Price and Schaffer[13] found that of the 39 melanomas in patients with LCMN that were reported in large studies during the past 2 decades, the melanoma had the following primary sites: 27 (69%) on the trunk, 3 (8%) on the head/neck, 1 (2%) on an extremity, 3 (8%) in the CNS; 2 (5%) in the retroperitoneum; and 3 cases (8%) with the primary site unknown.

Although the number of satellite nevi is associated with risk of NCM, it does not seem to confer an increased risk for developing cutaneous melanoma.[26] Beyond CMN diameter and localization, the impact of CMN color, thickness, and surface characteristics on melanoma risk remains to be determined.

2. The lifetime risk of melanoma (cutaneous and extracutaneous) in CMN larger than 20 cm PAS is probably less than 5%.

Statistical data[30,31] regarding melanoma risk are based on limited mean follow-up times, mostly between 5 and 10 years (for a review see[27]). This might contribute to an underestimation of the melanoma risk. On the other hand, smaller studies, especially if retrospective, are likely to exaggerate melanoma risk because of selection bias.[27] In addition, melanoma simulants, such as proliferative nodules, have probably been inadvertently classified as melanomas in some studies resulting in an overestimation of risk. For all the aforementioned reasons and for the necessity to distinguish between cutaneous and extracutaneous melanoma, it is currently not possible to estimate the true lifetime risk for a given patient developing cutaneous melanoma. According to data from the 2 latest cohort studies by Hale and colleagues[32] (mean follow-up, 5.3 years) and Kinsler and colleagues[14] (mean follow-up, 9.2 years), the absolute risk of melanoma appears to be quite low. These studies reported that 0 of 170[32] and 2 of 122 (1.6%)[14] patients with LCMN (>20 cm PAS) developed cutaneous melanoma and 4 of 170 (2.4%)[32] and 2 of 122 (1.6%)[14] developed extracutaneous melanomas.

When attempting to extrapolate lifetime risk of melanoma from studies that had limited follow-up times, it is important to factor in the observation that LCMN-associated cutaneous and extracutaneous melanomas tend to arise most commonly early in life (mean age at diagnosis, 15.5 years; median age, 7 years[27]). The 39 melanomas reported in one of the aforementioned reviews[13] were diagnosed at a median age of 3.5 years (range, birth–58 years). This is not to say that melanomas do not develop in older patients with LCMN; in fact, numerous cases of CMN-associated melanomas have been observed in older patients.[29,30,33]

To help better predict and define melanoma risk, it is imperative for future studies to take into account CMN size (ie, risk may differ in CMN with a maximum diameter of 20, 40, and 60 cm PAS), differentiating between cutaneous and extracutaneous melanoma and taking into account other factors such as thickness and nodularity of the CMN. Furthermore, the outcomes of cutaneous melanomas, whether fatal or nonfatal, should be stated.

3. A significant proportion of cutaneous melanoma in CMN arises deep to the dermoepidermal junction.

There is a wide range of benign and malignant tumors that may arise within CMN (**Table 1**). CMN-associated cutaneous melanomas may arise from epidermal melanocytes or from melanocytes located in the dermis or in deeper structures such as the subcutis and fascia. The former type resembles conventional melanoma in terms of clinical appearance and histology (superficial spreading or nodular type); this type rarely arises before puberty and may develop in CMN of any size, including small CMN. The latter type is more characteristic of LCMN. It clinically presents as an enlarging cutaneous nodule, often in childhood or early infancy. Histologically, it usually

Table 1 CMN-associated tumors			
	Cutaneous Melanocytic Proliferations	Melanocytic Proliferations of the CNS	Other CMN-Associated Tumors
Benign	• CMN • Proliferative nodule	• Leptomeningeal melanocytosis • Melanocytoma of the CNS (intermediate dignity)	• Neurofibroma • Lipoma (subcutaneous, in some cases leptomeningeal)
Malignant	Cutaneous melanoma • Classical melanoma arising from epidermal or uppermost dermal layers (mostly after puberty) • Deeply situated dermal or subcutaneous melanoma[a] (often in childhood, mostly CMN >40 cm)	• CNS melanoma	• Rhabdomyosarcoma • Liposarcoma • Malignant peripheral nerve sheath tumor • Neuroblastoma

[a] In some cases situated as deep as the fascia, muscle, and retroperitoneum.

consists of small monomorphous cells (melano-blastoma).[34,35] This type of melanoma is easier to detect via palpation than by visual inspection.

The impact of surgery on the risk of cutaneous melanoma remains a controversial issue. An intuitive argument is that the reduction in the number of nevomelanocytic cells (ie, nevomelanocytic burden) should stochastically reduce the risk for developing cutaneous melanoma within the CMN.[36] Superficial treatment modalities are therefore (at least theoretically) less effective than complete resections at reducing cutaneous melanoma risk. Conversely, Kinsler and Bulstrode[19] have claimed that surgical intervention may adversely affect the behavior of residual nevomelanocytic cells, and this may in fact increase the risk for melanoma. Based on this theory, the investigators recommend against routine surgery of CMN. The authors are of the opinion that Kinsler and colleagues' supposition requires consideration but that currently available data do not justify their view against prophylactic excision of LCMN. Regarding treatments aimed at eliminating the superficial component of CMN, there is no conclusive evidence-based data showing any benefit or harm vis-à-vis melanoma risk. In addition, it remains unproved that superficially treated areas (eg, after curettage) may hinder a timely diagnosis of melanoma arising from deeper structures. The heart of the question regarding any contemplated intervention is whether the magnitude of melanoma risk reduction warrants routinely recommending it to patients.[37] However, the answer to this question remains unknown and will likely remain controversial for the foreseeable future.[26]

QUESTION 4: CAN THE CMN BE REMOVED?

Although the medical indications for surgical intervention vis-à-vis melanoma risk reduction remain debatable, its potential to improve cosmesis and psychosocial well-being is irrefutable. For many families and physicians, the predominant reason to operate on a CMN is aesthetic improvement. With this in mind, clinicians need to carefully evaluate the therapeutic armamentarium and select one procedure or a combination of procedures that will likely have the greatest impact on improving aesthetics while still preserving and maintaining normal function. Several detailed reviews on the subject of therapeutic options for CMN have already been published.[13,38–41] CMN therapy was also a key topic of discussion during the 2011 International CMN Expert Meeting in Tübingen, Germany.[42] Based on the published reviews and expert experiences, which are often reflected by images obtained before and after

therapeutic intervention, it becomes immediately apparent that there is more than one way to "skin a CMN." The choice of a treatment method depends on size, localization, CMN surface structure, and, most importantly, the expertise and experience of the surgeon. Therefore, it should come as no surprise that the answer to the question of how best to treat a given CMN is tightly linked to available resources and the treating physician's expertise. It is also important to recognize situations in which it may be better to "stand there and do nothing." In other words, in certain circumstances it may be prudent to refrain from subjecting patients to the surgical removal of CMN, for example, in patients with symptomatic NCM, in CNS melanoma, or in cases in which the intervention is likely to result in a loss of function.

At present, staged excision down to the fascia with flap reconstruction after previous tissue expansion of adjacent normal skin represents the mainstay of therapy for LCMN of the trunk, scalp, and forehead.[38,39,42] Tissue expanders can be implanted beginning at the age of 3 months, and, with proper parent education, the consecutive filling/expansion procedure can usually be performed safely at home.[38] Repeated rounds of tissue expansions may be performed in 3 to 6 monthly intervals. In CMN of the upper extremity, large expanded transposition flaps from abdomen/flank/back may yield better aesthetic and functional results.[43] Free tissue transfer and expanded pedicle flaps represent alternative options for CMN located on the lower extremity.[44]

Conventional plastic surgery without using tissue expanders may still be a good choice for the removal of LCMN. This is easier to accomplish if performed during the first 1 to 2 years of life while the skin adjacent to the CMN is amenable to considerable mobilization.[42,45] Although primary wound closure is preferred, both aesthetically and functionally, circumstances may arise in which split-thickness skin grafting or application of artificial skin substitutes cannot be avoided or may prove necessary. It is imperative that all surgical interventions be planned in such a manner as to avoid functional compromise of the area repaired. However, even the best intended surgeries might not eventuate in the desired aesthetic results or might impair normal mechanical function such as restriction of mobility of the involved area. In facial CMN, even an eye-catching nevus might be preferable to an impairment of mimical function or of the integrity of the aesthetic units by scar tension.

Neonatal dermabrasion and curettage represent surgical modalities that mainly remove the superficial layers of the skin. Although it may prove difficult to achieve excellent cosmetic results on very thick and deeply penetrating CMN, these procedures can yield acceptable cosmetic results if performed on appropriately selected CMN such as those with a high nevomelanocytic burden in the superficial layers of the skin.[46,47] These methods are currently being used most frequently in Europe, with dermabrasion being preferred in German-speaking countries and neonatal curettage being preferred in Belgium. One of the major limitations of these procedures is that they need to be performed early in life because the best results are obtained when the procedures are started within the first 4 to 8 weeks of birth. In giant CMN, up to 3 to 4 rounds of treatment may be required. Partial repigmentation is a common finding after superficial treatments, especially if performed on deeply penetrating CMN and if therapy starts later in infancy.

Laser therapy may represent a treatment option, especially for small and medium-sized CMN, including facial CMN. August and colleagues[48] treated 55 patients with medium-sized CMN under local anesthesia (mean age, 18 years). The mean number of laser treatments was between 5 and 6, separated by 3-month intervals. Carbon dioxide laser treatment was most effective for head and neck nevi with a papillomatous (mammillated) surface, whereas flat (macular) truncal CMN responded best to frequency-doubled Nd:YAG laser therapy. In giant CMN, carbon dioxide laser has been used with varying results, including cases with a satisfactory pigment reduction, but hypertrophic scarring may be a complication. Laser-induced scarring seems to be more frequent on the extremities, especially lower arms and limbs and on the anterior trunk.[48–51] Partial repigmentation with a speckled appearance is quite common after laser treatment.

Parents or patients (if old enough) need to consider a couple of general issues before deciding for or against surgical intervention. First, most LCMN tend to lighten during the first decade of life; in fair skinned-children the degree of lightening can be quite remarkable.[19] Therefore, the potential for cosmetically disturbing scars or speckled repigmentation must be weighed against the possibility of the CMN becoming lighter in color over time. The same consideration has to be made regarding superficial treatments because the repigmentation after the procedure may result in a similar color as would have occurred had the CMN been allowed to undergo spontaneous lightening. Second, psychological studies have revealed that 3 out of 4 older children and adolescents with a CMN prefer a scar over the original nevus.[26,52] With that said, 1 in 4 patients or parents regret their decision of considering surgical intervention.[26] Obviously, satisfaction surveys administered to patients and families may be inherently biased in favor of the actual decisions that they made for themselves in real life.[19] Future studies need to be designed to factor in this potential source of bias.

QUESTION 5: WHERE CAN CMN-AFFECTED INDIVIDUALS OR THEIR FAMILY MEMBERS FIND HELP?

Much of the anxiety present in individuals affected by a CMN stems from a lack of transparent and reliable information and from the scarcity of clinicians experienced in the management of CMN and/or NCMs. Once the emotional shock of giving birth to a child with a CMN has subsided, families are confronted with numerous management decisions and the need to find experienced clinicians and surgeons. Regular dermatologic follow-up consultations should be arranged and should aim at (1) surveillance for melanoma by inspection, palpation, and possibly imaging methods, for example, positron emission tomography for certain diagnostic purposes (this is important even after excision/dermabrasion because melanoma can develop from residual cells); (2) surveillance for NCM by periodic neurologic examinations; (3) reinforcing prevention issues such as UV protection; (4) reinforcing the importance of joining support groups; (5) determining how the patients and their families are adjusting to their life and if psychological intervention may be of benefit; (6) providing coping strategies; and (7) photodocumenting the clinical course (eg, general or partial spontaneous lightening of the CMN) and reinforcing the importance to register at the International CMN Registry (http://www.nevus.org/login.php) and update this registration regularly.

In addition to medical consultations, most families have a strong desire to share their own experiences and/or hear the experiences of others who have undergone a similar predicament. Nowadays the Internet is a major source of information, allowing anyone to rapidly acquire knowledge on rare diseases while at the same time providing a portal that allows one to find others similarly affected.[53] The Internet has provided a means for patients, families, and physicians to cooperate and interact much more efficiently, clearly a tremendous benefit to all who are involved. CMN support groups have been founded in several countries, and the parents of a newborn child with a CMN should be encouraged to visit the Web sites of these groups (**Table 2**) and to organize or visit gatherings of CMN families (eg, the biennial Nevus Outreach Conferences

Table 2	
CMN support groups	
Country	**Web Site**
United States	http://www.nevus.org/ http://www.nevusnetwork.org/
Great Britain	http://www.caringmattersnow. co.uk/
France	http://www.naevus.fr/ http://www.naevus2000france europe.org/
Germany, Austria, Switzerland	http://www.naevus-netzwerk. de/
Spain	http://www.asonevus.org/
Portugal	http://www.associacaonevo portugal.org/index.html
The Netherlands	http://www.nevusnetwerk.nl/
Australia	http://www.nevussupport.com/
Italy	http://www.nevogigante.it/

[http://www.nevus.org/our-conferences_id562.html? page_id=562]). The added benefit to many of these patient/parent-driven support groups is that they often foster collaborations between the support groups and interested expert clinicians, surgeons, psychologists, neurologists, and a host of other researchers with the mutual aim of trying to continuously improve the quality of life of a person with a CMN. The fruits of these collaborative efforts are already visible with the publication of several important studies using data obtained from Internet-based patient advocacy group registries[21,25,29] or from data derived from direct cooperation between patient groups and their physicians.[14,19,28,53] In addition, in 2011, these collaborations were instrumental in organizing the first international CMN expert meeting, which resulted in some remarkable outcomes.[42] First, it resulted in the creation of a task force whose mission is to unify currently existing CMN/NCM databases into one collaborative and prospective international CMN/NCM registry. Second, it set the groundwork for an initiative that aims to create a CMN/NCM tissue repository, which could someday be accessed for research purposes. Third, this meeting also lead to the formation of the Nevus Science Group, a network of expert scientists who are interested in addressing the many unresolved issues pertaining to CMN and NCM. It is reasonable to speculate that all the aforementioned efforts should start providing important insights into the CMN etiology, pathogenesis, and therapy in the not too distant future.

REFERENCES

1. Kopf AW, Bart RS, Hennessey P. Congenital nevocytic nevi and malignant melanomas. J Am Acad Dermatol 1979;1(2):123–30.
2. DeDavid M, Orlow SJ, Provost N, et al. A study of large congenital melanocytic nevi and associated malignant melanomas: review of cases in the New York University Registry and the world literature. J Am Acad Dermatol 1997;36(3 Pt 1):409–16.
3. Krengel S, Scope A, Dusza SW, et al. New recommendations for the categorization of cutaneous features of congenital melanocytic nevi. J Am Acad Dermatol, in press.
4. Leech SN, Bell H, Leonard N, et al. Neonatal giant congenital nevi with proliferative nodules: a clinicopathologic study and literature review of neonatal melanoma. Arch Dermatol 2004;140(1):83–8.
5. van Houten AH, van Dijk MC, Schuttelaar ML. Proliferative nodules in a giant congenital melanocytic nevus—case report and review of the literature. J Cutan Pathol 2010;37(7):764–76.
6. Schaffer JV, Chang MW, Kovich OI, et al. Pigmented plexiform neurofibroma: distinction from a large congenital melanocytic nevus. J Am Acad Dermatol 2007;56(5):862–8.
7. Reyes-Mugica M, Gonzalez-Crussi F, Bauer BS, et al. Bulky naevocytoma of the perineum: a singular variant of congenital giant pigmented naevus. Virchows Arch A Pathol Anat Histopathol 1992;420(1):87–93.
8. Bastian BC, Xiong J, Frieden IJ, et al. Genetic changes in neoplasms arising in congenital melanocytic nevi: differences between nodular proliferations and melanomas. Am J Pathol 2002;161(4): 1163–9.
9. Kadonaga JN, Frieden IJ. Neurocutaneous melanosis: definition and review of the literature. J Am Acad Dermatol 1991;24(5 Pt 1):747–55.
10. Schaffer JV, Orlow SJ, Lazova R, et al. Speckled lentiginous nevus: within the spectrum of congenital melanocytic nevi. Arch Dermatol 2001;137(2): 172–8.
11. Vidaurri-de la Cruz H, Happle R. Two distinct types of speckled lentiginous nevi characterized by macular versus papular speckles. Dermatology 2006;212(1):53–8.
12. Torrelo A, de Prada I, Zambrano A, et al. Extensive speckled lentiginous nevus associated with giant congenital melanocytic nevus: an unusual example of twin spotting? Eur J Dermatol 2003;13(6):534–6.
13. Price HN, Schaffer JV. Congenital melanocytic nevi—when to worry and how to treat: facts and controversies. Clin Dermatol 2010;28(3):293–302.
14. Kinsler VA, Chong WK, Aylett SE, et al. Complications of congenital melanocytic naevi in children: analysis of 16 years' experience and clinical practice. Br J Dermatol 2008;159(4):907–14.

15. Ross AL, Sanchez MI, Grichnik JM. Molecular nevo-genesis. Dermatol Res Pract 2011;2011:463184.

16. Van Raamsdonk CD, Bezrookove V, Green G, et al. Frequent somatic mutations of GNAQ in uveal melanoma and blue naevi. Nature 2009;457(7229): 599–602.

17. Strauss RM, Newton Bishop JA. Spontaneous involution of congenital melanocytic nevi of the scalp. J Am Acad Dermatol 2008;58(3):508–11.

18. Ruiz-Maldonado R, Orozco-Covarrubias L, Ridaura-Sanz C, et al. Desmoplastic hairless hypopigmented naevus: a variant of giant congenital melanocytic naevus. Br J Dermatol 2003;148(6):1253–7.

19. Kinsler V, Bulstrode N. The role of surgery in the management of congenital melanocytic naevi in children: a perspective from Great Ormond Street Hospital. J Plast Reconstr Aesthet Surg 2009a; 62(5):595–601.

20. Marghoob AA, Dusza S, Oliveria S, et al. Number of satellite nevi as a correlate for neurocutaneous melanocytosis in patients with large congenital melanocytic nevi. Arch Dermatol 2004;140(2):171–5.

21. Agero AL, Benvenuto-Andrade C, Dusza SW, et al. Asymptomatic neurocutaneous melanocytosis in patients with large congenital melanocytic nevi: a study of cases from an Internet-based registry. J Am Acad Dermatol 2005;53(6):959–65.

22. Bett BJ. Large or multiple congenital melanocytic nevi: occurrence of neurocutaneous melanocytosis in 1008 persons. J Am Acad Dermatol 2006;54(5): 767–77.

23. Foster RD, Williams ML, Barkovich AJ, et al. Giant congenital melanocytic nevi: the significance of neurocutaneous melanosis in neurologically asymptomatic children. Plast Reconstr Surg 2001;107(4):933–41.

24. Bittencourt FV, Marghoob AA, Kopf AW, et al. Large congenital melanocytic nevi and the risk for development of malignant melanoma and neurocutaneous melanocytosis. Pediatrics 2000;106(4): 736–41.

25. Ka VS, Dusza SW, Halpern AC, et al. The association between large congenital melanocytic naevi and cutaneous melanoma: preliminary findings from an Internet-based registry of 379 patients. Melanoma Res 2005;15(1):61–7.

26. Slutsky JB, Barr JM, Femia AN, et al. Large congenital melanocytic nevi: associated risks and management considerations. Semin Cutan Med Surg 2010; 29(2):79–84.

27. Krengel S, Hauschild A, Schäfer T. Melanoma risk in congenital melanocytic naevi: a systematic review. Br J Dermatol 2006;155(1):1–8.

28. Kinsler VA, Birley J, Atherton DJ. Great Ormond Street Hospital for Children Registry for congenital melanocytic naevi: prospective study 1988-2007. Part 1—epidemiology, phenotype and outcomes. Br J Dermatol 2009;160(1):143–50.

29. Bett BJ. Large or multiple congenital melanocytic nevi: occurrence of cutaneous melanoma in 1008 persons. J Am Acad Dermatol 2005;52(5):793–7.

30. Lorentzen M, Pers M, Bretteville-Jensen G. The incidence of malignant transformation in giant pigmented nevi. Scand J Plast Reconstr Surg 1977; 11(2):163–7.

31. Swerdlow AJ, English JS, Qiao Z. The risk of melanoma in patients with congenital nevi: a cohort study. J Am Acad Dermatol 1995;32(4):595–9.

32. Hale EK, Stein J, Ben-Porat L, et al. Association of melanoma and neurocutaneous melanocytosis with large congenital melanocytic naevi—results from the NYU-LCMN registry. Br J Dermatol 2005; 152(3):512–7.

33. Yun SJ, Kwon OS, Han JH, et al. Clinical characteristics and risk of melanoma development from giant congenital melanocytic naevi in Korea: a nationwide retrospective study. Br J Dermatol 2012;166(1): 115–23.

34. Reed RB, Becker SW Sr, Becker SW Jr, et al. Giant pigmented nevi, melanoma, and leptomeningeal melanocytosis: a clinical and histopathological study. Arch Dermatol 1965;91:100–19.

35. Reed RJ. Giant congenital nevi: a conceptualization of patterns. J Invest Dermatol 1993;100:300S–12S.

36. Marghoob AA, Agero AL, Benvenuto-Andrade C, et al. Large congenital melanocytic nevi, risk of cutaneous melanoma, and prophylactic surgery. J Am Acad Dermatol 2006;54(5):868–70.

37. Kanzler MH. Management of large congenital melanocytic nevi: art versus science. J Am Acad Dermatol 2006;54(5):874–6.

38. Arneja JS, Gosain AK. Giant congenital melanocytic nevi. Plast Reconstr Surg 2009;124(Suppl 1):1e–13e.

39. Bauer BS, Corcoran J. Treatment of large and giant nevi. Clin Plast Surg 2005;32(1):11–8, vii.

40. Marghoob AA, Borrego JP, Halpern AC. Congenital melanocytic nevi: treatment modalities and management options. Semin Cutan Med Surg 2003;22(1): 21–32.

41. Tromberg J, Bauer B, Benvenuto-Andrade C, et al. Congenital melanocytic nevi needing treatment. Dermatol Ther 2005;18(2):136–50.

42. Krengel S, Breuninger H, Beckwith M, et al. Meeting report from the 2011 International Expert Meeting on Large Congenital Melanocytic Nevi and Neurocutaneous Melanocytosis, Tübingen. Pigment Cell Melanoma Res 2011;24(4):E1–6.

43. Margulis A, Bauer BS, Fine NA. Large and giant congenital pigmented nevi of the upper extremity: an algorithm to surgical management. Ann Plast Surg 2004;52(2):158–67.

44. Kryger ZB, Bauer BS. Surgical management of large and giant congenital pigmented nevi of the lower extremity. Plast Reconstr Surg 2008; 121(5):1674–84.

45. Rothfuss M, Schilling M, Breuninger H. Early excision of congenital melanocytic nevi under tumescent anesthesia and skin expansion by intracutaneous double butterfly sutures. J Dtsch Dermatol Ges 2009;7(5):427–33.

46. De Raeve LE, Roseeuw DI. Curettage of giant congenital melanocytic nevi in neonates: a decade later. Arch Dermatol 2002;138(7):943–7.

47. Rompel RH, Wehinger M, Möser J, et al. Konnatale Nävuszellnävi: Klinisches Bild und therapeutische Optionen. Pädiatr Praxis 2002;61:471–90 [in German].

48. August PJ, Ferguson JE, Madan V. A study of the efficacy of carbon dioxide and pigment-specific lasers in the treatment of medium-sized congenital melanocytic naevi. Br J Dermatol 2011;164(5):1037–42.

49. Horner BM, El-Muttardi NS, Mayou BJ. Treatment of congenital melanocytic naevi with CO2 laser. Ann Plast Surg 2005;55(3):276–80.

50. Michel JL, Caillet-Chomel L. Treatment of giant congenital nevus with high-energy pulsed CO2 laser. Arch Pediatr 2001;8(11):1185–94 [in French].

51. Michel JL. Laser therapy of giant congenital melanocytic nevi. Eur J Dermatol 2003;13(1):57–64.

52. Koot HM, de Waard-van der Spek F, Peer CD, et al. Psychosocial sequelae in 29 children with giant congenital melanocytic naevi. Clin Exp Dermatol 2000;25(8):589–93.

53. Krengel S, Breuninger H, Hauschild A, et al. Installation of a network for patients with congenital melanocytic nevi in German-speaking countries. J Dtsch Dermatol Ges 2008;6(3):204–8.

Dysplastic Nevi

Michele J. Farber, MD[a], Edward R. Heilman, MD[b,c],
Robert J. Friedman, MD, MSc (Med)[d,*]

KEYWORDS

- Dysplastic nevi • Melanoma • Genetic mutation • Cytologic atypia

KEY POINTS

- The dysplastic nevus has been the subject of much debate in terms of its clinical and histologic definitions as well as its biologic potential.
- Dysplastic nevi are acquired melanocytic lesions that often mimic melanoma clinically and portend an increased risk for melanoma, although it is highly unusual that dysplastic nevi themselves eventuate into melanoma.
- Management of patients with dysplastic nevi and dysplastic nevus syndrome should include vigilant follow up, thorough physical examination, and timely biopsy of suspicious lesions.

INTRODUCTION

Dysplastic nevi have been a subject of much debate since their original description in 1978.[1,2] Although some question the biological potential of dysplastic nevi themselves, several studies have shown that the presence of dysplastic nevi confers a substantial risk for melanoma.[3–5] In addition to predisposing patients to melanoma, dysplastic nevi have been shown to harbor genetic mutations, indicating their position on a continuum between banal nevi and melanoma. Dysplastic nevi are also clinically relevant as mimickers of melanoma, despite dysplastic nevi themselves only rarely progressing to melanoma, and can be quite challenging diagnostically. Given the controversy surrounding dysplastic nevi, this article reviews the history, epidemiology, biology and genetics, clinical features, histopathologic features, and management guidelines for patients with these lesions.

HISTORY

Dysplastic nevi were first described by Clark and colleagues[6] in 1978, when they used the term "B-K mole syndrome" after 2 of the patients presenting with this previously unrecognized condition in families affected by familial malignant melanoma. By this first definition, dysplastic nevi were distinctive melanocytic nevi that could be distinguished by their clinical and histologic features. Around the same time, Lynch and colleagues[7] described this phenotype as familial atypical multiple mole melanoma syndrome. With further research, and the recognition that this entity can be sporadic in addition to familial,[8] additional names were proposed including dysplastic nevus and dysplastic nevus syndrome, atypical mole (and syndrome), and Clark nevus (and syndrome).[8,9] The histopathologic classification of these lesions has been equally confusing and debated. Different proposed terminology has included nevus with architectural disorder, pagetoid melanocytic proliferation, atypical melanocytic proliferation, and intraepithelial melanocytic neoplasia.[10–13]

In an attempt to resolve some of the debate and set forth management guidelines for this clinical entity, the National Institutes of Health (NIH) Consensus Development Conference was held in 1992. A panel of experts at this meeting concluded

[a] Jefferson Medical College, Thomas Jefferson University, 1020 Walnut Street, Philadelphia, PA 19107, USA;
[b] Department of Dermatology, State University of New York, Downstate Medical Center, 450 Clarkson Avenue, Brooklyn, NY 11203, USA; [c] Department of Pathology, State University of New York, Downstate Medical Center, 450 Clarkson Avenue, Brooklyn, NY 11203, USA; [d] Department of Dermatology, NYU School of Medicine, 562 First Avenue, New York, NY 10016, USA
* Corresponding author.
E-mail address: rfriedmanmdceo@hotmail.com

Dermatol Clin 30 (2012) 389–404
doi:10.1016/j.det.2012.04.004

that the dysplastic nevus is a distinct clinicopathologic entity that can be distinguished clinically and histopathologically from banal nevi. The Conference also recommended that these lesions be called atypical moles rather than dysplastic nevi, citing a lack of consensus on the definition of dysplasia. In addition, they proposed that the familial syndrome in melanoma-prone families be termed familial atypical mole and melanoma syndrome, which they defined as: (1) occurrence of melanoma in 1 or more first- or second-degree relatives; (2) a large number of melanocytic nevi, usually over 50, some of which are atypical and variable in size; and (3) some melanocytic nevi showing specific histopathologic features. Furthermore, this panel proposed a histopathologic definition as "nevus with architectural disorder" and suggested also including information on the degree of cytologic atypia.[10]

These recommendations, however, have not been fully accepted. According to a survey of the fellows of the American Academy of Dermatology, a majority prefer the nomenclature dysplastic nevus to atypical mole.[14] Dysplastic nevus and dysplastic nevus syndrome are the most commonly used terms used in the literature. These names are also useful because they incorporate the histopathologic characteristics of the lesions.[3,8] As such, the term dysplastic nevus is used throughout this article.

EPIDEMIOLOGY

The prevalence of dysplastic nevi depends on whether the diagnosis is based on clinical or histopathologic criteria. Clinically, dysplastic nevi have been reported to range in prevalence from 2% to 18% in the Caucasian population.[4,15–17] Similarly, the histopathologic finding of melanocytic dysplasia has been reported at a prevalence of approximately 10%.[18] However, dysplastic nevi are found with much higher frequency in patients with a history of melanoma, with researchers reporting a prevalence of 34% to 59% in this population.[5,19–21] The variation in prevalence rates potentially reflects the differing diagnostic criteria used for dysplastic nevi as well as the interplay of genetic and environmental factors; dysplastic nevi as well as the dysplastic nevus syndrome phenotype have been reported with higher frequency in people who are chronically sun exposed in comparison with those who do not have chronic sun exposure.[22]

Several studies have shown that dysplastic nevi confer an increased risk of melanoma. Several retrospective case-control studies have confirmed this association, with risk increasing based on the number of dysplastic nevi. Estimates of melanoma risk range from between 2- and 12-fold in patients with dysplastic nevi. Although other phenotypic factors, such as sun sensitivity, eye color, hair color, solar damage, freckles, and total number of nondysplastic nevi also influence melanoma risk, the relative risk of melanoma remains elevated when controlling for these characteristics.[5,19,20,22–29]

Prospective studies have also corroborated this finding. Compared with controls, patients with dysplastic nevi had a relative risk for melanoma of 47 to 92[30–33]; these figures exclude any personal or family history of melanoma, as these factors are associated with even higher melanoma risk in the setting of dysplastic nevi. Patients with dysplastic nevus syndrome are also at increased risk of melanoma. Marghoob and colleagues[34] examined the incidence of melanoma in patients with and without dysplastic nevus syndrome, and estimated a 10-year cumulative risk of newly diagnosed invasive melanomas of 10.7% in patients with dysplastic nevus syndrome compared with 0.62% in a control population. It is also important that, whereas a majority of studies quantified melanoma risk based on clinically identified dysplastic nevi, others showed that this association remains when dysplastic nevi are diagnosed histopathologically.[35]

Dysplastic nevi increase the risk of melanoma based on personal and family history. There is an approximately 100-fold increase in the incidence of melanoma in patients with a personal history of melanoma, more than 200-fold increase in those with at least 2 family members affected by melanoma, and more than 1200-fold increase in patients with both personal and family history of melanoma.[36] Other researchers have reported similar melanoma risk in patients with dysplastic nevi and a personal or family history of melanoma.[30,31,33,37] In patients with dysplastic nevi from melanoma-prone families (2 or more family members with melanoma), Tucker and colleagues[37] reported that approximately 50% of people develop melanoma by age 50 years and approximately 82% develop melanoma by age 72 years. These patients also present with melanoma at younger ages, with approximately 10% of melanoma cases in this cohort occurring before age 20 years.

Although dysplastic nevi are associated with a significant risk for melanoma, most dysplastic nevi themselves do not eventuate into melanoma.[3,4] Melanomas may arise in association with dysplastic nevi on histopathology,[36–38] but an association does not indicate dysplastic nevi as precursor lesions to melanoma. The presence of dysplastic nevi is better used in the clinical context as a phenotypic marker of patients who are at increased risk for melanoma and thus need closer follow-up.

CLINICAL FEATURES

Dysplastic nevi are acquired melanocytic lesions that frequently share some of the same clinical features as melanoma.[39] As such, many have suggested that the ABCD (Asymmetry, Border irregularity, Color variegation, and Diameter >6 mm) rule of melanoma can be useful for identifying dysplastic nevi, with the degree of each of these features differentiating these 2 entities. Although a useful algorithm for identifying suspicious melanocytic lesions, this overlap in criteria results in a tendency to overdiagnose melanoma. Dysplastic nevi can also simulate other types of pigmented lesions and can often be very difficult to diagnose clinically.[39,40]

Dysplastic nevi were initially defined by Clark and colleagues[6] as moles that were greater than 5 mm in diameter, irregular in outline, and variable in color. These researchers also noted that these lesions were flat and were also markedly variable from one another. Subsequent groups have set forth more specific criteria for dysplastic nevi, with Kelly and colleagues[41] classifying lesions as clinically dysplastic if they had a macular component and showed at least 3 of the following 5 clinical features: irregularly distributed pigmentation, ill-defined border, irregular border, background of erythema, size greater than 5 mm. Tucker and colleagues[5] used similar clinical features to define dysplastic nevi, emphasizing that these lesions should be greater than 5 mm in diameter, flat or containing a flat component, and should display at least 2 additional features: variable pigmentation, irregular or asymmetric outline, and indistinct borders.

Dysplastic nevi are conspicuously heterogeneous in appearance, with several clinical subtypes. The most common are: (1) the lentiginous variant with a flat surface and a homogeneous dark brown to black color; (2) the fried-egg or sunnyside-up variant that has a darker or lighter center as compared with the periphery, and can be either macular or papular (raised center and a flat periphery); (3) a targeted variant, with concentric annular zones varying in pigment shade; (4) seborrheic keratosis–like or mammillated variant, with a verrucous or cobblestone surface and often dark-brown pigmentation; (5) erythematous type that is pink to red in color; and (6) melanoma stimulant that exhibits the ABCD features of melanoma (**Figs. 1–5**).[42,43]

Patients with dysplastic nevi tend to have multiple moles, the majority of which are not dysplastic.[39] In terms of distribution, dysplastic nevi are most

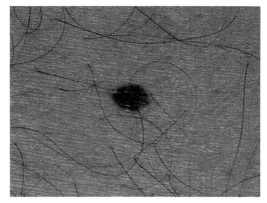

Fig. 1. A lentiginous variant of a dysplastic nevus. (*Courtesy of* Jason B. Lee, MD, Department of Dermatology and Cutaneous Biology, Thomas Jefferson University Hospital.)

frequently found on the trunk, particularly the upper back, but they can be present anywhere on the skin, including sun-protected areas such as the scalp, breasts, and buttocks. Dysplastic nevi typically become clinically apparent at puberty and are more predominant in people younger than 30 to 40 years than in older populations. However, people older than 40 years can present with new dysplastic nevi.[4]

Because these patients tend to have numerous nevi, the clinical differentiation between dysplastic nevi and dysplastic nevus syndrome is also important, as the latter portends a markedly higher risk for developing melanoma. Although debated, the phenotype for this syndrome commonly includes having more than 100 melanocytic nevi, including at least 1 clinically dysplastic nevus as well as at least 1 nevus larger than 8 mm in diameter.[42,44] This syndrome can be sporadic or familial, with

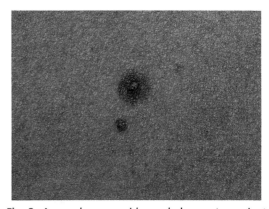

Fig. 2. A papular sunnyside-up darker-center variant of a dysplastic nevus. (*Courtesy of* Jason B. Lee, MD, Department of Dermatology and Cutaneous Biology, Thomas Jefferson University Hospital.)

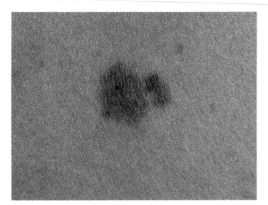

Fig. 3. A papular sunnyside-up lighter-center variant of a dysplastic nevus. (*Courtesy of* Jason B. Lee, MD, Department of Dermatology and Cutaneous Biology, Thomas Jefferson University Hospital.)

different classifications based on the degree of family and personal history of dysplastic nevi and melanoma. However, classifying familial dysplastic nevus syndrome based on history without examining family members can be inaccurate.[45]

HISTOLOGIC FEATURES

It is not necessary to perform a biopsy of a dysplastic nevus unless there is clinical suspicion for melanoma. Although dysplastic nevi can be diagnosed based on clinical features, they are occasionally difficult to distinguish from melanoma without histopathologic confirmation. It is therefore crucial that one is able to distinguish dysplastic nevi from melanoma histopathologically, to properly manage patients with each of these conditions.

Many debate over the histopathologic criteria for diagnosing dysplastic nevi. The 1992 NIH Consensus Conference defined the histopathologic

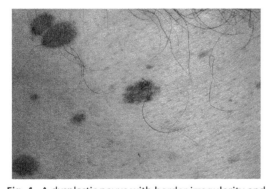

Fig. 4. A dysplastic nevus with border irregularity and marked color variegation on a background of multiple nevi. (*Courtesy of* Jason B. Lee, MD, Department of Dermatology and Cutaneous Biology, Thomas Jefferson University Hospital.)

features of dysplastic nevi as: (1) architectural disorder with asymmetry; (2) subepidermal fibroplasia; and (3) lentiginous melanocytic hyperplasia with spindle or epithelioid melanocytes aggregating in nests of variable size and forming bridges between adjacent rete ridges. Another important feature was intraepidermal melanocytes extending singly and in nests beyond the main dermal component. Although cytologic atypia was sometimes present histopathologically, it was not determined to be a defining characteristic of dysplastic nevi (**Figs. 6–10**).[10]

Subsequent studies have aimed to confirm the validity and reproducibility of the histopathologic features of dysplastic nevi. In 1993, the European Organization for the Research and Treatment of Cancer Malignant Melanoma Cooperative Group compared dysplastic nevi with other melanocytic nevi (including common nevi, and in situ and invasive melanoma) and demonstrated a set of features to reliably distinguish dysplastic nevi. These characteristics included the presence of marked junctional proliferation of single and variably shaped nests of melanocytes often with bridging between nests, melanocytes with large and variably pleomorphic nuclei, irregular nests, and a lymphohistiocytic infiltrate within the epidermis. These criteria were 86% sensitive and 91% specific for diagnosing dysplastic nevi if at least 3 of the aforementioned features were present.[46] Additional important architectural characteristics of dysplastic nevi included asymmetry, irregular epidermal hyperplasia or atrophy, diffuse lamellar fibroplasia in the dermis, and a bandlike perivascular lymphocytic infiltrate.[3] Others have corroborated these criteria; in an analysis of specific histopathologic diagnostic criteria in 62 dysplastic nevi, Steijlen and colleagues[18] found that the most discriminating features of dysplastic nevi were dustlike melanin pigment, irregular nevoid nests, markedly increased junctional activity, and large melanocytic nuclei. These investigators determined that dysplastic nevi could be reproducibly diagnosed using a combination of 2 or more of these criteria along with presence of a lymphocytic infiltrate.

As addressed by the NIH Consensus Conference, dysplastic nevi can have features of cytologic atypia in addition to defining architectural features (**Fig. 11**). The Dysplastic Nevus Panel examined a random sample of melanocytic lesions (including common nevi, dysplastic nevi, and melanoma), grading the degree of atypia in each lesion based on the size of the nucleus, variability in shape and size of the nucleus, chromatin staining, and features of the nucleolus and cytoplasm. This study showed that melanocytic dysplasia can be

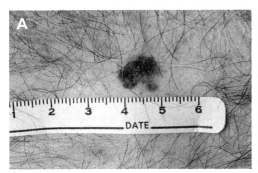
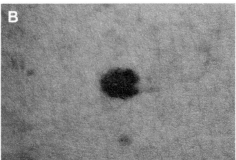

Fig. 5. (A) A melanoma-stimulant variant dysplastic nevus with asymmetry, border irregularity, color variegation, and diameter greater than 6 mm. These lesions can be difficult to distinguish clinically from melanoma (compare with B). (B) A melanoma in situ. Clinical context can provide important diagnostic clues, as this was a new lesion in a patient with very few total nevi. (Courtesy of Jason B. Lee, MD, Department of Dermatology and Cutaneous Biology, Thomas Jefferson University Hospital.)

reproducibly graded using preset criteria, reporting an intraclass correlation coefficient of 0.67 and a Pearson correlation coefficient ranging from 0.67 to 0.84.[47]

However, it is still debated whether cytologic atypia is a necessary diagnostic criterion for dysplastic nevi.[48] In addition, architectural disorder and cytologic atypia, when present, are not always positively correlated with one another.[49] To provide a more cohesive approach, Shea and colleagues[49] proposed classifying dysplastic nevi based on both cytologic and architectural features, incorporating architectural disorder and cytologic atypia into a scoring system for delineating mild, moderate, and severe dysplastic nevi based on overall score. Subsequently, Pozo and colleagues[50] found that no architectural features consistently distinguished mild from moderate dysplastic nevi, although severely dysplastic nevi could be accurately differentiated from mild and moderate dysplastic nevi based on 2 architectural features (junctional symmetry and location of suprabasilar melanocytes) and 3 nuclear variables (pleomorphism, heterogeneous chromatin, and nucleolar prominence). As such, this group proposed categorizing dysplastic nevi as high-grade (severe dysplastic nevi) and low-grade (mild and moderate dysplastic nevi).

The clinical relevance of dysplastic nevi lies in their association with increased rates of developing melanoma. Initial studies indicate that pathologic grade relates to melanoma risk. Arumi-Uria and colleagues[51] showed that the likelihood of having personal history of melanoma increased with the grade of dysplastic nevi, and similarly, Shors and colleagues[35] showed that the relative risk of melanoma was greater among patients having dysplastic nevi that were moderate or severe. These studies shed some light onto the

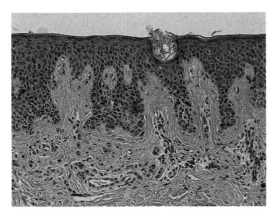

Fig. 6. Histopathologic image of routine dysplastic nevus with lentiginous melanocytic hyperplasia. There are enlarged melanocytes aggregating in nests along the bases and sides of the elongated rete ridges (hematoxylin and eosin stain, original magnification ×100).

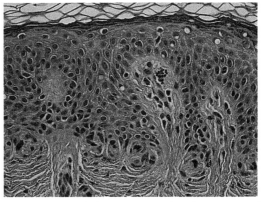

Fig. 7. Histopathologic image showing nests of enlarged melanocytes along the bases of the rete. Some of the melanocytes contain hyperchromatic and pleomorphic nuclei (hematoxylin and eosin stain, original magnification ×200).

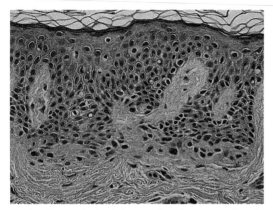

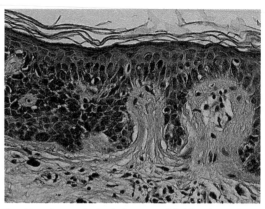

Fig. 8. Histopathologic image showing nests of melanocytes tend towards confluence and form bridges between adjacent rete. Note the random cytologic atypia of the melanocytes (hematoxylin and eosin stain, original magnification ×200).

Fig. 10. Histopathologic image exhibiting lentiginous melanocytic hyperplasia with subepidermal concentric eosinophilic fibroplasia (hematoxylin and eosin stain, original magnification ×200).

significance of histologic diagnosis of dysplastic nevi. However, there is still controversy regarding the criteria for histologic grading of dysplastic nevi,[3] and assessment of melanoma risk based on histologic grade is subject to interreader variability.

Although there are specific and reproducible histologic criteria for dysplastic nevi, they can sometimes still be difficult to differentiate from melanoma. In a study examining interobserver variation in pathologists' diagnoses, Brochez and colleagues[52] found that dysplastic nevi were the most common false-positive lesion diagnosed as melanoma, with 17.6% of dysplastic nevi diagnosed as melanoma in situ and 3.2% of dysplastic nevi in the study diagnosed as invasive melanoma when compared with a reference diagnosis by a panel of experts. In addition, melanomas were misdiagnosed in 12% of cases as dysplastic nevi. Others found that misdiagnosis is most frequent

when comparing lesions at extremes of the spectrum, for example, severely dysplastic nevi and melanoma in situ, and concluded that dysplastic nevi and melanomas can be reliably distinguished outside of these limits.[53] Arguably the most clinically relevant differentiation is between a severe dysplastic nevus and a melanoma, and the misdiagnosis of these lesions underscores the difficulty in managing the patient with dysplastic nevi.

In light of this diagnostic difficulty, some have suggested guidelines to distinguish dysplastic nevi and melanoma histopathologically. Dysplastic nevi are relatively symmetric as compared with melanomas, have uniformly elongated rete ridges

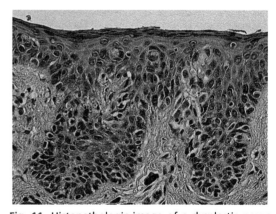

Fig. 11. Histopathologic image of a dysplastic nevus exhibiting moderate atypia. (1) The nests are poorly formed and the melanocytes are not cohesive. (2) Solitary melanocytes extend to higher levels of the epidermis. (3) Some melanocytes contain enlarged and pleomorphic nuclei with abundant cytoplasm. (4) Some of these cells have nuclei with prominent nucleoli (hematoxylin and eosin stain, original magnification ×200).

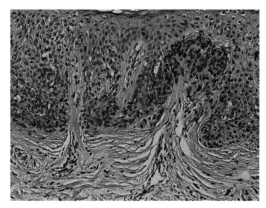

Fig. 9. Histopathologic image with prominent subepidermal lamellar fibroplasia (hematoxylin and eosin stain, original magnification ×200).

whereas melanomas show irregular thickening and thinning of the epidermis, and cytologic atypia, when present in dysplastic nevi, is more random, whereas cytologic atypia in melanomas tends to be uniform. Melanomas also tend to show more pigmentary incontinence, and there is a lack of maturation of cells in the dermis, whereas dysplastic nevi often display maturation with cells becoming smaller as they approach the base of the lesion. Specific concerning features for melanoma include pagetoid proliferation with scatter of lesional melanocytes between benign keratinocytes, continuous lentiginous proliferation extending between rete ridges, and presence of mitotic figures. In addition, the diagnosis of melanoma should be considered if the cytologic atypia is 50% or greater.[3]

PATHOGENESIS AND ETIOLOGY: GENETICS AND BIOLOGY

Given the increased incidence of melanoma in patients with dysplastic nevi, it is possible that some of the genetic mutations causing melanoma may play a role in the pathogenesis of dysplastic nevi. As discussed in this section, genetic mutations in dysplastic nevi have been found in both familial and sporadic types of this condition.

Patients from melanoma-prone families frequently present with the dysplastic nevus phenotype, which has been attributed to an autosomal dominant mode of inheritance.[7,54] Specific melanoma susceptibility genes in familial melanoma include the tumor suppressor gene cyclin-dependent kinase inhibitor 2A (CDKN2A) at the 9p21 locus, which encodes cell-cycle control proteins p16[INK4A] and p14[ARF], and the oncogene CDK4.[55-57] Mutations in CDKN2A are present in 20% to 40% of cases of melanoma-prone families[56-58] and germline mutations in CDKN2A are present in approximately 2% of all melanoma cases,[59] whereas CD4 mutations are more rare.[57] Demonstrating the genetic relationship between dysplastic nevi and familial melanoma, Goldstein and colleagues[60] performed a genetic segregation/linkage analysis of 20 American melanoma-prone families and found evidence of a gene-covariate interaction between the CDKN2A gene and presence of dysplastic nevi. Although penetrance of CDKN2A is incomplete, penetrance is more likely in patients who also have dysplastic nevi. Bishop and colleagues[61] showed that people with dysplastic nevus syndrome and a family history of melanoma were 3 times more likely have mutations in CDKN2A than those without this phenotype. Although the dysplastic nevus phenotype did not definitively identify those with CDKN2A mutations, specific clinical characteristics predicting gene

carrier status were nevi on the buttocks, nevi on the feet, a total of more than 100 nevi, and at least 2 clinically dysplastic nevi. Expression of the phenotype is likely modified by other genes that cosegregate with CDKN2A. Also noteworthy is that one study examining patients from families with atypical mole syndrome found no mutations in CDKN2A, ARF, CDK4, PTEN, or BRAF,[62] indicating the heterogeneity of underlying genetic mutations in dysplastic nevi, currently unknown mutations, as well as the likely interplay with environmental factors.

Several groups have demonstrated deletions at p16 in both familial and sporadic dysplastic nevi, which is encoded by CDKN2A.[63-65] Sini and colleagues[65] found hemizygous deletions at the 9p21 locus, which contains the p16 gene, in 55% to 62% of melanomas and dysplastic nevi. This genetic alteration is rare in common melanocytic nevi, indicating that the 9p21 locus may play a role in melanocytic transformation. Silencing of p16 with mutations at both alleles was found in many of the melanomas in this study but in none of the nevi, indicating that loss of heterozygosity may be required for tumorigenesis. Others have also demonstrated point mutations in p16 and also in p53 in addition to hemizygous p16 deletions in dysplastic nevi from patients with no known family history of dysplastic nevus syndrome.[66]

Several researchers have examined possible explanations for increased genetic mutations in patients with dysplastic nevi. One explanation is that cells are highly sensitive to ultraviolet radiation in this population. It has been shown that lymphoid cells cultured in vitro from patients with hereditary dysplastic nevus syndrome are hypermutable when exposed to ultraviolet radiation.[67] This finding was corroborated by other researchers who demonstrated increased hypermutability to ultraviolet light in fibroblasts and lymphocytes from patients with dysplastic nevus syndrome.[68-70] These patients may also have a decreased ability to repair DNA damage induced by ultraviolet light.[69,71] This hypermutability could be due to alterations in melanogenesis; Salopek and colleagues[72] showed that dysplastic nevi have significantly higher levels of pheomelanin than common melanocytic nevi or normal skin, and pheomelanin was found to be toxic to cells after ultraviolet light exposure whereas eumelanin was found to be photoprotective.

Microsatellite instability is another factor potentially contributing to the increased rate of genetic mutations in patients with dysplastic nevi. Hussein and colleagues[73] found that melanomas and dysplastic nevi both had an increased frequency of microsatellite instability, which was significantly higher than in banal melanocytic nevi. In addition, the frequency of microsatellite instability correlated with the degree of atypia in dysplastic nevi. Other groups confirmed that microsatellite instability was more frequent in dysplastic nevi than in banal melanocytic nevi,[74] and also showed that the frequency of microsatellite instability was higher in dysplastic nevi from patients with a personal or family history of melanoma, suggesting that there is a relationship between microsatellite instability and melanoma risk.[75]

Dysplastic nevi contain many mutations of the same genes also seen in melanomas, including those in oncogenes and tumor suppressor genes, as well as cell growth and apoptotic regulators.[72,76–85] However, many of these mutations alone are likely not adequate for promoting tumorigenesis. For example, BRAF mutations are common in dysplastic nevi and melanoma[86–88] but are also seen with similar frequency in benign melanocytic nevi.[86] Many experts posit that the similar genetic mutations in dysplastic nevi and melanoma place dysplastic nevi along a continuum between banal nevi and melanoma.[1,3,81] Further research is needed to fully elucidate how these mutations relate to the pathogenesis of dysplastic nevi, as well as the genetic signatures that promote senescence in dysplastic nevi versus progression in melanoma.

CLINICAL MANAGEMENT

Patients with dysplastic nevi or dysplastic nevus syndrome can be challenging to manage clinically. Most patients with dysplastic nevi can be cared for by any dermatologist, and generally only those with a significant family history of melanoma or a large number of nevi require referral to a pigmented-lesion clinic. The general approach to care for patients with dysplastic nevi includes: (1) acquiring a personal and family history of dysplastic nevi, melanoma, and evolving lesions; (2) performing thorough physical examinations on a regular basis; (3) using diagnostic aids such as dermoscopy, total body photography, and digital imaging devices to facilitate early detection of melanoma; (4) taking biopsy of any suspicious lesions; (5) counseling patients on preventive measures including sun avoidance and sun protection; and (6) removing nevi when there is clinical suspicion of melanoma or to improve cosmesis.

Personal and Family History

Patients with dysplastic nevi are at increased risk of melanoma.[3] When taking a personal history, it is important to gather information on any history of skin or other cancer, prior excisions of nevi, episodes of sunburn, ultraviolet-radiation exposure, or immunosuppression.[4,34] Because dysplastic nevi can be sporadic or part of familial syndromes, it is also important to take a thorough history of melanoma and dysplastic nevi in first-degree and second-degree relatives. In addition, given that the risk of melanoma increases with the number of family members affected by melanoma,[42] a thorough history is vital for assessing a patient's relative risk of melanoma and resultant need for follow-up examinations. A complete history is also useful for identifying family members who may also need screening for melanoma.

Although family histories play an important role in caring for patients with dysplastic nevi, there are several limitations of which one should be aware. First, patients occasionally report misinformation about family history. In a study including 1910 participants, Weinstock and Brodsky[89] found that only 17% of reported family history of melanomas could confirmed by medical records. This degree of inaccuracy is not typically reported for other types of cancer. In addition, family history does not always distinguish patients who have predisposing genetic mutations. Bishop and colleagues[61] found a poor correlation between abnormal phenotype and germline mutations in CDKN2A; although patients with dysplastic nevus syndrome had CDKN2A mutations 3 times more frequently than those without this phenotype, there was enough overlap between gene carriers and noncarriers to suggest that phenotypic abnormalities alone were not useful for identifying gene carriers. Because there is no widely available genetic test for CDKN2A mutations, these findings underscore the importance of frequent follow-up in patients from melanoma-prone families.

To identify melanoma as early as possible, it is vital to screen patients with dysplastic nevi and dysplastic nevus syndrome. The frequency of screening in patients with dysplastic nevi depends on the relative risk of developing melanoma. Current guidelines base risk assessment on family history of dysplastic nevi and melanoma as well as phenotypic characteristics, as these factors can predict increased likelihood of developing melanoma.[4,10] Specific phenotypic traits that can guide clinical management of patients with dysplastic nevi include an abundance of banal nevi, blonde or red hair, fair complexion, tendency to develop sunburn, and inability to tan.[34]

In patients from melanoma-prone families, screening should be performed every 3 to 6 months initially, which then can be increased to 6 to 12 months if the patient and physician agree that the patient's nevi have remained stable over time. This cohort includes patients with a family history of melanoma in a first-degree or second-degree relative as well as those with the dysplastic nevus phenotype.[4] In patients with few moles including 1 to 2 dysplastic nevi, screening can be performed at 6- to 12-month intervals. Because melanoma is exceedingly rare in the pediatric population,[90] as are histologically proven dysplastic nevi,[91] it is not necessary to begin screening until the late teenage years or early twenties. However, in the small subset of patients from melanoma-prone families, with melanoma in 2 or more relatives in the same branch, screening should begin earlier, as melanoma risk begins around age 10 years in this cohort.[37] Because melanoma risk increases with age, these patients will require lifelong follow-up.

Frequent follow-up provides the opportunity to educate patients on the importance of preventive measures, such as use of sunscreen and sun avoidance. Sun protection is particularly important in patients at risk for melanoma, such as those with dysplastic nevi, because it has been proved to prevent melanoma.[92] Another important element of each follow-up visit is questioning patients regarding and examining for change in any lesions. However, it is important to be aware that dysplastic nevi are dynamic lesions, and a change does not always herald malignancy. While some have noted dysplastic nevi to be stable over time,[93] a historical cohort study of 153 patients over a period of 5 years found that 51% of all evaluated dysplastic nevi showed clinical signs of change. Dysplastic nevi became more or less clinically atypical, or even disappeared, with no correlation to personal or family history of melanoma, sex, or total number of nevi. It was most common that a change in a dysplastic nevus was in the direction of reduced atypia.[94] Tools such as total body photography and dermoscopy can help to identify lesions showing suspicious change and also limit biopsies of benign lesions (see later discussion).

Physical Examination

Dysplastic nevi and melanoma can be present anywhere on the skin, including sun-protected and sun-exposed areas. Therefore, patients with dysplastic nevi require a thorough physical examination of the entire cutaneous surface, including the scalp, intertriginous folds, and interdigital and interphalangeal web spaces. In addition, those with dysplastic nevus syndrome may also require an ophthalmologic examination, as this syndrome increases risk for ocular melanoma and cutaneous melanoma.[95] In a case-control study, Bataille and colleagues[96] found that patients with dysplastic

nevus syndrome had a lifetime risk of 1 in 200 of developing ocular melanoma. In a subsequent literature review, it was reported that dysplastic nevus syndrome is the strongest link between cutaneous melanoma and ocular melanoma.[97,98] There is still debate regarding the utility and cost-effectiveness of ocular examinations in patients with dysplastic nevi; some experts have suggested yearly ophthalmologic examinations for all patients with dysplastic nevus syndrome,[4] whereas others only recommend routine examinations in specific situations, which include patients with strong expression of the dysplastic nevus syndrome phenotype, patients with dysplastic nevus syndrome and nevi of the iris, and patients with dysplastic nevus syndrome with a personal history of cutaneous melanoma.[97]

Diagnostic Aids for Melanoma

Patients with dysplastic nevi and particularly dysplastic nevus syndrome may have numerous nevi, frequently amounting to more than 100 moles. Although dysplastic nevi frequently simulate melanoma clinically, dysplastic nevi themselves only rarely progress to melanoma.[1–4] To limit biopsies of benign lesions, it is important that the clinician use all available tools to differentiate benign from suspicious lesions and to identify lesions exhibiting evolution over time.

Dermoscopy has been shown to significantly improve diagnostic accuracy in identifying melanoma when compared with unassisted examination, although the diagnostic performance depends on examiner experience.[99] Several algorithms have been devised to facilitate dermoscopic identification of melanoma from other skin lesions, including pattern analysis, the ABCD (Asymmetry, Border, Color, Dermoscopic features) rule of dermoscopy, Menzies surface microscopy scoring system, epiluminescence microscopy 7-point checklist, and the CASH (Color, Architecture, Symmetry, Homogeneity) system. To investigate the reliability and reproducibility of each of these diagnostic algorithms, 40 experienced dermoscopists evaluated 108 dermoscopic images as part of the Consensus Net Meeting on Dermoscopy using pattern analysis, the ABCD rule, the Menzies method, and the 7-point checklist.[100] Although all methods were similarly sensitive in identifying melanomas, with sensitivity ranging from 82.6% to 85.7%, pattern analysis had significantly higher specificity for melanoma, at 83.4% compared with 70% to 71.5%. In addition, although there was poor interobserver agreement on individual dermoscopic criteria, the interobserver agreement was good for overall management decisions when taking into account all dermoscopic features for each individual lesion. This finding reinforces the utility of using a diagnostic algorithm to improve the accuracy of melanoma identification with dermoscopy, and shows that pattern analysis may yield the best overall diagnostic performance.[100]

A specific dermoscopic system to classify dysplastic nevi was proposed by Hofmann-Wellenhof and colleagues[101] based on structural features and pigment distribution. In terms of structural features, this group noted that dysplastic nevi could be reticular, globular, or homogeneous (structureless), or a combination of the aforementioned types. These investigators also described several pigment distributions, including central hypopigmentation or hyperpigmentation, eccentric hypopigmentation or hyperpigmentation, and multifocal hypopigmentation or hyperpigmentation. In addition to classifying dysplastic nevi, it is also important that one is able to distinguish these lesions from melanoma dermoscopically. Salopek and colleagues[40] found that identifying 4 or more colors was a useful threshold for distinguishing melanomas from dysplastic nevi based on sensitivity and specificity. Familiarity with specific dermoscopic criteria for melanoma can also help to differentiate these entities. Statistically significant and specific criteria for identifying new melanomas include: (1) red, blue, gray, or white color; (2) moderate to marked border irregularity; and (3) multiple homogeneous areas, particularly when variable in size or when more than 25% of the lesion is involved. Other specific and statistically significant criteria for identifying early melanoma include: (1) pigment network ending abruptly; (2) white scarlike areas; (3) depigmented areas; and (4) a whitish veil. Although variably shaped brown globules and black dots are highly specific for melanoma, their presence or absence is not a reliable distinguishing factor between melanoma and dysplastic nevi.

Particularly for patients with multiple nevi or dysplastic nevus syndrome, other technologies may be necessary to augment the physical examination. Total body photography can be an extremely useful tool for identifying evolving lesions. Using photography has been shown to improve diagnosis of subtly changing melanocytic lesions that do not meet clinical criteria for melanoma, thus facilitating early diagnosis, and also limiting unneeded biopsies of clinically suspicious lesions that are stable over time.[102] Combining total body photography and dermoscopy can be very powerful clinically; although change in a nevus can be a clue to malignancy, only a small proportion of new or changed nevi are actually melanoma. Using dermoscopy to evaluate evolving or suspicious lesions identified by photography has been shown to promote early detection of melanoma and to limit biopsies of benign lesions.[103,104]

Other modalities to augment the physical examination include reflectance confocal microscopy, which uses a low-power laser beam focused on the skin surface to allow imaging of the epidermis and even into the dermis, depending on the wavelength of the laser beam. This method, however, is not widely available and is limited by cost.[105] The newest screening tools are computer-assisted dermoscopic imaging systems. Recently approved by the Food and Drug Administration for clinical use, MelaFind is a multispectral digital dermoscope that uses computer analysis to recommend lesions for either biopsy or later follow-up. MelaFind was found to be highly sensitive in identifying small-diameter melanomas (<6 mm).[106] Monheit and colleagues[107] later found that MelaFind was 98.2% sensitive in differentiating melanomas from other pigmented skin lesions, and also had a lower biopsy rate in comparison with experienced dermoscopists. MelaFind may be very useful in monitoring patients with dysplastic nevi and differentiating these lesions from melanomas.

Genetics and Genetic Counseling

Mutations in CDKN2A are present in 20% to 40% of cases of melanoma-prone families.[56–58] In addition, the dysplastic nevus syndrome phenotype can indicate increased likelihood of gene penetrance in patients from these families.[61] Given this high rate of mutations and the fact that a majority of patients with this mutation will develop melanoma,[37] genetic screening is a potentially useful tool in these patients.

At present in the United States, the consensus of the Melanoma Genetics Consortium is that genetic testing should not be routinely offered unless an individual has a family member with a mutation identified as part of a research study. The reasons for this are that a positive result may not alter prevention and surveillance strategies, and genetic testing may have negative psychological consequences.[108] However, genetic testing is commonplace in other countries; in Italy genetic screening is offered to patients with a history of melanoma in 2 or more family members in the same branch. This practice is justified based on an average CDKN2A mutation rate of 33% in Italian melanoma-prone families, with the mutation rate increasing based on the number of affected family members.[109] The implications for genetic testing in the United States may change as further studies elucidate the factors affecting CDKN2A penetrance and as new technologies improve the management of these patients.

SURGICAL AND OTHER MANAGEMENT

Dysplastic nevi can be diagnosed clinically and only need to be removed when there is suspicion for melanoma.[5,33,34] Although dysplastic nevi portend a higher risk for melanoma, dysplastic nevi themselves rarely progress to melanoma. In a prospective follow-up of melanoma-prone families for more than 20 years, Tucker and colleagues[93] showed that most dysplastic nevi either remain stable or regress, and few showed change suspicious of melanoma. As such, they recommended careful surveillance as the best method of identifying melanomas in their early stages, also noting that prophylactic excision of dysplastic nevi is not an effective treatment given the frequency of melanomas that arise de novo.[93] In further support of the surveillance approach, Kelly and colleagues[41] performed a prospective study of 278 patients with 5 or more dysplastic nevi and determined that excising all 5838 dysplastic nevi from participating patients at the outset of their study would have prevented only 3 melanomas, noting that two-thirds of the melanomas were de novo lesions. Kelly and colleagues also determined that the cost of prophylactic excision would be far greater than routine clinical follow-up. Prophylactic excision therefore cannot be justified in light of its ineffective risk reduction, cost, and associated morbidity.

When dysplastic nevi are concerning for melanoma, there are several options for biopsy. The recommendation for lesions suspicious for melanoma is an excision with 1- to 3-mm margins as well as a deep margin of subcutaneous fat. However, other biopsy techniques such as shave or incisional biopsy may be appropriate depending on the clinical scenario, mainly if the suspicion for melanoma is low or excisional biopsy is unreasonable based on anatomic location.[110,111] A shave biopsy has been shown to provide accurate diagnosis of dysplastic nevi. Although shave biopsies can be superficial, using deep shaves or saucerization can allow sampling of the deep margin.[111] Investigating the efficacy of biopsy techniques, Armour and colleagues[112] examined 63 specimens from patients with a clinical diagnosis of dysplastic nevi, and compared histopathological concordance between shave and punch biopsies with later elliptical excisions. These investigators showed that 95.5% of shave biopsies were concordant with later excision, but punch biopsies were concordant in only 70.7% of cases, concluding that shave biopsies allow accurate diagnosis of dysplastic nevi. When choosing a biopsy technique, the primary concern is that it provides a representative sample of the lesion in question and adequate tissue for accurate histopathologic diagnosis.[111]

Another management issue arises when surgically removed dysplastic nevi are incompletely excised. Emerging evidence indicates that it may not be necessary to reexcise all cases of dysplastic nevi that have positive margins on histopathology. In a prospective study of patients with a history of a prior biopsy, Goodson and colleagues[113] showed that patients with previously biopsied mildly to moderately dysplastic nevi had only a 3.6% rate of recurrence of at 2 years of follow-up. There was no statistically significant association between a positive margin and rate of recurrence in their study, indicating that it is likely unnecessary to reexcise dysplastic nevi when incompletely excised. Most notably, none of the lesions in this study were found to progress to melanoma, reinforcing the notion that dysplastic nevi do not need routine biopsy. Other researchers corroborated this finding, noting that no melanomas occurred in patients with incompletely excised dysplastic nevi when followed for a mean of more than 6 years.[114] However, neither of these studies report specifically on severe dysplastic nevi. Further data are necessary to guide appropriate management of these lesions, particularly because severely dysplastic nevi are most difficult to definitively distinguish from melanoma on histopathology, and dermatopathologists often recommend reexcision of severely dysplastic nevi if there is uncertainty.

To prevent scarring from surgery, or for patients concerned about the cosmetic appearance of dysplastic nevi, researchers have sought alternative methods of removal. Such approaches consist of topical therapies including tretinoin with and without hydrocortisone, 5-fluorouracil, imiquimod, systemic isotretinoin, and laser ablation.[115–123] None of these have consistently shown efficacy in treating dysplastic nevi. Laser ablation may potentially induce melanoma, and is not recommended until further studies examine its safety in this domain.[124,125]

PREVENTING DYSPLASTIC NEVI

Dysplastic nevi result from the interplay of genetic and environmental factors.[22,126] Therefore environmental factors, mainly sun protection, are the controllable contributors to dysplastic nevi. Regular sunscreen use has been proved to prevent melanoma; Green and colleagues[127] conducted a randomized study of 1621 adults, asking one group to apply sunscreen daily and the other to apply sunscreen at their own discretion for a period of 5 years. A reduction in melanomas was found in the group that used sunscreen regularly, with 11 new primary melanomas in the group using regular sunscreen and 22 melanomas among the group assigned to discretionary use, including a substantial reduction in invasive melanomas with regular sunscreen use. Although the role of sun protection in the development of dysplastic nevi has not been specifically examined, regular sunscreen use has been shown to prevent the development of new nevi in addition to melanoma.[128] In light of these findings, one can speculate that regular use of sunscreen and sun-protective clothing is likely to prevent dysplastic nevi. Regardless, sun protection is essential for any patient with dysplastic nevi because it does reduce the risk of melanoma.

FUTURE OUTLOOK

Patients with dysplastic nevi and dysplastic nevus syndrome in particular can be extremely difficult to manage. The physician is often weighing concern over potentially unnecessary biopsy with possibly missing a melanoma, and the dermatopathologist has a similar dilemma of classifying a lesion as simply dysplastic or as melanoma. As technologies such as computer-assisted digital dermoscopy and reflectance confocal microscopy become more widely available, it may be possible in the near future to distinguish confidently between dysplastic nevi and melanoma on clinical grounds alone. Further research will also be useful in elucidating the pathogenesis and genetic signatures of dysplastic nevi, particularly in dysplastic nevus syndrome. At present, patients with dysplastic nevi can be effectively managed with vigilant follow-up, total body skin examinations augmented by dermoscopy and photography, biopsy of suspicious lesions, and sun protection.

REFERENCES

1. Clark WH Jr, Elder DE, Guerry D IV, et al. A study of tumor progression: the precursor lesions of superficial spreading and nodular melanoma. Hum Pathol 1984;15(12):1147–65.
2. Clark WH Jr, Ackerman AB. An exchange of views regarding the dysplastic nevus controversy. Semin Dermatol 1989;8(4):229–50.
3. Elder DE. Dysplastic naevi: an update. Histopathology 2010;56(1):112–20.
4. Naeyaert JM, Brochez L. Dysplastic nevi. N Engl J Med 2003;349(23):2233–40.
5. Tucker MA, Halpern A, Holly EA, et al. Clinically recognized dysplastic nevi. A central risk factor for cutaneous melanoma. JAMA 1997;277(18):1439–44.
6. Clark WH Jr, Reimer RR, Greene M, et al. Origin of familial malignant melanomas from heritable melanocytic lesions. 'The B-K mole syndrome'. Arch Dermatol 1978;114(5):732–8.
7. Lynch HT, Frichot BC 3rd, Lynch JF. Familial atypical multiple mole-melanoma syndrome. J Med Genet 1978;15(5):352–6.
8. Elder DE, Goldman LI, Goldman SC, et al. Dysplastic nevus syndrome: a phenotypic association of sporadic cutaneous melanoma. Cancer 1980;46(8):1787–94.
9. Ackerman AB, Milde P. Naming acquired melanocytic nevi. Common and dysplastic, normal and atypical, or Unna, Miescher, Spitz, and Clark? Am J Dermatopathol 1992;14(5):447–53.
10. Diagnosis and treatment of early melanoma. NIH consensus development conference. January 27-29, 1992. Consens Statement 1992;10(1):1–25.
11. Frankel KA. Intraepithelial melanocytic neoplasia: a classification by pattern analysis of proliferations of atypical melanocytes. Am J Dermatopathol 1987;9(1):80–1.
12. Sina B, Wood C. Atypical melanocytic proliferations. Am J Dermatopathol 1991;13(3):317–9.
13. Urso C, Giannini A, Bartolini M, et al. Histological analysis of intraepidermal proliferations of atypical melanocytes. Am J Dermatopathol 1990;12(2):150–5.
14. Tripp JM, Kopf AW, Marghoob AA, et al. Management of dysplastic nevi: a survey of fellows of the American Academy of Dermatology. J Am Acad Dermatol 2002;46(5):674–82.
15. Crutcher WA, Sagebiel RW. Prevalence of dysplastic naevi in a community practice. Lancet 1984;1(8379):729.
16. Lee G, Massa MC, Welykyj S, et al. Yield from total skin examination and effectiveness of skin cancer awareness program. Findings in 874 new dermatology patients. Cancer 1991;67(1):202–5.
17. Nordlund JJ, Kirkwood J, Forget BM, et al. Demographic study of clinically atypical (dysplastic) nevi in patients with melanoma and comparison subjects. Cancer Res 1985;45(4):1855–61.
18. Steijlen P, Bergman W, Hermans J, et al. The efficacy of histopathological criteria required for diagnosing dysplastic naevi. Histopathology 1988;12(3):289–300.
19. Grob J, Gouvernet J, Aymar D, et al. Count of benign melanocytic nevi as a major indicator of risk for nonfamilial nodular and superficial spreading melanoma. Cancer 1990;66(2):387–95.
20. Holly EA, Kelly JW, Shpall SN, et al. Number of melanocytic nevi as a major risk factor for malignant melanoma. J Am Acad Dermatol 1987;17(3):459–68.
21. Ng PC, Barzilai DA, Ismail SA, et al. Evaluating invasive cutaneous melanoma: is the initial biopsy representative of the final depth? J Am Acad Dermatol 2003;48(3):420–4.

22. Bataille V, Grulich A, Sasieni P, et al. The association between naevi and melanoma in populations with different levels of sun exposure: a joint case-control study of melanoma in the UK and Australia. Br J Cancer 1998;77(3):505–10.

23. Augustsson A, Stierner U, Rosdahl I, et al. Common and dysplastic naevi as risk factors for cutaneous malignant melanoma in a Swedish population. Acta Derm Venereol 1991;71(6):518–29.

24. Garbe C, Büttner P, Weiß J, et al. Associated factors in the prevalence of more than 50 common melanocytic nevi, atypical melanocytic nevi, and actinic lentigines: multicenter case-control study of the central malignant melanoma registry of the German Dermatological Society. J Invest Dermatol 1994;102(5):700–5.

25. Garbe C, Krüger S, Stadler R, et al. Markers and relative risk in a German population for developing malignant melanoma. Int J Dermatol 1989;28(8): 517–23.

26. Halpern AC, Guerry DP IV, Elder DE, et al. Dysplastic nevi as risk markers of sporadic (non-familial) melanoma: a case-control study. Arch Dermatol 1991;127(7):995–9.

27. MacKie RM, Aitchison TC, Freudenberger T. Risk factors for melanoma. Lancet 1989;2(8668):928.

28. Roush GC, Nordund JJ, Forget B, et al. Independence of dysplastic nevi from total nevi in patients with melanoma and comparison subjects. Cancer Res 1985;45:1855–61.

29. Swerdlow A, English J, MacKie R, et al. Benign melanocytic naevi as a risk factor for malignant melanoma. Br Med J (Clin Res Ed) 1986; 292(6535):1555–9.

30. MacKie R, McHenry P, Hole D. Accelerated detection with prospective surveillance for cutaneous malignant melanoma in high-risk groups. Lancet 1993;341(8861):1618–20.

31. Rigel DS, Rivers JK, Friedman RJ, et al. Risk gradient for malignant melanoma in individuals with dysplastic naevi. Lancet 1988;331(8581):352–3.

32. Schneider JS, Moore DH, Sagebiel RW. Risk factors for melanoma incidence in prospective follow-up: the importance of atypical (dysplastic) nevi. Arch Dermatol 1994;130(8):1002–7.

33. Tiersten A, Grin C, Kopf A, et al. Prospective follow-up for malignant melanoma in patients with atypical-mole (dysplastic-nevus) syndrome. J Dermatol Surg Oncol 1991;17(1):44–8.

34. Marghoob AA, Kopf AW, Rigel DS, et al. Risk of cutaneous malignant melanoma in patients with 'classic' atypical-mole syndrome: a case-control study. Arch Dermatol 1994;130(8):993–8.

35. Shors A, Kim S, White E, et al. Dysplastic naevi with moderate to severe histological dysplasia: a risk factor for melanoma. Br J Dermatol 2006;155(5): 988–93.

36. Halpern AC, Guerry DP, Elder DE, et al. A cohort study of melanoma in patients with dysplastic nevi. J Invest Dermatol 1993;100:346S–9S.

37. Tucker MA, Fraser MC, Goldstein AM, et al. Risk of melanoma and other cancers in melanoma-prone families. J Invest Dermatol 1993;100:350S–5S.

38. Skender-Kalnenas TM, English DR, Heenan PJ. Benign melanocytic lesions: risk markers or precursors of cutaneous melanoma? J Am Acad Dermatol 1995;33(6):1000–7.

39. Salopek TG, Friedman RJ. Dysplastic nevi. In: Rigel DS, Friedman RJ, Dzubow LM, et al, editors. Cancer of the skin. Philadelphia: Saunders; 2005. p. 203–19.

40. Salopek TG, Kopf AW, Stefanato CM, et al. Differentiation of atypical moles (dysplastic nevi) from early melanomas by dermoscopy. Dermatol Clin 2001;19(2):337–45.

41. Kelly JW, Yeatman JM, Regalia C, et al. A high incidence of melanoma found in patients with multiple dysplastic naevi using photographic surveillance. Med J Aust 1997;167:191–4.

42. Hofman-Wellenhof R, Soyer HP. Atypical (dysplastic) nevus. In: Soyer HP, Argenziano G, Hofman-Wellenhof R, et al, editors. Color atlas of melanocytic lesions of the skin. New York: Springer; 2007. p. 87–96.

43. Friedman RJ, Farber MJ, Warycha MA, et al. The 'dysplastic' nevus. Clin Dermatol 2009;27(1):103–15.

44. Kopf AW, Friedman RJ, Rigel DS. Atypical mole syndrome. J Am Acad Dermatol 1990;22(1):117–8.

45. Crijns MB, Vink J, Van Hees CL, et al. Dysplastic nevi: occurrence in first-and second-degree relatives of patients with 'sporadic' dysplastic nevus syndrome. Arch Dermatol 1991;127(9):1346–51.

46. De Wit P, Van't Hof-Grootenboer B, Ruiter D, et al. Validity of the histopathological criteria used for diagnosing dysplastic naevi: an interobserver study by the pathology subgroup of the EORTC malignant melanoma cooperative group. Eur J Cancer 1993;29(6):831–9.

47. Weinstock MA, Barnhill RL, Rhodes AR, et al. Reliability of the histopathologic diagnosis of melanocytic dysplasia. Arch Dermatol 1997;133(8):953–8.

48. Ackerman A, Mihara I. Dysplasia, dysplastic melanocytes, dysplastic nevi, the dysplastic nevus syndrome, and the relation between dysplastic nevi and malignant melanomas. Hum Pathol 1985;16(1):87–91.

49. Shea CR, Vollmer RT, Prieto VG. Correlating architectural disorder and cytologic atypia in Clark (dysplastic) melanocytic nevi. Hum Pathol 1999; 30(5):500–5.

50. Pozo L, Naase M, Cerio R, et al. Critical analysis of histologic criteria for grading atypical (dysplastic) melanocytic nevi. Am J Clin Pathol 2001;115(2): 194–204.

51. Arumi-Uria M, McNutt NS, Finnerty B. Grading of atypia in nevi: correlation with melanoma risk. Mod Pathol 2003;16(8):764–71.

52. Brochez L, Verhaeghe E, Grosshans E, et al. Inter-observer variation in the histopathological diagnosis of clinically suspicious pigmented skin lesions. J Pathol 2002;196(4):459–66.

53. Duncan LM, Berwick M, Bruijn JA, et al. Histopathologic recognition and grading of dysplastic melanocytic nevi: an interobserver agreement study. J Invest Dermatol 1993;100:318S–21S.

54. Bale SJ, Chakravarti A, Greene M. Cutaneous malignant melanoma and familial dysplastic nevi: evidence for autosomal dominance and pleiotropy. Am J Hum Genet 1986;38(2):188–96.

55. Begg CB, Orlow I, Hummer AJ, et al. Lifetime risk of melanoma in CDKN2A mutation carriers in a population-based sample. J Natl Cancer Inst 2005; 97(20):1507–15.

56. Bishop DT, Demenais F, Goldstein AM, et al. Geographical variation in the penetrance of CDKN2A mutations for melanoma. J Natl Cancer Inst 2002;94(12):894–903.

57. Goldstein AM, Struewing JP, Chidambaram A, et al. Genotype-phenotype relationships in US melanoma-prone families with CDKN2A and CDK4 mutations. J Natl Cancer Inst 2000;92(12):1006–10.

58. Ruiz A, Puig S, Malvehy J, et al. CDKN2A mutations in Spanish cutaneous malignant melanoma families and patients with multiple melanomas and other neoplasia. J Med Genet 1999;36(6): 490–3.

59. Bishop DT, Demenais F, Iles MM, et al. Genome-wide association study identifies 3 loci associated with melanoma risk. Nat Genet 2009;41(8): 920–5.

60. Goldstein AM, Martinez M, Tucker MA, et al. Gene-covariate interaction between dysplastic nevi and the CDKN2A gene in American melanoma-prone families. Cancer Epidemiol Biomarkers Prev 2000; 9(9):889–94.

61. Bishop JA, Wachsmuth RC, Harland M, et al. Genotype/phenotype and penetrance studies in melanoma families with germline CDKN2A mutations. J Invest Dermatol 2000;114(1):28–33.

62. Celebi J, Ward K, Wanner M, et al. Evaluation of germline CDKN2A, ARF, CDK4, PTEN, and BRAF alterations in atypical mole syndrome. Clin Exp Dermatol 2005;30(1):68–70.

63. Hashemi J, Linder S, Platz A, et al. Melanoma development in relation to non-functional p16/INK4A protein and dysplastic naevus syndrome in Swedish melanoma kindreds. Melanoma Res 1999;9(1):21–30.

64. Park WS, Vortmeyer AO, Pack S, et al. Allelic deletion at chromosome 9p21 (p16) and 17p13 (p53) in microdissected sporadic dysplastic nevus. Hum Pathol 1998;29(2):127–30.

65. Sini MC, Manca A, Cossu A, et al. Molecular alterations at chromosome 9p21 in melanocytic naevi and melanoma. Br J Dermatol 2008; 158(2):243–50.

66. Lee JY, Dong SM, Shin MS, et al. Genetic alterations of p16INK4a and p53 genes in sporadic dysplastic nevus. Biochem Biophys Res Commun 1997;237(3):667–72.

67. Perera MI, Um K, Greene MH, et al. Hereditary dysplastic nevus syndrome: lymphoid cell ultraviolet hypermutability in association with increased melanoma susceptibility. Cancer Res 1986;46(2): 1005–9.

68. Jung EG, Bohnert E, Boonen H. Dysplastic nevus syndrome: Ultraviolet hypermutability confirmed in vitro by elevated sister chromatid exchanges. Dermatologica 1986;173(6):297–300.

69. Moriwaki SI, Tarone RE, Tucker MA, et al. Hypermutability of UV-treated plasmids in dysplastic nevus/familial melanoma cell lines. Cancer Res 1997; 57(20):4637–41.

70. Seetharam S, Waters HL, Seidman MM, et al. Ultraviolet mutagenesis in a plasmid vector replicated in lymphoid cells from a patient with the melanoma-prone disorder dysplastic nevus syndrome. Cancer Res 1989;49(21):5918–21.

71. Abrahams PJ, Houweling A, Cornelissen-Steijger PD, et al. Impaired DNA repair capacity in skin fibroblasts from various hereditary cancer-prone syndromes. Mutat Res 1998;407(2):189–201.

72. Salopek TG, Yamada K, Ito S, et al. Dysplastic melanocytic nevi contain high levels of pheomelanin: quantitative comparison of pheomelanin/eumelanin levels between normal skin, common nevi, and dysplastic nevi. Pigment Cell Res 1991;4(4):172–9.

73. Hussein MR, Sun M, Tuthill RJ, et al. Comprehensive analysis of 112 melanocytic skin lesions demonstrates microsatellite instability in melanomas and dysplastic nevi, but not in benign nevi. J Cutan Pathol 2001;28(7):343–50.

74. Rubben A, Bogdan I, Grussendorf-Conen EI, et al. Loss of heterozygosity and microsatellite instability in acquired melanocytic nevi: towards a molecular definition of the dysplastic nevus. Recent Results Cancer Res 2002;160:100–10.

75. Birindelli S, Tragni G, Bartoli C, et al. Detection of microsatellite alterations in the spectrum of melanocytic nevi in patients with or without individual or family history of melanoma. Int J Cancer 2000; 86(2):255–61.

76. Ahmed AA, Nordlind K, Hedblad M, et al. Interleukin (IL)-1 alpha- and -1 beta-, IL-6-, and tumor necrosis factor-alpha-like immunoreactivities in human common and dysplastic nevocellular nevi and malignant melanoma. Am J Dermatopathol 1995;17(3):222–9.

77. Elder DE, Herlyn M. Antigens associated with tumor progression in melanocytic neoplasia. Pigment Cell Res 1992;(Suppl 2):136–43.

78. Ewanowich C, Brynes RK, Medeiros L, et al. Cyclin D1 expression in dysplastic nevi: an immunohisto-chemical study. Arch Pathol Lab Med 2001;125(2): 208–10.

79. Fleming MG, Howe SF, Candel AG. Immunohisto-chemical localization of cytokines in nevi. Am J Dermatopathol 1992;14(6):496–503.

80. Lazzaro B, Strassburg A. Tumor antigen expression in compound dysplastic nevi and superficial spreading melanoma defined by a panel of nevo-melanoma monoclonal antibodies. Hybridoma 1996;15(2):141–6.

81. Meier F, Satyamoorthy K, Nesbit M, et al. Molecular events in melanoma development and progression. Front Biosci 1998;3:D1005–10.

82. Moretti S, Martini L, Berti E, et al. Adhesion mole-cule profile and malignancy of melanocytic lesions. Melanoma Res 1993;3(4):235–9.

83. Nanney LB, Coffey RJ, Ellis DL. Expression and distribution of transforming growth factor-α within melanocytic lesions. J Invest Dermatol 1994; 103(5):707–14.

84. Platz A, Ringborg U, Grafström E, et al. Immunohisto-chemical analysis of the N-ras p21 and the p53 proteins in naevi, primary tumours and metastases of human cutaneous malignant melanoma: increased immunopositivity in hereditary melanoma. Melanoma Res 1995;5(2):101.

85. Wang Y, Rao U, Mascari R, et al. Molecular analysis of melanoma precursor lesions. Cell Growth Differ 1996;7(12):1733–40.

86. Pollock PM, Harper UL, Hansen KS, et al. High frequency of BRAF mutations in nevi. Nat Genet 2003;33(1):19–20.

87. Uribe P, Wistuba II, González S. BRAF mutation: a frequent event in benign, atypical, and malignant melanocytic lesions of the skin. Am J Dermatopa-thol 2003;25(5):365–70.

88. Yazdi AS, Palmedo G, Flaig MJ, et al. Mutations of the BRAF gene in benign and malignant melano-cytic lesions. J Invest Dermatol 2003;121(5): 1160–2.

89. Weinstock MA, Brodsky GL. Bias in the assess-ment of family history of melanoma and its associ-ation with dysplastic nevi in a case-control study. J Clin Epidemiol 1998;51(12):1299–303.

90. Schmid-Wendtner MH, Berking C, Baumert J, et al. Cutaneous melanoma in childhood and adoles-cence: an analysis of 36 patients. J Am Acad Der-matol 2002;46(6):874–9.

91. Haley JC, Hood AF, Chuang TY, et al. The frequency of histologically dysplastic nevi in 199 pediatric patients. Pediatr Dermatol 2000;17(4): 266–9.

92. Robinson JK, Bigby M. Prevention of melanoma with regular sunscreen use. JAMA 2011;306(3): 302–3.

93. Tucker MA, Fraser MC, Goldstein AM, et al. A natural history of melanomas and dysplastic nevi. Cancer 2002;94(12):3192–209.

94. Halpern AC, Guerry DP IV, Elder DE, et al. Natural history of dysplastic nevi. J Am Acad Dermatol 1993;29(1):51–7.

95. Rodriguez-Sains R. Ocular findings in patients with dysplastic nevus syndrome. Ophthalmology 1986; 93(5):661–5.

96. Bataille V, Sasieni P, Cuzick J, et al. Risk of ocular melanoma in relation to cutaneous and iris naevi. Int J Cancer 1995;60(5):622–6.

97. Hurst EA, Harbour JW, Cornelius LA. Ocular mela-noma: a review and the relationship to cutaneous melanoma. Arch Dermatol 2003;139(8):1067–73.

98. Van Hees C, De Boer A, Jager M, et al. Are atypical nevi a risk factor for uveal melanoma? A case-control study. J Invest Dermatol 1994; 103(2):202–5.

99. Kittler H, Pehamberger H, Wolff K, et al. Diagnostic accuracy of dermoscopy. Lancet Oncol 2002;3(3): 159–65.

100. Argenziano G, Soyer HP, Chimenti S, et al. Dermo-scopy of pigmented skin lesions: results of a consensus meeting via the internet. J Am Acad Dermatol 2003;48(5):679–93.

101. Hofmann-Wellenhof R, Blum A, Wolf IH, et al. Dermoscopic classification of Clark's nevi (atyp-ical melanocytic nevi). Clin Dermatol 2002;20(3): 255–8.

102. Feit NE, Dusza SW, Marghoob AA. Melanomas de-tected with the aid of total cutaneous photography. Br J Dermatol 2004;150(4):706–14.

103. Banky JP, Kelly JW, English DR, et al. Incidence of new and changed nevi and melanomas detected using baseline images and dermoscopy in patients at high risk for melanoma. Arch Dermatol 2005; 141(8):998–1006.

104. Lucas CR, Sanders LL, Murray JC, et al. Early mela-noma detection: nonuniform dermoscopic features and growth. J Am Acad Dermatol 2003;48(5):663–71.

105. Goodson AG, Grossman D. Strategies for early melanoma detection: approaches to the patient with nevi. J Am Acad Dermatol 2009;60(5):719–35.

106. Friedman RJ, Gutkowicz-Krusin D, Farber MJ, et al. The diagnostic performance of expert der-moscopists vs a computer-vision system on small-diameter melanomas. Arch Dermatol 2008; 144(4):476–82.

107. Monheit G, Cognetta AB, Ferris L, et al. The perfor-mance of MelaFind: a prospective multicenter study. Arch Dermatol 2011;147(2):188–94.

108. Kefford RF, Newton Bishop JA, Bergman W, et al. Counseling and DNA testing for individuals

perceived to be genetically predisposed to melanoma: a consensus statement of the Melanoma Genetics Consortium. J Clin Oncol 1999;17(10): 3245–51.

109. Bruno W, Ghiorzo P, Battistuzzi L, et al. Clinical genetic testing for familial melanoma in Italy: a cooperative study. J Am Acad Dermatol 2009; 61(5):775–82.

110. Sober AJ, Chuang TY, Duvic M, et al. Guidelines of care for primary cutaneous melanoma. J Am Acad Dermatol 2001;45(4):579–86.

111. Tran KT, Wright NA, Cockerell CJ. Biopsy of the pigmented lesion—when and how. J Am Acad Dermatol 2008;59(5):852–71.

112. Armour K, Mann S, Lee S. Dysplastic naevi: to shave, or not to shave? A retrospective study of the use of the shave biopsy technique in the initial management of dysplastic naevi. Australas J Dermatol 2005;46(2):70–5.

113. Goodson AG, Florell SR, Boucher KM, et al. Low rates of clinical recurrence after biopsy of benign to moderately dysplastic melanocytic nevi. J Am Acad Dermatol 2010;62(4):591–6.

114. Kmetz EC, Sanders H, Fisher G, et al. The role of observation in the management of atypical nevi. South Med J 2009;102(1):45–8.

115. Bondi EE, Clark WH Jr, Elder D, et al. Topical chemotherapy of dysplastic melanocytic nevi with 5% fluorouracil. Arch Dermatol 1981;117(2):89–92.

116. Duke D, Byers HR, Sober AJ, et al. Treatment of benign and atypical nevi with the normal-mode ruby laser and the Q-switched ruby laser: clinical improvement but failure to completely eliminate nevomelanocytes. Arch Dermatol 1999;135(3):290–6.

117. Dusza SW, Delgado R, Busam KJ, et al. Treatment of dysplastic nevi with 5% imiquimod cream, a pilot study. J Drugs Dermatol 2006;5(1):56–62.

118. Edwards L, Jaffe P. The effect of topical tretinoin on dysplastic nevi: a preliminary trial. Arch Dermatol 1990;126(4):494–9.

119. Edwards L, Meyskens F, Levine N. Effect of oral isotretinoin on dysplastic nevi. J Am Acad Dermatol 1989;20(2):257–60.

120. Halpern AC, Schuchter LM, Elder DE, et al. Effects of topical tretinoin on dysplastic nevi. J Clin Oncol 1994;12(5):1028–35.

121. Meyskens FL Jr, Edwards L, Levine NS. Role of topical tretinoin in melanoma and dysplastic nevi. J Am Acad Dermatol 1986;15(4):822–5.

122. Somani N, Martinka M, Crawford RI, et al. Treatment of atypical nevi with imiquimod 5% cream. Arch Dermatol 2007;143(3):379–85.

123. Stam-Posthuma J, Vink J, Le Cessie S, et al. Effect of topical tretinoin under occlusion on atypical naevi. Melanoma Res 1998;8(6):539–48.

124. Stratigos AJ, Dover JS, Arndt KA. Laser treatment of pigmented lesions—2000: how far have we gone? Arch Dermatol 2000;136(7):915–21.

125. Zipser MC, Mangana J, Oberholzer PA, et al. Melanoma after laser therapy of pigmented lesions—circumstances and outcome. Eur J Dermatol 2010; 20(3):334–8.

126. Kelly JW, Rivers JK, MacLennan R, et al. Sunlight: a major factor associated with the development of melanocytic nevi in Australian schoolchildren. J Am Acad Dermatol 1994;30(1):40–8.

127. Green AC, Williams GM, Logan V, et al. Reduced melanoma after regular sunscreen use: randomized trial follow-up. J Clin Oncol 2011;29(3): 257–63.

128. Gallagher RP, Rivers JK, Lee TK, et al. Broad-spectrum sunscreen use and the development of new nevi in white children: a randomized control trial. JAMA 2000;283(22):2955–60.

New Approaches to Melanoma Prevention

June K. Robinson, MD[a],*, Mary Kate Baker, MPH[b],
Joel J. Hillhouse, PhD[b]

KEYWORDS

- Tanning attitude • Melanoma • Tanning

KEY POINTS

- Skin cancer, which is caused by exposure to ultraviolet radiation, is a major public health concern. Intentional tanning remains a modifiable risk factor.
- Parents and physicians can modify the behavior of teen and young adults using strategies based on harm reduction.
- The most likely indoor tanners are women between the ages of 20 and 30 who do so to enhance their appearance or to reduce stress. By suggesting alternatives that address these motivations, the woman may choose to change the behavior. Sunless tanning is a popular alternative for achieving the tanned look without the risks of exposure to harmful UVR. Stress relief may be obtained through regular exercise.

Over the past several decades in the United States, national programs have primarily targeted white people for sun protection educational programs; however, people's attitudes about having a tan have not significantly changed. During this same period in developed countries, indoor tanning has become an increasingly common source of ultraviolet radiation (UVR) exposure.[1–3] Broad-spectrum UVR has long been recognized as the highest risk category of carcinogen by the International Agency for Research on Cancer, and UVR-emitting tanning devices were elevated to this category in 2009.[4] UVR exposure is the primary environmental etiologic factor for both melanoma and nonmelanoma skin cancers.[5–7] People who deliberately tan often do so with natural light via sunbathing and/or with artificial light from tanning beds.

Melanoma is the second most common cancer in individuals aged 15 to 29 years, accounting for 11% of all malignant neoplasms in this age group.[8]

The incidence rate of melanoma is increasing at a disturbing rate of 2.7% per year among young non-Hispanic white women.[9] Although the causes for this trend are multifactorial, the observed rise of melanoma in women, particularly in the truncal skin, suggests deliberate exposure to UVR sources as a plausible etiology.[8,10,11]

SCOPE OF INDOOR TANNING

More than 30 million people in the United States, of which 2.3 million are adolescents, tan indoors annually.[12] Studies show that 25% to 40% of young women have used indoor tanning in the past year, with the prevalence of use among women in their late teens and early twenties estimated at more than 35%.[13–15] The median number of indoor tanning visits for women in this age group is 40 to 50 per year.[16] Mothers often accompany their daughters during the first tanning experience, thus, giving permission for underage tanning and

[a] Department of Dermatology, Northwestern University Feinberg School of Medicine, 676 North St Clair Street, Suite 1260, Chicago, IL 60611, USA; [b] Department of Community & Behavioral Health, East Tennessee State University College of Public Health, 807 University Parkway, Johnson City, TN 37614, USA
* Corresponding author.
E-mail address: June-robinson@northwestern.edu

Dermatol Clin 30 (2012) 405–412
doi:10.1016/j.det.2012.04.006
0733-8635/12/$ – see front matter © 2012 Elsevier Inc. All rights reserved.

establishing a pattern of regular tanning that carries over into young adulthood.[17] Fifty or more hours of sunbed use are associated with a 3 times greater risk of developing melanoma.[10]

Indoor tanning beds and booths have a widespread presence beyond indoor tanning salons, with facilities now located within gyms, beauty salons, and even people's homes. Across 116 cities in the United States, the overall mean number of commercial tanning facilities per city (mean = 41.8) was much higher than the overall mean number of Starbucks (mean = 19) and McDonald's (mean = 29.6) in these same locations.[18]

Tanning Attitudes

Part of the popularity of indoor tanning may be because tanned skin is portrayed as attractive and desirable in popular culture. Appearance-enhancing factors are consistently found to strongly motivate intentions to achieve a tan, overriding the knowledge and perception of the remote threat of developing skin cancers women may hold.[19–22] The contradiction between people knowing that UVR exposure causes skin cancer and holding the belief that having a tan makes a person look healthy and/or attractive may be explained by the strong evidence that people have at least 2 cognitive systems.[23] One system involves conscious, controlled, and focused effort in processing stimuli and produces explicit beliefs and attitudes. The other system is rapid, effortless, automatic application of implicit knowledge, beliefs, attitudes, and skills stored through repeated exposures in long-term memory. The first system may "know" that UVR exposure causes skin cancer, yet the second admires and compliments the person with a "nice tan." Cognitive dissonance of this magnitude can be resolved either by conscious decision making or by implicit attitudes. When people are engaged in thinking through decisions and have cognitive resources, motivation, knowledge, and opportunity to ponder the pros and cons of different actions, then the action is often different from the impulsive action not entirely under conscious control.[24] Implicit attitudes are more likely to influence behavior when cognitive processing capacity is low owing to fatigue, anxiety, or cognitive overload. For example, when a teen is invited to go along with others to the pool to be with friends, the anxiety over fitting in with the peer group may stifle the nagging thought of not having sunscreen. Among teens, impulsive actions are often more common than carefully weighing the pros and cons of a behavior and making a thoughtful decision about engaging in tanning.

At-risk Population

The most likely indoor tanners were women between the ages of 20 and 30 who had skin types that would become slightly burned with a moderate tan or not burned with a good tan 1 week after 1-hour exposure to sunlight (ie, skin types III or IV on the Fitzpatrick Skin Type Classification Scale).[16,25] Among adult women, those who have tanned indoors were more likely to have unhealthier diets, smoke, drink alcohol, and lack correct information on the safety of indoor tanning compared with women who did not engage in indoor tanning.[3] Both adult men and women were most likely to have engaged in this activity while younger than 30.[16]

In younger populations of teens, which are also often predominantly composed of girls, indoor tanners were more likely to engage in other risk-seeking behaviors, such as smoking, drinking, and recreational drug use[25,26] and had less healthy lifestyle choices[27] compared with those who had never used tanning beds/booths. The clustering of addictive behaviors, such as smoking and drinking, with indoor tanning may reflect general risk-taking behavior rather than addiction.[28] Given the young age at initiation, high prevalence of use, and other correlated risk-taking behaviors, young women who tan indoors are an ideal group to target for health promotion messages.

Promoting Behavioral Change

Behavioral economics suggests that promoting healthy alternatives that serve a similar function as an unhealthy behavior but with no greater effort or cost can reduce unhealthy behavior. People indoor tan for 2 primary reasons: physical appearance and stress reduction. Thus, alternatives that address these motivations could be effective in promoting behavior change.[16,29] Secondary reasons for indoor tanning are to prevent sunburn when engaging in outdoor activities and to ensure adequate vitamin D.

When counseling patients, it helps to consider the patient's perspective of the benefit of tanning. Is the patient tanning to look good for an event, such as the prom or a wedding? Is the patient a regular tanner who tans year round and uses tanning to improve mood and relieve stress? The range of tanning types extends from event tanners through spontaneous mood tanners to regular tanners.[16] Physicians can open a dialogue with the patient when taking a history by using open-ended questions, such as how does having a tan make you feel? The conversation allows the physician to take a patient-centered approach, and frame a harm reduction message that evolves from the patient's responses. There are a number of ready alternatives to the secondary reasons for tanning that the physician can provide. Sunburns can be prevented more effectively with use of sunscreen than with a tan, especially in those who have difficulty tanning. Patients who are concerned about vitamin D production can be encouraged to eat foods high in vitamin D (ie, salmon, fortified orange juice) and/or advised to take oral supplements.

Event Tanning

The event tanner is primarily motivated by appearance. Such patients may be receptive to using sun protection to prevent early aging of the skin. For such tanners, a physician could suggest forgoing tanning and allocating the tanning funds to other ways of enhancing appearance such as clothing, a manicure, or a makeover with a new hairstyle and cosmetics. The physician may also suggest substituting sunless tanning for UV tanning as a harm reduction strategy. The event tanner patient may see this as a worthwhile opportunity to look good and boost self-confidence. The dermatologist who is familiar with the various types of sunless tanning can help guide the patient's choice.

Non-UVR tanning products, also known as sunless tanning products, including lotions, spray-on tans, and bronzers, are popular alternatives for achieving a tanned look without the risks of exposure to harmful UVR. Sunless tanning lotions and spray-on tans contain the Food and Drug Administration–approved active ingredient dihydroxyacetone (DHA) in a concentration ranging from 3% to 5%, which preferentially reacts with basic amino acids in the stratum corneum of the skin to form dark brown compounds that deepen the skin's color.[30] Bronzing cosmetics, in the form of powders, moisturizers, or foundations, contain water-soluble dyes to instantaneously give the skin a tanned look and are easily removed by cleansing the area of application but may also be removed by perspiration and may stain clothing.[31]

The use of non-UVR tanning products as an alternative to a UVR-induced tan has been explored in only a few studies. Recently, Pagota and colleagues[32] demonstrated that education about and promotion of sunless tanning products in a population of sunbathers resulted in significantly increased rates of use of these products and decreased rates of sunbathing, which persisted for 1 year after the intervention. In another study, 73% of tanning bed users who received spray-on tan treatments at indoor tanning salons reported decreased use or intention to use indoor tanning beds.[33] There is possible benefit in promoting non-UVR tanning products as an effective

and safer alternative to UVR-induced tanning for the purpose of achieving a tanned look.

Although a few studies have explored the prevalence and predictors of use of non-UVR tanning product use in the United States,[13,34–37] the role of these products as an effective substitute to indoor tanning remains largely uncharacterized among the high-risk population of indoor tanners. Preliminary evidence suggests that indoor tanners who adopt sunless tanning subsequently reduce intentional tanning.[33] The major deterrent to using spray-on tanning is the perception that the color conferred by this method of tanning is not natural. Very few participants commented on cost as a significant barrier to using spray-on tans in the open-response answer choices of the survey. A 2004 investigation of US tanning businesses offering non-UVR tanning services determined the median prices for these options ranged from $26.00 to $87.50 per session, whereas the price for a UVR tanning session was significantly less expensive at $13.50.[31]

Combining appearance-based strategies may be more effective with event tanners than a single educational intervention. An intervention consisting of the use of a sunless tanning lotion along with education on photoaging and viewing of a personal UV facial photograph resulted in greater exercise of sun protection behaviors compared with the group that underwent the same intervention without addition of the sunless tanning lotion.[37] Effective interventions are typically of low intensity and can be performed during the physician visit. Messages targeting appearance are most effective in late-adolescent females, with techniques including self-guided booklets, a video on photoaging, 30-minute peer counseling sessions, and UV facial photography to demonstrate the extent of skin damage from UV exposure. To reduce risk for skin cancer, the US Preventive Services Task Force recommends counseling persons aged 10 to 24 years with fair skin to minimize exposure to UVR.[38]

Spontaneous Mood Tanners

Women may tan inconsistently for short periods of perhaps 1 season and often do so to help them relax or to feel good about themselves.[39] For those who engage in tanning to relax, physicians may suggest other healthy alternatives that create similar immediate consequences to intentional tanning. Exercise classes, such as Pilates and spinning, are sources of stress relief, and yoga has proven efficacious for stress reduction.[40–43] A widely available healthy alternative, such as yoga, gives patients an opportunity to try something that may be new to them that is consistent with seeking a healthy lifestyle. Although sunless tanning is not a source of stress reduction, it may be used in combination with other means of stress reduction to help tanners feel good about themselves.

Regular Tanners

Regular tanners, who tan frequently throughout the year, often discuss how tanning makes them feel relaxed with feelings of tranquility. Some may even report euphoria. Tanning might reduce stress because of a direct physiologic effect of UVR[44–47] and/or because the act itself is relaxing (ie, lying down in a warm, quiet place). Regular tanners may respond to suggestions for ways to relieve stress, such as regular exercise, and ways to promote relaxation, such as yoga.

The likelihood of a behavior being adopted depends on (1) the reinforcing value of that behavior relative to alternatives, (2) the cost of engaging in the behavior relative to alternatives, and (3) the relative availability of the behavior and its alternatives.[39,48] "Behavioral substitution" occurs over time as one behavior declines and another replaces it. For example, as use of the nicotine patch increases, cigarette smoking declines. According to behavioral economics, behavioral substitution of indoor tanning could be facilitated by increasing the costs of indoor tanning and increasing the availability and desirability of alternatives. As the costs of sunbathing and indoor tanning (eg, perceived risk for skin cancer, skin damage, sunburns, as well as the monetary cost of a session of tanning) accumulate, the use of alternatives, such as spray-on tanning, that produce the same outcome with fewer costs should increase.

Legislative Actions

In July 2010, a 10% federal tax on indoor tanning became the first legislative step affecting the monetary costs of the behavior. The impact of the tax on consumer behavior has yet to be determined. Only 26% of Illinois salons reported experiencing fewer clients after implementation of the tax, and distinguishing the impact of the tax from the current economic climate as the source of decline was difficult.[49] Furthermore, 78% of tanning salon owners reported that clients did not seem to care about the tax. The effect of tobacco taxation on smoking led to the hypothesis that because of the limited income of younger clients, a price increase may be a greater deterrent for younger than for older clients[50]; however, this may not be the case for indoor tanning, whose use has steadily increased in the past 2 decades.[2] Tanning salon operators frequently reported that the salon's younger and first-time clients were less likely than its older clients to notice or care about the increased prices resulting from the tax.[49] These results may indicate that the demand for indoor tanning services is perhaps insensitive to a 10% tax level.

Before October 2011, Howard County, Maryland, was the only jurisdiction in the United States to ban indoor tanning for minors. However, California recently became the first state in the United States to ban commercial indoor tanning for anyone younger than 18; the law went into effect in January 2012. This legislation is likely to have a dramatic impact on teen tanning, and other states may soon follow California's lead.

Tanning Dependence

Physicians should be particularly concerned for individuals who tan regularly and frequently, even after receiving information about tanning's serious harmful effects; this may be indicative of pathologic behavior, often termed "tanning dependence" in the literature. The dual process model indicates that dependence behaviors are influenced by both rational decisions and implicit cognitions (ie, unconscious affects that influence a person's behavior). Recent research indicates that individuals who are more motivated by dependence processes in their tanning behaviors have a weaker relationship between their intentions (ie, rational decisions) and behavior (ie, what they actually do).[51]

Initial explorations into tanning dependence[52–61] have modified existing screening instruments to estimate the prevalence of dependence. Using a modified version of a common alcohol-screening questionnaire, the CAGE,[62] has reported prevalence rates range from 12% to 55%. The 4 items from the CAGE were modified to reflect tanning behavior.[52] For example, the item "Have you ever felt that you need to cut down on your drinking, but still continue?" is adapted to, "Have you ever tried to stop tanning, but still continue?" The item, "Have people annoyed you by criticizing your drinking?" became "Do you ever get annoyed when people tell you not to tan?" and, "Have you ever felt guilty about drinking?" became "Do you ever feel guilty that you tan too much?" The last item, "Have you ever had an eye-opener—a drink first thing in the morning to steady your nerves or get rid of a hangover?" transitioned to "When you wake up in the morning, do you want to tan?" It should be noted this last item does not convey the same sense of chemical dependency in the original CAGE (ie, to steady the nerves by using the substance).

Others have adapted items from the *Diagnostic and Statistical Manual of Mental Disorders*, 4th edition (DSM-IV), criteria for substance use disorders to diagnose tanning abuse and dependence using the 5 dependency criteria of tolerance, withdrawal, loss of control, compulsive use, and continued use despite adverse consequences. Some items do not translate flawlessly from substance use disorders to tanning, because tanning is not generally illegal (with the exception of underage tanning in California), nor does it seem to impair performance of activities in the same way many substances do (**Table 1**).[63] The most recent study on tanning dependence adapted items from the Structured Clinical Interview for DSM Disorders (SCID),[63] which focus on opiate abuse and dependence to determine if participants met criteria for tanning abuse or dependence. Results indicated that the prevalence of tanning abuse was 10.8%, and the prevalence of dependence was 5.4% in a sample of college students (mean age = 21.8 years).[64] These rates are congruent with past year prevalence rates for other forms of substance abuse and dependence from national surveys (eg, alcohol dependence = 5.9%).[65] Indoor tanning frequency in dependent tanners was more than 10 times the rate of participants with no diagnosis.

From a physiologic standpoint, a small clinical study recently demonstrated that frequent users of tanning beds exhibited brain activity similar to that observed in people addicted to drugs or alcohol.[66] Regional cerebral blood flow did not increase when tanners were exposed to filtered UVR, suggesting the tanners could distinguish real UVR from the sham solely on the basis of subjective response. Moreover, the study participants had less desire to tan after exposure to UVR than when compared with the sham UVR, suggesting UVR had a rewarding effect. Further research on dependence in relation to indoor tanning is needed.

Table 1
DSM-IV criteria for substance dependence

DSM-IV Criteria	Original Question	Modification for Tanning
Tolerance	Need for markedly increased of amounts of substance to achieve intoxication or desired effect	Do you feel that you need to spend more and more time in the sun or tanning bed to maintain your tan?
Withdrawal	Withdrawal symptoms if use of substance is decreased or stopped	Do you feel unattractive or anxious to tan if you do not maintain your tan?
Loss of control	Substance often taken in larger amounts or over a longer period than intended Persistent desire or unsuccessful efforts to cut down or control substance use	Do you think that you should stop tanning or decrease the time you spend tanning? Have you tried to stop tanning, but still continue?
Compulsive use	Important social, occupational, or recreational activities are given up or reduced because of substance use	Have you ever missed a social engagement, work, school, or other recreational activities because you went to the beach or tanning salon instead?[a]
Continued use despite adverse consequences	Substance use is continued despite having a persistent or recurrent physical or psychological problems that are likely to have been caused or exacerbated by the substance	Have you ever gotten into trouble at work, with family, or with friends because of tanning?[a] Do you continue to tan despite knowing that it is bad for your skin (can cause wrinkles, premature aging, sun spots, and so forth)? Have you ever had a skin cancer, or do you have a family history of skin cancer?

Abbreviation: DSM-IV, Diagnostic and Statistical Manual Mental Disorders, 4th edition.
[a] Items with poor correlation with substance dependency responses because tanning is not illegal nor does it impair performance of activities of daily living.

SUMMARY

Skin cancer is a major public health concern, and tanning remains a modifiable risk factor. In the near future, laws and taxes are likely to be ineffective in stemming tanning.[67] Multidimensional influences, including psychosocial, individual, environmental, and policy-related factors, create the milieu for the individual to engage in tanning. Parents and physicians can modify the behavior of teens and young adults using strategies based on harm reduction. Environmental and policy-related factors similar to those used to contain the tobacco industry in the United States in the 20th century need to be created. Federal regulations can restrict direct advertising and the excise tax can be increased to a prohibitive amount. Social networking may assist with affect regulation.

REFERENCES

1. Robinson JK, Rigel DS, Amonette R. Trends in sun exposure knowledge, attitudes and behaviors: 1986-1996. J Am Acad Dermatol 1997;37:179–86.
2. Robinson JK, Kim J, Rosenbaum S, et al. Indoor tanning: knowledge, attitudes, behavior, and information sources among young adults from 1988 to 2007. Arch Dermatol 2008;144:484–8.
3. Cokkinides VE, Weinstock MA, O'Connell MC, et al. Use of indoor tanning sunlamps by US youth, ages 11-18 years, and by their parent or guardian caregivers: prevalence and correlates. Pediatrics 2002; 109(6):1124–30.
4. International Agency for Research on Cancer Working Group on artificial ultraviolet (UV) light, skin cancer. The association of use of sunbeds with cutaneous malignant melanoma and other skin cancers: a systematic review. Int J Cancer 2007;120(5): 1116–22.
5. Armstrong BK, Kricker A. The epidemiology of UV induced skin cancer. J Photochem Photobiol B 2001;63(1–3):8–18.
6. Madan V, Lear JT, Szeimies RM. Non-melanoma skin cancer. Lancet 2010;375(9715):673–85.
7. Narayanan DL, Saladi RN, Fox JL. Ultraviolet radiation and skin cancer. Int J Dermatol 2010;49(9): 978–86.
8. Herzog C, Pappo A, Bondy M, et al. Malignant melanoma: cancer epidemiology in older adolescents and young adults. National Cancer Institute, SEER AYA monograph; 2007. p. 53–63. Available at: http://seer.cancer.gov/publications/aya/5_melanoma.pdf. Accessed September, 2011.
9. Purdue MP, Freeman LB, Anderson WF, et al. Recent trends in incidence of cutaneous melanoma among U.S. Caucasian young adults. J Invest Dermatol 2008;128(12):2905–8.
10. Lazovich D, Vogel RI, Berwick M, et al. Indoor tanning and risk of melanoma: a case-control study in a highly exposed population. Cancer Epidemiol Biomarkers Prev 2010;19(6):1557–68.
11. Cust AE, Armstrong BK, Goumas C, et al. Sunbed use during adolescence and early adulthood is associated with increased risk of early-onset melanoma. Int J Cancer 2011;128(10):2425–35.
12. Indoor Tanning Association. About indoor tanning. Available at: http://www.theita.com/?page=Indoor_Tanning. Accessed September 12, 2011.
13. Choi K, Lazovich D, Southwell B, et al. Prevalence and characteristics of indoor tanning use among men and women in the United States. Arch Dermatol 2010;146(12):1356–61.
14. Cokkinides V, Weinstock M, Lazovich D, et al. Indoor tanning use among adolescents in the US, 1998 to 2004. Cancer 2009;115(1):190–8.
15. Demko CA, Borawski EA, Debanne SM, et al. Use of indoor tanning facilities by white adolescents in the United States. Arch Pediatr Adolesc Med 2003; 157(9):854–60.
16. Hillhouse J, Turrisi R, Shields AL. Patterns of indoor tanning use: implications for clinical interventions. Arch Dermatol 2007;143(12):1530–5.
17. Baker MK, Hillhouse JJ, Liu X. The effect of initial indoor tanning with Mother on current tanning patterns. Arch Dermatol 2010;146(12):1427–8.
18. Hoerster KD, Garrow RL, Mayer JA, et al. Density of indoor tanning facilities in 116 large U.S. cities. Am J Prev Med 2009;36(3):243–6.
19. Cafri G, Thompson JK, Jacobsen PB, et al. Investigating the role of appearance-based factors in predicting sunbathing and tanning salon use. J Behav Med 2009;32(6):532–44.
20. Lazovich D, Forster J, Sorensen G, et al. Characteristics associated with use or intention to use indoor tanning among adolescents. Arch Pediatr Adolesc Med 2004;158(9):918–24.
21. Knight JM, Kirincich AN, Farmer ER, et al. Awareness of the risks of tanning lamps does not influence behavior among college students. Arch Dermatol 2002;138(10):1311–5.
22. Hillhouse JJ, Turrisi R, Kastner M. Modeling tanning salon behavioral tendencies using appearance motivation, self-monitoring and the theory of planned behavior. Health Educ Res 2000;15(4): 405–14.
23. Evans JS. Dual-processing accounts of reasoning, judgment, and social cognition. Annu Rev Psychol 2008;59:255–78.
24. Dovidio JF, Penner LA, Albrecht TL, et al. Disparities and distrust: the implications of psychological processes for understanding racial disparities in health and health care. Soc Sci Med 2008;67(3):478–86.
25. Schneider S, Kramer H. Who uses sunbeds? A systematic literature review of risk groups in developed

countries. J Eur Acad Dermatol Venereol 2009;24(6): 639–48.

26. Coups E, Phillips L. A more systematic review of correlates of indoor tanning. J Eur Acad Dermatol Venereol 2011;25(5):610–6.

27. O'Riordan DL, Field AE, Geller AC, et al. Frequent tanning bed use, weight concerns, and other health risk behaviors in adolescent females (United States). Cancer Causes Control 2006;17(5):679–86.

28. Bagdasarov Z, Banerjee S, Greene K, et al. Indoor tanning and problem behavior. J Am Coll Health 2008;56(5):555–61.

29. Danoff-Burg S, Mosher CE. Predictors of tanning salon use: behavioral alternatives for enhancing appearance, relaxing and socializing. J Health Psychol 2006;11(3):511–8.

30. Wittgenstein E, Berry HK. Reaction of dihydroxyacetone (DHA) with human skin callus and amino compounds. J Invest Dermatol 1961;36:283–6.

31. Fu JM, Dusza SW, Halpern AC. Sunless tanning. J Am Acad Dermatol 2004;50(5):706–13.

32. Pagota SL, Schneider KL, Oleski J, et al. The sunless study: a beach randomized trial of a skin cancer prevention intervention promoting sunless tanning. Arch Dermatol 2010;146(9):979–84.

33. Sheehan DJ, Lesher JL Jr. The effect of sunless tanning on behavior in the sun: a pilot study. South Med J 2005;98(12):1192–5.

34. Cokkinides VE, Brandi P, Weinstock MA, et al. Use of sunless tanning products among US adolescents aged 11 to 18 years. Arch Dermatol 2010;146(9): 987–92.

35. Brooks K, Brooks D, Dajani Z, et al. Use of artificial tanning products among young adults. J Am Acad Dermatol 2006;54(6):1060–6.

36. Stryker JE, Yaroch AL, Moser RP, et al. Prevalence of sunless tanning product use and related behaviors among adults in the United States: results from a national survey. J Am Acad Dermatol 2007;56(3): 387–90.

37. Mahler HIM, Kulik JA, Harrell J, et al. Effects of UV photographs, photoaging information, and use of sunless tanning lotion on sun protection behaviors. Arch Dermatol 2005;141(3):373–80.

38. Lin JS, Eder M, Weinmann S. Behavioral counseling to prevent skin cancer: a systematic review for the US Preventive Services Task Force. Ann Intern Med 2011;154:190–201.

39. Pagoto SL, Hillhouse J. Not all tanners are created equal: implications of tanning subtypes for skin cancer prevention. Arch Dermatol 2008;11:1505–8.

40. Satyapriya M, Nagendra HR, Nagarathna R, et al. Effect of integrated yoga on stress and heart rate variability in pregnant women. Int J Gynaecol Obstet 2009;104(3):218–22.

41. Smith C, Hancock H, Blake-Mortimer J, et al. A randomized comparative trial of yoga and relaxation to reduce stress and anxiety. Complement Ther Med 2007;15(2):77–83.

42. Granath J, Ingvarsson S, von Thiele U, et al. Stress management: a randomized study of cognitive behavioural therapy and yoga. Cogn Behav Ther 2006;35(1):3–10.

43. Michalsen A, Grossman P, Acil A, et al. Rapid stress reduction and anxiolysis among distressed women as a consequence of a three-month intensive yoga program. Med Sci Monit 2005;11(12):CR555–61.

44. Feldman SR, Liguori A, Kucenic M, et al. Ultraviolet exposure is a reinforcing stimulus in frequent indoor tanners. J Am Acad Dermatol 2004;51(1):45–51.

45. Kaur M, Liguori A, Lang W, et al. Induction of withdrawal-like symptoms in a small randomized, controlled trial of opioid blockade in frequent tanners. J Am Acad Dermatol 2006;54(4):709–11.

46. Levins PC, Carr DB, Fisher JE, et al. Plasma beta-endorphin and beta-lipoprotein response to ultraviolet radiation. Lancet 1983;2(8342):166.

47. Belon PE. UVA exposure and pituitary secretion. Variations of human lipotropin concentrations (beta LPH) after UVA exposure. Photochem Photobiol 1985;42(3):327–9.

48. Jaccard J. Attitudes and behavior: implications for attitudes toward behavioral alternatives. J Exp Soc Psychol 1981;17:286–307.

49. Jain N, Rademaker A, Robinson JK. Implementation of the federal excise tax on indoor tanning services in Illinois. Arch Dermatol 2012;(1):122–4.

50. Dellavalle RP, Schilling LM, Chen AK, et al. Teenagers in the UV tanning booth? Tax the tan. Arch Pediatr Adolesc Med 2003;157(9):845–6.

51. Baker MK, Hillhouse JJ, Turrisi R, et al. A dual process model of pathological tanning behavior. Poster session presented at the Appalachian Student Research Forum, Johnson City (TN), March 24, 2011.

52. Harrington CR, Beswick TC, Leitenberger J, et al. Addictive-like behaviours to ultraviolet light among frequent indoor tanners. Clin Exp Dermatol 2011; 36(1):33–8.

53. Heckman CJ, Egleston BL, Wilson DB, et al. A preliminary investigation of the predictors of tanning dependence. Am J Health Behav 2008;32(5):451–64.

54. Mosher CE, Danoff-Burg S. Indoor tanning, mental health, and substance use among college students: the significance of gender. J Health Psychol 2010; 15(6):819–27.

55. Nolan B, Feldman S. Ultraviolet tanning addiction. Dermatol Clin 2009;27:109–12.

56. Poorsattar S, Hornung R. UV light abuse and high-risk tanning behavior among undergraduate college students. J Am Acad Dermatol 2007;56(3):375–9.

57. Warthan MM, Uchida T, Wagner RF Jr. UV light tanning as a type of substance-related disorder. Arch Dermatol 2005;141(8):963–6.

58. Zeller S, Lazovich D, Forster J, et al. Do adolescent indoor tanners exhibit dependency? J Am Acad Dermatol 2006;54(4):589–96.

59. Pagoto SL, Schneider KL, Oleski J, et al. Design and methods for a cluster randomized trial of the Sunless Study: a skin cancer prevention intervention promoting sunless tanning among beach visitors. BMC Public Health 2009;9:50.

60. Nolan BV, Taylor SL, Liguori A, et al. Tanning as an addictive behavior: a literature review. Photodermatol Photoimmunol Photomed 2009;25(1):12–9.

61. van Steensel M. UV addiction: a form of opiate dependence. Arch Dermatol 2009;145:211.

62. Mayfield D, McLeod G, Hall P. The CAGE questionnaire: validation of a new alcoholism screening instrument. Am J Psychiatry 1974;131:1121–3.

63. First MH, Spitzer RL, Miriam G, et al. Structured clinical interview for DSM-IV axis I disorders–patient edition (SCID-I/P). New York: Biometrics Research Department, New York State Psychiatric Institute; 2002.

64. Baker MK, Hillhouse JJ, Turrisi R, et al. Skin cancer prevention in young women: evaluating a measure of pathological tanning. Poster session presented at the summit on cancer in Tennessee. Franklin (TN), June 16, 2011.

65. SAMHSA. 2001 National Household Survey on Drug Abuse 2010. Available at: http://www.oas.samhsa.gov/nhsda/2k1nhsda/vol2/appendixh_5.htm. Accessed June 1, 2011.

66. Harrington CR, Beswick TC, Graves M, et al. Activation of the mesostriatal reward pathway with exposure to ultraviolet radiation (UVR) vs. sham UVR in frequent tanners: a pilot study. Addict Biol 2012;17(3):680–6.

67. Mayer JA, Woodruff SI, Slymen DJ, et al. Adolescents' use of indoor tanning: a large-scale evaluation of psychosocial, environmental, and policy-level correlates. Am J Public Health 2011;101(5):930–8.

Dermatoscopy for Melanoma and Pigmented Lesions

Babar K. Rao, MD[a],*, Christine S. Ahn, BA[b]

KEYWORDS

- Noninvasive imaging • Skin imaging • Skin cancer detection • Dermoscopy
- Epiluminescence microscopy

KEY POINTS

- Dermatoscopy is a noninvasive tool that can improve the accuracy of diagnosing melanoma and pigmented lesions.
- The use of routine dermatoscopy can reduce the rate of excision of benign lesions.
- There are several diagnostic algorithms that are used by dermatologists.
- The optimal diagnostic approach to melanoma and pigmented lesions is a combination of clinical exam and different imaging techniques.

INTRODUCTION

Dermatoscopy, also known as dermoscopy, epiluminescence microscopy, incident light microscopy, and skin surface microscopy, is a noninvasive diagnostic technique that uses a magnifying device to observe skin lesions in vivo. Dermatoscopy allows for visualization of subsurface structures that are not otherwise visible to the naked eye, and also has established correlations to histopathologic structures (**Fig. 1**).

The use of dermatoscopy in the evaluation and diagnosis of pigmented lesions has increased over the last several decades, particularly for the early detection of melanoma. Despite the increased survival rates over the last 30 years, melanoma is one of the top 10 primary cancer sites, with the highest rates of incidence in the United States.[1] Among the public education initiatives and the advent of new technologies, dermatoscopy has emerged as an important noninvasive technique that improves the ability to detect melanoma at early stages associated with high rates of cure.[2]

This article reviews the history of dermatoscopy and the evolution of its use by dermatologists, the range of algorithms used to interpret dermatoscopic images, and the clinical efficacy and challenges of dermatoscopy in the management of melanoma and pigmented lesions.

HISTORY OF DERMATOSCOPY AND ITS USES

Dermatoscopy is the use of a microscope that allows dermatologists to visualize subsurface structures from the epidermis to the superficial papillary dermis that are not otherwise visible to the naked eye. Traditional dermatoscopes use nonpolarized light sources against an oil or alcohol interface to decrease light reflection, refraction, and diffraction, making the epidermis more translucent. Newer polarized light dermatoscopes have been developed that do not require a fluid interface.

The use of dermatoscopy has dated as far back as the seventeenth century, but it was not until the 1980s that studies showed the usefulness of dermatoscopy in the diagnosis of pigmented skin

Funding sources and conflicts of interest: Dr Rao has received speaking, stock, consulting support, and has served on the advisory board for Abbot, Galderma, CureMD, and Lucid. Ms Ahn has no funding sources or conflicts to disclose.

[a] Department of Dermatology, Robert Wood Johnson Medical School, University of Medicine and Dentistry of New Jersey, 1 World's Fair Drive, Suite 2400, Somerset, NJ 08873-1344, USA; [b] Department of Dermatology, Wake Forest School of Medicine, MS Box 2462, Medical Center Boulevard, Winston Salem, NC 27157, USA
* Corresponding author.
E-mail address: raobk@umdnj.edu

Dermatol Clin 30 (2012) 413–434
doi:10.1016/j.det.2012.04.005

Naked Eye Examination ⟹ Dermatoscopy ⟹ Biopsy

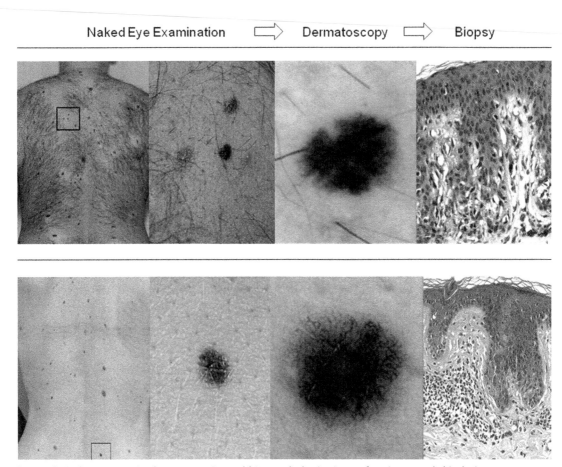

Fig. 1. Clinical macroscopic, dermatoscopic, and histopathologic views of a pigmented skin lesion.

lesions through the analysis of patterns.[3] In 1987, Pehamberger and colleagues[4] published the common dermatoscopic features of melanocytic and nonmelanocytic lesions, which has laid the foundation of diagnostic dermatoscopic methods. In 1989, Soyer and colleagues[5] correlated dermatoscopic structures to histopathologic structures, establishing dermatoscopy as a link between clinical and histopathologic views. In the same year, dermatoscopic terminology was defined at the First Consensus Conference on Skin Surface Microscopy in Hamburg, Germany to standardize the use of this technology.[6]

Worldwide interest in the use of dermatoscopy for the diagnosis of melanoma and pigmented lesions has increased over the past 2 decades. Between 1985 and 2009, the scientific output in dermatoscopy increased significantly, resulting in publications in high-impact dermatology journals including *Archives of Dermatology*, *Journal of the American Academy of Dermatology*, and *British Journal of Dermatology*. The largest proportion of dermatoscopy publications were from Italy (29%), followed by the United States (22%) and Austria (15%).[7]

In addition to increases in scientific output, the development of easier-to-use, handheld dermatoscopes, along with increased dermatoscopy training have led to the increased prevalence of its use by clinicians. The newer, polarized noncontact dermatoscopes that do not require fluid interface are convenient for clinicians because of the small size and portable nature of these devices. Although there are some differences among the dermatoscopes in the representation of certain colors such as the blue-white veil and pink or red, the capabilities of each device are complementary.[8]

Worldwide, the prevalence of the use of dermatoscopy has been studied through survey methods. In a survey of the practices of dermatoscopy among US dermatologists in 2001, 17% of responding dermatologists from the American Board of Medical Specialists Directory of Board Certified Medical Specialists reported using dermatoscopy to aid in clinical assessment, compared with 57% using a magnifying lens.[9] Since then, dermatoscopy practices have increased significantly, ranging from 51% of respondents in a survey of academic dermatology training programs to 70%

of survey respondents attending a dermatoscopy seminar at the American Academy of Dermatology's Summer Academy meeting in 2007. The most common reported reasons for using dermatoscopy across survey studies was the belief that it aided in the early detection of melanoma, led to fewer biopsies, and reduced patient anxiety. Current dermatoscopy users also rated the importance of dermatoscopy in the daily evaluation of skin lesions a mean of 7.4 on a scale of 1 to 10, with 1 representing no importance and 10 representing utmost importance. For dermatologists not using dermatoscopy, lack of training and the lack of usefulness were the most common reasons.[10–12]

In Australia, a survey assessing the prevalence and attitude toward dermatoscopy revealed that 98% of respondent dermatologists used dermatoscopy, of whom 95% received formal dermatoscopy training. Dermatologists who used dermatoscopy felt more confident with their clinical diagnosis with the addition of dermatoscopy (92%) and believed their diagnosis was more accurate than with the naked eye examination alone (86%). Furthermore, respondents believed that dermatoscopy enabled them to detect melanoma at earlier, curable stages (78%), and led to fewer biopsies (72%). A small percentage (3%) believed that dermatoscopy was not useful for the diagnosis of pigmented lesions, melanoma, or atypical nevi, and 12% believed that it was not useful for the diagnosis of nonpigmented lesions.[13]

In Europe, the use of dermatoscopy was documented in the Euromelanoma skin cancer prevention campaign. This campaign was a joint initiative of 20 European countries that was developed to screen for skin cancer. Among nearly 60,000 subjects screened, dermatoscopy was used to aid in 78% of clinical examinations for suspected melanoma.[14]

Since the first efforts to characterize dermatoscopic patterns in the 1980s, the use of dermatoscopy for melanoma and pigmented lesions has increased in prevalence worldwide. The major barrier to its use is the lack of training and understanding of the dermatoscopic diagnostic patterns and algorithms.

DERMATOSCOPIC DIAGNOSTIC ALGORITHMS

Various models are used to interpret dermatoscopic images of pigmented skin lesions. The primary goal of most of these algorithms is to distinguish between benign and malignant melanocytic lesions. The most widely used dermatoscopic algorithms are pattern analysis, the ABCD rule (asymmetry, border, color, and dermatoscopic structures), the

Menzies method, and the 7-point checklist. The virtual Consensus Net Meeting on Dermoscopy, an Internet meeting of 40 experienced dermatologists, evaluated the reproducibility and validity of these 4 algorithms by assessing diagnostic performance and interobserver and intraobserver agreement of 108 dermatoscopic images. The results of the consensus meeting showed that all 4 algorithms were valid ways to evaluate melanocytic lesions with dermatoscopy when used by experienced dermatologists.[15]

More recently, Henning and colleagues[16] described the CASH algorithm (color, architecture, symmetry, and homogeneity) for dermatoscopy, and Rao and colleagues described a simple and practical approach (ASAP) to dermatoscopy. This section reviews each dermatoscopic algorithm and the comparisons of diagnostic accuracy in the literature.

Pattern Analysis

Pattern analysis of pigmented lesions is a qualitative analysis that assesses the diagnostic value of all of the lesion parameters detectable on dermatoscopy. In 1987, Pehamberger and colleagues[4] analyzed more than 3000 pigmented lesions using dermatoscopy to define morphologic criteria that represented reliable markers of benign and malignant skin lesions. Each lesion was excised after dermatoscopic examination to verify the diagnosis through histopathologic examination of serial sections and to correlate dermatoscopic features to histopathologic features. This study established the dermatoscopic patterns for both melanocytic and nonmelanocytic pigmented lesions, and particularly for benign versus malignant growth patterns. The criteria in this study remain influential, serving as the basis for newer algorithms that simplify the dermatoscopic approach to pigmented lesions. Pattern analysis in some variation is still the most commonly used diagnostic method to evaluate dermatoscopic images, reportedly used in as many of 90% of respondents in a survey of dermatologists who use dermatoscopy.[12]

The criteria that were used to distinguish between benign and malignant growth patterns in pigmented skin lesions were based on the general appearance, the pattern of pigmentation, color, pigment network, the presence of globules and dots, depigmentation, and the margin of the pigmented skin lesion.[4] These criteria are defined as follows:

- General appearance: assessment of the general appearance of a lesion is based on the uniformity or heterogeneity of the lesion, the profile of the lesion (elevated or depressed relative to the surrounding skin), and the surface texture of the lesion.

- Pattern of pigmentation: this refers to the color and intensity of pigmentation, and specific pigmentation patterns such as a pigment network, dots, and globule.
- Color: colors seen on dermatoscopy are based on the location of melanin in the skin; from superficial to deep, black indicates melanin in the epidermis, light brown to dark brown indicates melanin at the dermoepidermal junction, gray indicates melanin at the papillary dermis, and steel blue indicates melanin in the reticular dermis.
- Pigment network: the pigment network is a subtle network of brown lines over the background tan color of skin, which result from the presence of melanin pigment in the epidermal basal cell layers that project to the skin surface in rete ridges. The appearance of the pigment network depends on the organization of the rete ridges. An irregular pigment network indicates disorderly spaced rete ridges.
- Brown globules: nests of melanin-containing melanocytes in the lower epidermis appear as brown globules. In benign lesions, they are uniform in size and distribution. In dysplastic or malignant pigmented lesions, brown globules vary in size and appear irregular in distribution.
- Black dots: melanin concentrated in cornified layers of the epidermis appears as black dots. In benign lesions, black dots are typically seen in the center of the lesion. In dysplastic or malignant lesions, black dots may spread out to the periphery.
- Depigmentation: absence of pigment and regression of pigment appear as areas of depigmentation relative to surrounding skin. In benign lesions, depigmentation may occur but appears regular and contained within the center of the lesion. In dysplastic or malignant lesions, depigmentation is irregular and may be found anywhere in the lesion.
- Margin of pigmented skin lesions: the margin of pigmentation can be regular or irregular, and can be well defined or thin out into the surrounding skin. Benign skin lesions have margins of gradually thinning out pigmentation. Malignant pigmented skin lesions have irregular borders and often show areas of abrupt pigmentation margins.

Pattern analysis of dermatoscopic morphologic features can distinguish between pigmented lesions that appear similar clinically but may range from benign to melanoma (**Table 1**). Pattern analysis is also useful in identifying benign nonmelanocytic pigmented lesions such as seborrheic keratosis, hemangioma, and malignant nonmelanocytic pigmented lesions such as pigmented basal cell carcinoma (**Figs. 2–4**).[4]

ABCD Rule

The ABCD rule of dermatoscopy was the second algorithm for dermatoscopy that was developed as a simplification of pattern analysis. The 4 criteria that comprise the algorithm are asymmetry, border, color, and dermatoscopic structural components. Among the 31 dermatoscopic criteria described in the pattern analysis method, these criteria were the most significant cofactors for diagnosing melanoma.[17] In this semiquantitative model, each of the 4 criteria is scored out of a variable number of maximum points and then applied to a formula that adjusts the points with conversion factors, yielding a total dermatoscopic score (TDS). According to this algorithm, lesions with TDS less than 4.75 are usually benign, a TDS between 4.80 and 5.45 is suggestive but not diagnostic of melanoma, and a TDS greater than 5.45 is highly suspicious of melanoma. Lesions with equivocal TDS (4.80–5.45) may be excised or followed to look for dermatoscopic changes over time (**Table 2**).[17] Each component of the ABCD rule is described as follows:

- Asymmetry: the asymmetry score is determined by visually dividing the lesion into 2 $90°$ axes to assess mirror symmetry in terms of contour, color, or structure (**Fig. 5**A). Asymmetry is scored from 0 to 2. A lesion with a score of 0 is symmetric in contour, color, and structure along both axes. A lesion is scored 1 point if there is asymmetry in contour, color, or structure in 1 axis, and 2 points if there is asymmetry in contour, color, or structure in both axes.
- Borders: the border score is determined by visually dividing the lesion into 8 sections (see **Fig. 5**B). The pigment pattern of each wedge is assessed for abrupt cutoff at the margins, rather than a gradual thinning of pigment network. Border is scored by the number of segments of the lesion with a sharp demarcation, ranging from 0 to 8.
- Colors: the 6 colors that comprise the color score of a lesion are red, white, light brown, dark brown, blue-gray, and black. As discussed earlier, the dermatoscopic appearance of black, brown, gray, and blue-gray indicates the location melanin in the lesion. In addition, red usually indicates an

inflammatory process, and white is seen with hyperkeratosis or scarring with regression. Color is scored by the number of these 6 colors present in the lesion, ranging from 1 to 6.

- Dermatoscopic structures: the dermatoscopic structure component is based on the presence of 5 specific structures, which include a pigment network, branched streaks, structureless or homogeneous areas, dots, and globules. The score is based on total number of different dermatoscopic structural components present in the lesion, ranging from 1 to 5.

The ABCD rule is largely intended to risk-stratify pigmented lesions. Therefore, diagnoses should not be based solely on the TDS. For lesions with TDS less than 4.75, it is important to supplement this numerical score with knowledge of known patterns of melanoma, such as pseudopods or white to blue-white colors, indicating regression areas. The presence of any known criteria of melanoma overrides a low TDS score and places the lesion at a higher risk of melanoma. In lesions with equivocal TDS, the presence of atypical vascular patterns such as milky red areas are considered to be high-risk criteria and the lesion should be managed accordingly. There are also some pigmented lesions that are not well diagnosed with the ABCD rule of dermatoscopy, often associated with false high TDS. Among these are dermatofibroma, actinic lentigo, pigmented actinic keratosis, and some types of melanocytic nevi.[17] Spitz nevi are an important subset of melanocytic lesions, which should be diagnosed with pattern analysis and not the TDS of the ABCD rule.

In an effort to simplify the ABCD rule, Blum and colleagues[18] reported on the diagnostic value of a modified ABC point list. In this version, points are given for asymmetry if there is asymmetry in at least 1 axis, for border if there is an abrupt cutoff of pigment network in at least one-quarter of the lesion, and for color if there are 3 or more colors or different structures present in the lesion. This method was comparable with the ABCD rule in sensitivity, specificity, and diagnostic accuracy.

7-Point Checklist

The 7-point checklist is a variation of pattern analysis that uses fewer criteria and a simplified point system. The criteria are divided into 3 major and 4 minor dermatoscopic criteria. These criteria are scored by whether they are absent or present. The presence of major criteria, which include an atypical pigment network, a blue-white veil, and

atypical vascular pattern, is given 2 points each (**Fig. 6**). For each of the minor criteria present, which include irregular streaks, irregular pigmentation, irregular dots/globules, and regression structures, 1 point is given (**Fig. 7**). A lesion with a total of 3 points or greater can be diagnosed as a melanoma with 95% sensitivity.[17]

Menzies Method

The Menzies method is a simplified algorithm based on 2 select criteria and pattern analysis specifically for positive features of melanoma. Similar to the ABCD rule, it combines the application of important, simplified criteria with pattern analysis. Lesions are divided into 2 categories, benign lesions and melanoma, based on asymmetry and color criteria alone. Unlike the ABCD rule, asymmetry in the Menzies method is determined by asymmetry in the pattern of the lesion, and does not take the contour into account. In addition, the color criterion of the Menzies method does not recognize white as a color.[17] In addition to these 2 criteria, the identification of any of the 9 positive features of melanoma is noted. In the scoring of the Menzies method, a lesion is benign if it shows symmetry of pattern within the lesion, and there is only 1 color present. In contrast, a lesion is considered a melanoma if there is asymmetry of pattern within the lesion, there is more than 1 color present, and there is 1 or more of any of the 9 positive dermatoscopic features of melanoma. These features include a blue-white veil, multiple brown dots, pseudopods, radial streaming, scarlike depigmentation, peripheral black dots/globules, multiple colors (5–6), multiple blue-gray dots, and a broad pigment network (**Fig. 8**).

3-Color Test

The 3-color test was reported in a study in which 3 dermatologists experienced with dermatoscopy evaluated 2 sets of lesions that consisted of melanoma and melanocytic nevi. In this analysis, the sensitivity and specificity of the 3-color dermatoscopy test for melanoma versus nevi were 92% and 51%, respectively.[19] Lesions were examined along with clinical features such as the age and sex of the patient, the diameter of the lesion, history of change, and features of asymmetry, irregularities, and multiple colors as seen on naked eye examination. The dermatoscopic features that were recorded included the presence of an irregular pigment network, the presence of a blue-white veil, and the number of colors present. Three or more colors seen on dermatoscopy had the greatest sensitivity (92%) for the diagnosis of melanoma when evaluated separately. The next

Table 1
Pattern analysis of pigmented lesions

Lesion Type	General Appearance	Surface	Pigment Pattern	Border	Depigmentation (Hypopigmentation)
Junctional nevus	Orderly; uniform	Skin surface preserved or smooth; no scales	Regular pigment network at periphery (usually blurred); brown globules equal size and regularly spaced along meshes of pigment network; Intense uniform pigmentation in center pigment network; black dots may occur in center of lesion	Regular; simple outline, pigment network thins out at periphery; no pseudopods; no radial streaming	Usually absent
Compound nevus	Orderly	Skin surface coarse; hyperkeratotic, smooth			Regular; well defined
Lentigo maligna melanoma in situ	Polymorphous; multiple patterns	Skin surface preserved; flat	Prominent but highly irregular pigment network, often obscured by uniform pigmentation; black dots at periphery	Pigment network stops abruptly at edge; no pseudopods, radial streaming may be present	White and pink regions of depigmentation with irregular outline
Lentigo maligna melanoma invasive	Polymorphous; multiple patterns	Skin surface preserved in flat areas; loss of normal skin surface in nodular areas	Highly irregular, prominent pigment network, black dots at periphery; loss of pigment network in nodular areas	Pigment network stops abruptly at edge; pseudopods and radial streaming	White and pink regions of depigmentation with irregular outline
Dysplastic nevus (I and II)	Polymorphous	I: Flat II: Macular with papular component; skin surface not preserved; irregular	I: Prominent pigment network, focally irregular; brown globules of variable size haphazardly spaced; patches of uniform hyperpigmentation; black dots II: No pigment network; irregular brown globules aggregated in center or periphery; irregular depigmentation; black dots, target lesionlike appearance	Irregular, semicircular extensions at periphery; focally pigment network stops abruptly at periphery; peripheral aggregation of brown globules; no radial streaming	I: Not frequent II: Irregular, center, and periphery

Superficial spreading melanoma	Polymorphous; multiple patterns	Skin surface not preserved; slightly elevated, irregular	Irregular, prominent pigment network; brown to black globules of variable size haphazardly spaced; intensely colored patches; black dots at periphery; areas of uniform pigmentation varying in size and ranging in color (blue-gray to black)	Pigment network irregular, stops abruptly at the edge; pseudopods and radial streaming	Bizarre; pink or white
Nodular melanoma	Polymorphous or uniform	Skin surface not preserved; nodular, smooth, or hyperkeratotic	Usually uniformly pigmented; thin rim of prominent and irregular pigment network at periphery; black dots at peripheral areas of uniform pigmentation from gray, blue, brown, to black	Pigment network irregular, stops abruptly at the edge, pseudopods either black or blue; radial streaming	White and pink regions with irregular outline; often speckled with black and blue dots
Angioma	Monomorphous; orderly	Skin surface not preserved; papular	No pigment pattern	Regular; well defined	Absent
Pigmented basal cell carcinoma	Polymorphous	Skin surface not preserved; macular or papular; irregular	No pigment pattern except black dots; telangiectasia	Irregular; no pigment network; no pseudopods; no radial streaming; telangiectasia	Irregular
Seborrheic keratosis	Polymorphous	Skin surface not preserved; verrucous, horny plugs	No pigment pattern except black dots and streaks of pigment; brownish appearance	Irregular	Absent

Adapted from Pehamberger H, Steiner A, Wolff K. In vivo epiluminescence microscopy of pigmented skin lesions. I. Pattern analysis of pigmented skin lesions. J Am Acad Dermatol 1987;17:571–83.

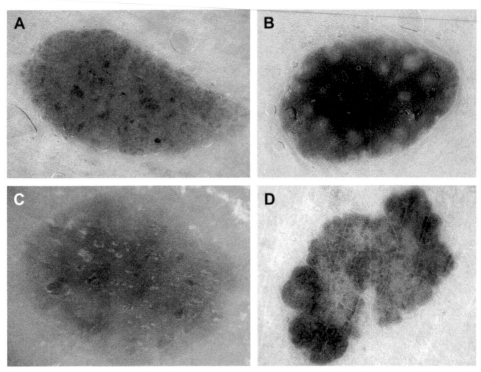

Fig. 2. Dermatoscopic pattern analysis features of seborrheic keratosis include networklike structures (*A*), multiple milialike cysts (*B*), comedolike openings (*C*), and sharply demarcated or moth-eaten borders (*D*).

most sensitive variable was the history of change in the lesion as reported by the patient (86% of melanomas).[19] However, the 3-color test was reevaluated by Blum and colleagues,[20] and reported a lower sensitivity (77%) and specificity of 90%. Depending on the thickness of the lesion, early melanomas may show only 1 or 2 colors. Thus, in the absence of other dermatoscopic criteria for melanoma such as asymmetry, border, or dermatoscopic structures, the 3-color test is not sensitive enough to detect early melanomas.

CASH Algorithm

The CASH (color, architecture, symmetry, homogeneity) algorithm is a semiquantitative model that differs from previous dermatoscopic algorithms by incorporating architectural order or disorder into the characterization of benign versus malignant melanocytic neoplasms.[16] The rationale behind the addition of architectural organization is that benign melanocytic nevi grow in a controlled manner and tend to maintain a well-organized,

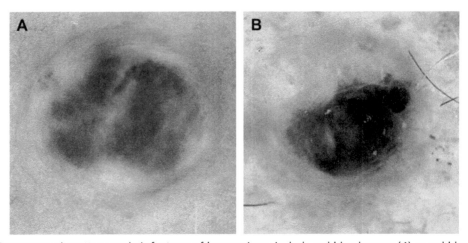

Fig. 3. Dermatoscopic pattern analysis features of hemangioma include red-blue lacunas (*A*) or red-blue to red-black diffuse homogeneous areas (*B*).

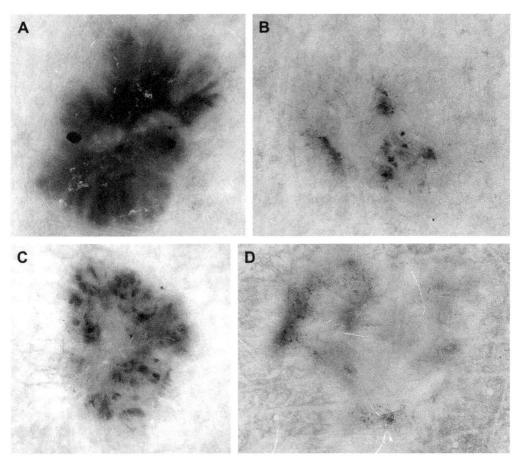

Fig. 4. Dermatoscopic pattern analysis features of basal cell carcinoma include spoke wheel areas (*A*), absent pigment network (*B*), multiple blue-gray globules (*C*), and arborizing vessels (*D*).

Table 2
ABCD rule

Criteria	Description	Score
(A) Asymmetry	0 in a symmetric lesion, 1 point for the presence of asymmetry in 1 axis, 2 points for asymmetry in both axes	0–2
(B) Borders	1 point for each eighth of the lesion where there is an abrupt cutoff of pigment at the peripheral margin	0–8
(C) Colors	1 point for presence of each color: red, white, light brown, dark brown, blue-gray, black	1–6
(D) Dermoscopic structural components	1 point for presence of each specific dermoscopic structural components: pigment network, branched streaks, structureless or homogeneous areas, dots, globules	1–5

Score:
TDS = (A × 1.3) + (B × 0.1) + (C × 0.5) + (D × 0.5)
TDS <4.75, usually benign
= 4.8–5.45, suggestive but not diagnostic of melanoma
>5.45, highly suspicious of melanoma

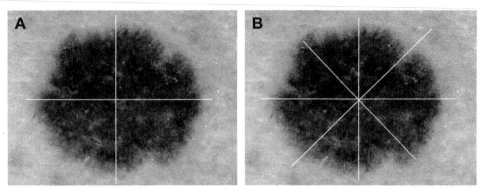

Fig. 5. Measuring asymmetry and border in the ABCD rule. When measuring asymmetry, the lesion is visually divided into two 90° axes. The axes should be oriented in a way that maximizes any existing symmetry (A). Borders are assessed by visually dividing the lesion into 8 segments and counting the number of segments that contain abrupt cutoff of pigment (B).

orderly architecture. Malignant melanocytes proliferate autonomously and do not grow in a structured, orderly pattern. The color, symmetry, and homogeneity components of the CASH algorithm have overlapping criteria with the ABCD rule. The total CASH score ranges from 2 to 17, and a cutoff score was set at 8 points to yield 98% sensitivity

and 68% specificity for differentiating melanoma from dysplastic or melanocytic nevi.[16] Each component of the CASH algorithm is described as follows:

- Color: the same colors from the ABCD rule comprise the color score for the CASH

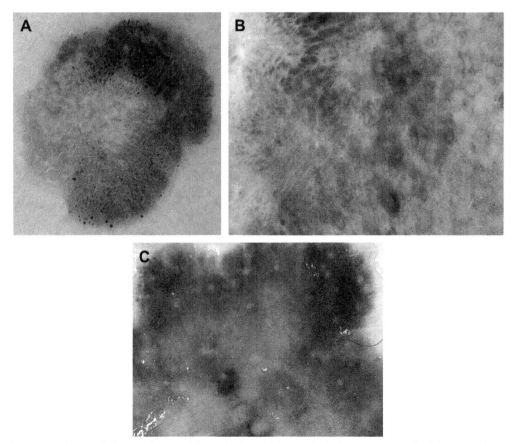

Fig. 6. Major criteria of the 7-point checklist, which include atypical pigment networks (A), atypical vascular patterns (B), and a blue-white veil (C).

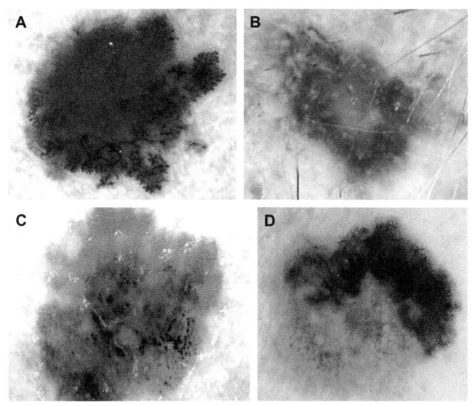

Fig. 7. Minor criteria of the 7-point checklist, which include irregular streaks (pseudopods or radial streaming) (*A*), irregular pigmentation (*B*), irregular dots or globules (*C*), and regression areas (*D*).

algorithm (light brown, dark brown, black, red, white, and blue). The score ranges from 1 to 6, with 1 point for each color present.

- Architecture: architectural order is determined by the uniformity and distribution of structures. In benign lesions, the pigment network is uniform in pigment and spatial arrangement. If dots or globules are present, they appear similar in size, shape, and color. Dots tend to be centrally located, and globules tend to be symmetrically distributed. When there is architectural disorder, the pigment network and other pigment patterns often do not resemble benign patterns, and streaks, radial streaming, or pseudopods may be present. Architecture is scored on a scale from 0 to 2, with 0 points for no or mild architectural disorder, 1 point for moderate disorder, and 2 points for marked architectural disorder (**Fig. 9**).
- Symmetry: symmetry is evaluated and scored in the same method as the ABCD rule, ranging from 0 to 2, with 0 points for no asymmetry and 2 points for biaxial asymmetry (see **Fig. 5A**).

- Homogeneity: homogeneity/heterogeneity is scored on a scale from 1 to 7. The presence of any of 7 dermatoscopic structures is given 1 point. These structures include a pigment network, dots/globules, streaks/pseudopods, blue-white veil, regression structures, blotches, and polymorphous blood vessels.

ASAP to Pigmented Lesions

The ASAP algorithm is a practical dermatoscopic approach to the management of pigmented lesions. Many dermatoscopic algorithms involve calculations of indices that help observers distinguish between melanoma and benign melanocytic nevi. Instead of requiring a scoring system like other diagnostic algorithms, the ASAP method focuses on simple patterns to determine whether a lesion should be biopsied or not, rather than whether a lesion is benign or malignant.

The dermatologist using the ASAP approach looks for known benign patterns, known malignant patterns, and suspicious features in an otherwise benign pattern. On dermatoscopy, if a lesion has a common, known benign pattern with no suspicious features, then a biopsy is unnecessary. If

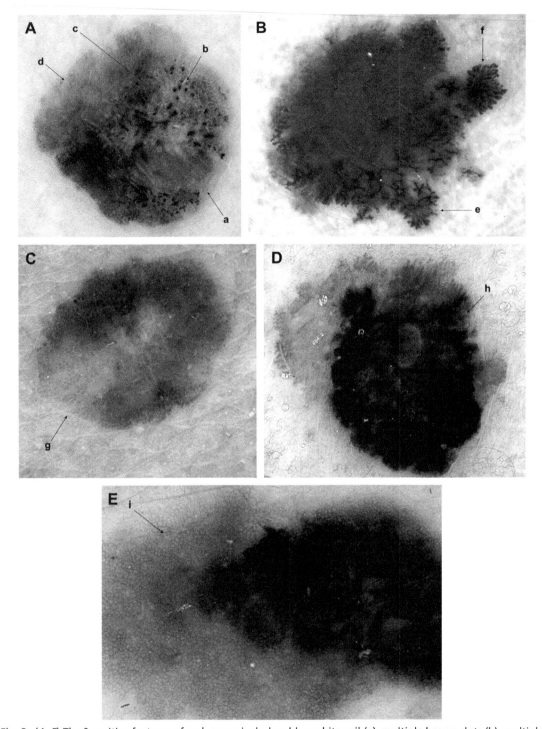

Fig. 8. (*A–E*) The 9 positive features of melanoma include a blue-white veil (a), multiple brown dots (b), multiple colors (5 or 6) (c), radial streaming (d), pseudopods (e), peripheral black dots/globules (f), scarlike depigmentation (g), multiple blue/gray dots (h), and a broad pigment network (i).

a lesion has a known malignant pattern or has suspicious features, then a biopsy is necessary. For lesions with unknown patterns, the lesion should also be biopsied (**Fig. 10**).

This approach requires knowledge of the common benign and malignant patterns of melanocytic nevi. Each known pattern is associated with specific diagnoses that guide the dermatologist toward the

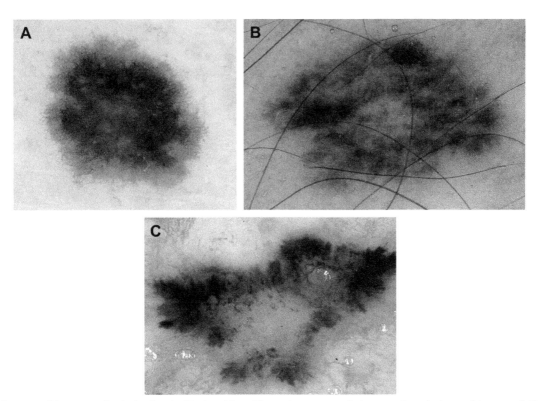

Fig. 9. Architecture criteria in the CASH algorithm. These dermatoscopic images show lesions with no or little architectural disorder (A), moderate architectural disorder (B), and marked architectural disorder with central hypopigmentation, radial streaming, and asymmetry (C).

clinical decision to biopsy or not. The common known patterns of benign pigmented lesions are reticular, globular, reticuloglobular, homogeneous brown, homogeneous blue, starburst patterns (Table 3), as well as the patterns of seborrheic keratosis and hemangioma (see Figs. 2 and 3), which do not require biopsy. The known malignant patterns, which require biopsy, are derived from pattern

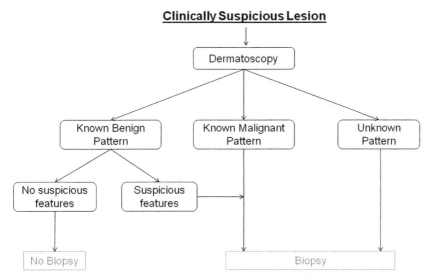

Fig. 10. A flowchart for the ASAP approach to clinically suspicious lesions. If a lesion has a known benign dermatoscopic pattern and no suspicious features are present, no biopsy is necessary. If a lesion has a known benign pattern but there is a suspicious feature present, a biopsy is performed. For lesions with known malignant patterns or unknown patterns, removal or biopsy is performed.

Table 3
Common benign patterns of melanocytic nevi and associated differential diagnoses

Pattern	Description	Differential Diagnosis	
Reticular pattern	Grids of brown lines over a diffuse light-brown background	Junction nevi Dysplastic nevi	
Reticuloglobular	A mixture of a pigment network and dots and globules	Compound nevi Dysplastic nevi	
Globular	Dots and globules	Intradermal nevi Congenital nevi	
Homogeneous brown	Brown pigmentation with no visible reticular or globular pattern	Congenital nevi Dysplastic nevi	
Homogeneous blue	No pigment pattern, uniformly steel blue	Blue nevi	
Starburst	Regular, prominent pigment pattern with a regular radial pattern	Spitz nevi	

analysis features of melanoma. These positive features are also used in the Menzies method (see **Fig. 8**).

- Reticular patterns: reticular pigment networks appear as grids of brown lines over a diffuse light-brown background. They are seen in junctional and dysplastic nevi, and are characterized as typical and atypical. Typical pigment networks are evenly distributed and extend to the periphery of the lesion.
- Globular patterns: globular patterns are seen commonly in intradermal and congenital nevi. These patterns are characterized as regular and irregular. In regular globular patterns, the dots and globules appear the same in size and are uniformly dispersed throughout the lesion.
- Reticuloglobular patterns: this pattern comprises both reticular and globular pattern features, and is frequently found in compound or dysplastic nevi.
- Homogeneous brown patterns: melanocytic nevi that have a homogeneous brown pigment network are common in junctional, congenital, or dysplastic nevi.
- Homogeneous blue patterns: a homogeneous blue pattern is seen in blue nevi.
- Starburst patterns: the distinct starburst pattern of some melanocytic nevi is seen in Spitz/Reed nevi, where pigmented streaks are symmetrically distributed at the periphery. These pigmented lesions are an exception in that they are difficult to manage with high confidence based on clinical examination alone. Because of uncertainty, the recommendation for Spitz/Reed nevi is biopsy.

Dysplastic nevi with reticular, reticuloglobular, or homogeneous brown patterns may further show pattern variants. Typical pattern variants of dysplastic nevi include peripheral or central hyperpigmentation or hypopigmentation, patchy hyperpigmentation or hypopigmentation, patchy network, and peripheral globules. Lesions that show these variations in reticular and reticuloglobular patterns do not require biopsy (**Table 4**).

The known malignant patterns include a blue-white veil, irregular vascular pattern, atypical pigment network, irregular pigmentation, multiple (5–6) colors, regression, irregular streaks, or irregular dots and globules (see **Fig. 8**). In any context, the presence of any of these known, positive features of melanoma on dermatoscopy should lead the clinician to perform a biopsy.

Comparison of Methods of Dermatoscopic Diagnosis

Many studies have sought to assess the accuracy of the different models of dermatoscopic algorithms in terms of sensitivity, specificity, and diagnostic accuracy.[16,21–23] In an Internet Consensus Meeting of 40 expert dermatologists, the reproducibility and validity of pattern analysis, the ABCD rule, the Menzies method, and the 7-point checklist were compared. All of the methods allowed for better sensitivity in distinguishing melanoma versus benign melanocytic lesions. Of all diagnostic methods in this study, pattern analysis had the best diagnostic performance, with a sensitivity of 83.7% and a positive likelihood ratio of 5.1.[15] However, across 6 studies on the diagnostic accuracy of dermatoscopic algorithms, the CASH algorithm, 7-point checklist, and Menzies method have shown the highest levels of sensitivity in the literature, and pattern analysis was shown to have the lowest range of sensitivity (**Table 5**).

Despite the lower sensitivity of pattern analysis reported in studies, studies have shown that pattern analysis enhances the diagnostic accuracy of dermatologists in predicting histologic atypia in melanocytic nevi compared with clinical examination alone. In contrast, the diagnostic performance of dermatoscopy using the ABCD rule was similar to that of clinical diagnosis alone (30% accuracy).[24] In addition, pattern analysis was the most reliable method for teaching dermatoscopy to dermatology residents after undergoing a teaching program with both formal lessons and interactive CD-ROM lessons on dermatoscopy. In the comparison of pattern analysis, the ABCD rule, and the 7-point checklist, pattern analysis yielded the highest mean diagnostic accuracy (68.7%), followed by the ABCD rule (56.1%), and the 7-point checklist (53.4%). In terms of teaching dermatoscopic features of melanoma to dermatology residents, pattern analysis is likely the most reliable method, because it is the most comprehensive and allows for the assessment of both melanocytic and nonmelanocytic lesions.[25]

Each dermatoscopic algorithm has shown varying levels of diagnostic accuracy in different studies, depending on the type of lesions being studied and the level of experience of the observing dermatologist. The ASAP approach has not yet been evaluated in a retrospective study; however, studies have shown that using dermatoscopy based on the decision to biopsy or not results in significant improvement in sensitivity.[26]

Although some studies have reported sensitivity levels as high as 98% achieved by the CASH algorithm, a prospective study by Haenssle and

Table 4
Global pattern variants of dysplastic nevi

Variation of Reticular or Reticuloglobular Pattern

Reticular or reticuloglobular pattern with:
(A) Peripheral hyperpigmentation
(B) Peripheral hypopigmentation

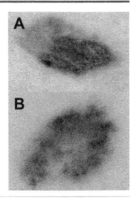

Reticular or reticuloglobular pattern with
(A) Central hyperpigmentation
(B) Central hypopigmentation

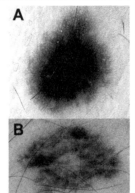

Reticular or reticuloglobular pattern with
(A) Patchy hyperpigmentation
(B) Patchy hyperpigmentation and hypopigmentation

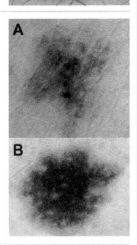

Reticular or reticuloglobular pattern with patchy network

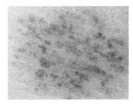

Reticular or reticuloglobular pattern with peripheral globules

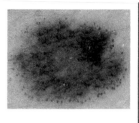

colleagues[27] reinforces the fact that these algorithms are meant to support, not supplant, clinical judgment. The 7-point checklist was studied in a 10-year prospective surveillance of patients at high risk for melanoma. In this long-term study, the sensitivity, specificity, and diagnostic accuracy of the 7-point checklist were assessed. A total of 688 patients were screened at regular intervals by naked eye examination, the 7-point checklist, and digital dermatoscopy follow-up. Based solely on the 7-point checklist threshold of at least 3 points, the study achieved a sensitivity of 62%, which was lower than any of the reported levels (76%–95%) in previous retrospective studies.[18,22,23,28] Of 127 melanomas, 48 lesions had scores less than 3 points, and thus would not have been detected with the 7-point checklist alone. The use of complementary information such as lesional history or dynamic changes detected through digital dermatoscopy were responsible for diagnosing these melanomas that were missed through the algorithm alone.[27]

DERMATOSCOPY IN CLINICAL PRACTICE

This section discusses how dermatoscopy affects clinical decision-making overall and in specific settings such as patients with high risks of melanoma or patients with multiple clinically equivocal nevi. The impact of training on the use of dermatoscopy and important limitations and pitfalls of dermatoscopy are also reviewed.

Clinical Implications

Dermatoscopy influences clinical practice by guiding management decisions. Dermatoscopy can improve the ability to determine whether or not a lesion should undergo biopsy. In prospective studies on the clinical impact of dermatoscopy, the addition of dermatoscopy to naked eye examination was associated with a significant reduction in the number of pigmented skin lesions excised for diagnostic verification, and an increased sensitivity between 10% and 27%.[29–32] The diagnostic accuracy of classifying lesions as melanoma or

---

Table 5
Comparison of sensitivity, specificity, and diagnostic accuracy of dermoscopy algorithms

Dermoscopy Diagnostic Algorithm	Sensitivity (%)	Specificity (%)	Diagnostic Accuracy (%)
Pattern analysis	68[22]–91[28]	83.4[15]–90[28]	76.8[22]
ABCD rule	77.5[22]–90.5[18]	66[28]–80.4[22]	78.1[18]–79.0[22]
7-point checklist	76[23]–95[28]	57[23]–87[18]	64[28]–88.1[18]
Menzies method	84.6[22]–95.2[18]	38[23]–77.8[18]	81.1[22]–83.3[18]
CASH algorithm	87[23]–98[16]	67[23]–68[16]	81[16]

---

nonmelanoma was also significantly higher when dermatoscopy was used to aid the naked eye examination.[33] The relative diagnostic odds ratio for melanoma was 15.6 for dermatoscopy compared with naked eye examination ($P = .016$), and sensitivity for melanoma was higher with dermatoscopic examination (90%, compared with 74% with naked eye examination alone).[34]

Dermatoscopy also plays a significant role in the management of high-risk patients from families with melanoma. In a prospective study in the Netherlands, 132 consecutive patients with familial history of melanoma were recruited, and predermatoscopy and postdermatoscopy diagnoses and management decisions for 49 suspicious pigmented lesions were made by expert dermatologists. Dermatoscopy did not affect the sensitivity of diagnoses but resulted in 42% fewer excisions, increasing the specificity of diagnosis from 53% to 75% ($P = .031$). Thus, even in high-risk groups, dermatoscopy resulted in a significant reduction in the number of unnecessary excisions.[35]

Patients with multiple equivocal nevi also present a challenge to dermatologists, because the unnecessary excision of multiple lesions is undesired. In a study of patients with multiple irregular nevi, dermatoscopists evaluated the lesions based only on morphologic features and then evaluated the lesion relative to other nevi from the same patient. In the first morphologic approach, 55.1% of the overall recommendations were for excision, whereas the comparative approach lowered the number of excisions at a rate of 41%. The 2 lesions that were determined to be melanomas were recommended for excision regardless of the approach. Thus, in patients with multiple equivocal nevi, dermatoscopy is beneficial when used to evaluate morphology and to compare these features in the context of other lesions on the same patient. This situation does not change the sensitivity of diagnosing melanomas and may result in lower rates of excisions.[36]

In addition to melanocytic pigmented skin lesions, the use of dermatoscopy improves the diagnostic accuracy for all types of pigmented lesions, including nonmelanocytic. In a study by Rosendahl and colleagues,[37] 463 consecutively excised pigmented skin lesions were analyzed, of which 47% were nonmelanocytic. When melanocytic lesions were compared with nonmelanocytic lesions, the improvement achieved by dermatoscopy was higher for nonmelanocytic lesions than for melanocytic. A simple algorithm based on pattern analysis reached a sensitivity of 98.6% for basal cell carcinomas, 86.5% for pigmented squamous cell carcinomas, and 79.3% for melanoma. These levels may be considered adequate for the detection of both melanoma and nonmelanoma skin cancer.

Training

The efficacy of dermatoscopy is dependent on the training and experience of the physician. Although the diagnostic accuracy of melanoma is significantly higher when clinical examination is aided by dermatoscopy, dermatoscopy by untrained or less experienced examiners is equivalent or inferior to clinical examination.[38,39] The most common reason for not using dermatoscopy among nonusers is the lack of training. Despite the increase in dermatology training programs in the United States that used dermatoscopy between 2001 and 2009, most respondents (85.9%) would prefer additional training in dermatoscopy.[11]

In a study comparing dermatoscopic diagnoses made by an experienced dermatologist, a clinician with minimal training, and computer-aided analyses, the inexperienced clinician had a lower sensitivity (69%) than experienced dermatologists (92%) and computer analyses (92%). Dermatologists regardless of experience achieved higher specificity than the computer analysis (74%).[40] In a meta-analysis, dermatoscopy was more accurate than clinical examination alone for the diagnosis of melanoma among experienced users, and had a higher discriminating power than clinical examination, with an odds ratio of 76 (16 for clinical examination), and positive likelihood ratio of 9 (3.7 for clinical examination).[41]

Training and regular clinical use of dermatoscopes can improve diagnostic accuracy of melanoma and pigmented lesions. In a prospective study, 6 dermatologists were studied before and after a 10-month period of dermatoscopy training with a modified pattern analysis diagnostic algorithm. The number of melanomas that were left undiagnosed decreased from 18 to 5, and the number of potentially left unexcised decreased from 18 to 3. The numbers of benign lesions that were excised was unchanged after the 10-month period, suggesting that training increased the sensitivity but not the specificity of melanoma diagnosis.[42]

Although dermatoscopy has become incorporated into many dermatology training programs, studies have investigated the efficacy of other training courses that can teach dermatoscopy to dermatologists who have already completed postgraduate training. When inexperienced dermatologists were assessed before and after a short-term formal training course in dermatoscopy, the use of dermatoscopy before training did not lead to better diagnostic accuracy. After the course, the sensitivity, negative predictive value, and diagnostic accuracy of dermatoscopic diagnoses improved significantly, validating the benefit of a short, formal course in dermatoscopy for the early detection of melanoma.[43] There is also evidence that Internet-based courses may serve as a teaching tool in dermatoscopy. Among inexperienced dermatologists, there was considerable improvement in the diagnosis of melanoma with dermatoscopy before and after an Internet-based training course. When the ABCD rule, Menzies method, and pattern analysis were used, the improvements in sensitivity and diagnostic accuracy were significant. Specificity of melanoma diagnosis was not affected after the training for any of the dermatoscopic algorithms.[44]

Challenges and Pitfalls

As with all diagnostic tools, there are limitations to dermatoscopy. The effective use of dermatoscopy relies on the presence of classic features of pattern analysis that allow trained dermatoscopists to make an accurate diagnosis. However, melanomas may present in numerous other ways with uncharacteristic dermatoscopic appearances, otherwise known as the featureless melanoma. These lesions often lack the melanoma-specific criteria, making it difficult for dermatologists to detect. These difficult-to-diagnose presentations of melanoma are reported at a prevalence of 5% to 10%. Early melanomas with uncharacteristic clinical and dermatoscopic appearances often have similar dermatoscopic features to benign melanocytic lesions, even when evaluated with pattern analysis, the ABCD rule, and the 7-point checklist. In a retrospective study of such lesions, the diagnostic accuracy of all 3 methods was inadequate, and the investigators could not identify any dermatoscopic feature or patterns of features that reliably differentiated between melanomas and benign melanocytic lesions at the time of initial presentation. Thus, dermatoscopy depends on the presence of classic dermatoscopic features, and is limited in the diagnosis of very early and most featureless melanomas.[45] To address this problem, studies have been conducted to characterize dermatoscopic features of difficult-to-diagnose melanoma and to assess the usefulness of short-term surveillance with dermatoscopy to detect minimal changes as the melanoma develops.[46]

For featureless lesions, studies have reported on some of the clues, especially dermatoscopic vascular patterns, that help recognize these lesions.[47] A combined clinicodermatoscopic approach is supported by most studies. In 2007, Puig and colleagues[48] evaluated 93 difficult-to-diagnose melanomas by dividing the lesions into 3 categories: melanomas lacking specific criteria of melanocytic or nonmelanocytic tumors, melanomas showing features of nonmelanocytic tumors, and melanomas showing features of melanocytic nevi. For each category, features are described that may help increase the clinical suspicion for these lesions.

- Melanoma without specific melanocytic criteria or nonmelanocytic tumor: among the studied lesions, 10 were amelanotic melanoma and 6 were hypomelanotic melanoma. Vascular structures were a key feature of amelanotic melanoma. The features most commonly seen were polymorphous vascular patterns, mainly composed of dotted and linear irregular vessels or milky globules. There were also remnants of pigmentation in areas of regression and ulceration. More than half of these lesions had patient-reported history of change.
- Melanomas with specific nonmelanocytic features: melanomas that showed specific features of 3 different nonmelanocytic lesions were identified: angiomalike melanoma, basal cell carcinomalike melanoma, and solar lentigo/seborrheic keratosislike melanoma. For angiomalike melanoma, red to purple lacunar structures were present in all lesions. Compared with angiomas, these structures were ill defined and linear vessels were visible inside. In basal cell carcinomalike melanoma, the characteristics of basal cell carcinoma

were observed, leading to surgical excision. Solar lentigo/seborrheic keratosislike melanoma showed benign features such as fingerprintlike structures, milialike cysts, and comedo openings. Compared with solar lentigo/seborrheic keratosis, these melanomas had variable blue-gray colors.

- Melanomas with specific benign melanocytic features: the melanomas with specific criteria of benign melanocytic nevi presented with features of Clark nevi, congenital or dermal nevi, or Spitz nevi. Clark nevuslike melanomas comprised more than 50% of difficult-to-diagnose melanomas in the series. There were variable amounts of regression and peripheral hyperpigmentation in these lesions. In addition, some lesions showed uniform or central hyperpigmentation, multifocal hyperpigmentation and hypopigmentation, and central hypopigmentation. Congenital nevuslike melanoma had blue homogeneous pigmentation with a history of change, which prompted excision. In the Spitz-like melanoma, starburst patterns of streaks, globules, or reticulation were seen. Similar to basal cell carcinoma, the features of spitzoid lesions prompted the removal of these lesions.

In another study to determine the predictive dermatoscopic features of amelanotic and hypomelanotic melanoma, lesions were collected from hospital-based clinics from 5 continents. The significant positive predictors of melanoma (compared with benign melanocytic lesions and nonmelanocytic lesions) were blue-white veils, scarlike depigmentation, multiple blue-gray dots, irregularly shaped depigmentation, 5 or 6 colors, predominant central vessels, red-blue color, and peripheral light-brown structureless areas of greater than 10% of the lesion area. The most significant negative predictors of melanoma were comma vessels, milialike cysts, symmetric pigmentation pattern, blue-gray globules irregular in size or distribution, multiple blue-gray globules, arborizing small diameter vessels, and symmetric shape. Of the vascular-related features, the most predictive of melanoma were central vessels, hairpin vessels, milky red-pink areas, more than 1 shade of pink, combination of dotted and linear irregular vessels, and linear irregular vessels. This study proposed a model for distinguishing malignant from nonmalignant lesions that lack pigment. In a point system, 1 point was added or deducted for the presence of each positive or negative feature, respectively. With a total nonnegative score ($\geq$0), there was high sensitivity (97%) and a low specificity (47%) for the diagnosis of melanoma. If the total score was greater than or equal to 1, a higher

specificity was achieved (79%) but sensitivity decreased (69%). For truly amelanotic melanomas, diagnosis is largely dependent on the appearance of vascular patterns, which can be visualized only on dermatoscopy.[49]

Sequential digital dermatoscopy imaging (SDDI) has been shown to be helpful in diagnosing featureless or incipient melanoma. In this method, lesions are monitored with dermatoscopy over short-term intervals (3 or 4 months) to observe changes over time. Changes within such a short time frame mostly occur in malignant lesions only, because benign lesions are largely biologically senescent. In a 3-month interval program, the specificity for the diagnosis of melanoma is reportedly 83% and in 1 study, approximately 17% of atypical benign lesions showed change by that time. Shortening the SDDI interval to 6 weeks does not seem to provide any advantage. In a study of 1331 suspicious lesions, 31% of melanomas eventually diagnosed had not changed at 6 weeks.[50] In a series of incipient or early featureless melanomas, more than half of melanomas and nevi (61.8%) showed no specific dermatoscopic features for melanoma after 1.5 to 4.5 months. After 4.5 to 8 months, 45% showed no specific dermatoscopic features, and after 8 months, 35.1% still showed no specific features. With longer follow-up, the changes that occurred were spreading and enlarging of the lesion asymmetrically, with concurrent architectural and color changes.[51]

Dermatoscopy is a valuable tool that aids in the diagnosis of early melanoma and other pigmented lesions. There are rules of clinical management, which have been reported in the literature and which provide recommendations for avoiding missing or misdiagnosing difficult-to-diagnose melanomas[52,53]:

- Dermatoscopy should not only be used for clinically suspicious lesions.
- Biopsy should be performed in lesions lacking a clinical-dermatoscopic correlation.
- Biopsy should be performed in lesions with unspecific pigment pattern.
- Biopsy should be performed in lesions with spitzoid features.
- Biopsy should be performed in lesions with extensive regression features.
- In patients with multiple nevi, biopsy should be performed in lesions that change after short-term follow-up.
- Biopsy should be performed in pink lesions with an atypical vascular pattern.

Future Directions

Despite the advances in diagnostic accuracy of melanoma, the prevalence of the disease continues to increase. Public health initiatives have shifted from education about the ABCDs of melanoma to the message of a new or changing skin lesion to promote and facilitate early diagnosis of skin cancer.[54]

The use of dermatoscopy has been evaluated in the primary care setting, where many skin lesions are first seen. Dermatoscopy can be used as a referral tool for primary care providers, which may assist in the clinical decision to refer to a dermatologist. Some studies suggest the use of teledermatoscopy as a referral tool, which involves the use of a Web-based referral service so that general practitioners and an expert remote dermatologist can access patient images. This strategy may be valuable because of specialty access issues, because the median wait time to see a dermatologist for a changing mole is 26 days in the United States.[55] In a study of 660 referred lesions from primary providers, 75% had no suspicious dermatoscopic structures, indicating a significant potential to reduce the number of biopsies, as well as health care costs and wait times.[56]

However, the accuracy of teledermatoscopy has been inconsistent. Studies have reported teledermatoscopy leading to improper management of up to 30% of equivocal melanomas.[57] According to one, the diagnostic accuracy rates for teledermatology were inferior to clinic dermatology, and the use of teledermatoscopy in particular did not significantly change teledermatology diagnostic accuracy rates. Furthermore, the rate of appropriate management was significantly worse for teledermatology than for clinic dermatology and up to 7 of 36 index melanomas would have been mismanaged through teledermatology. Thus, teledermatology and teledermatoscopy should be used with caution for patients with suspected malignant lesions.[58]

Reflectance confocal microscopy is an emerging noninvasive examination tool for the evaluation of skin lesions. Although the features of skin lesions under confocal microscopy are still being characterized, it is intended as an adjunct to clinical examination of suspicious lesions that are clinically equivocal and featureless on dermatoscopy. Confocal microscopy allows the observer to visualize each layer of the skin on a cellular level. The use of confocal microscopy has already been described for nodular melanomas, which have historically been identified as the melanomas that predominantly have nonspecific global dermatoscopic patterns. Distinctive dermatoscopic and confocal features were seen in nodular melanomas compared with superficial spreading melanomas, which may be helpful in the differential diagnosis of these lesions.[59]

SUMMARY

Dermatoscopy improves clinicians' accuracy in diagnosing melanoma and pigmented lesions by as much as 30% over naked eye examination alone. The use of routine dermatoscopy has improved the ratio of malignant to benign excised melanocytic lesions, from the predermatoscopy period (1997), the shift phase (1998), to the dermatoscopy period (1999 and on).[60]

All of the diagnostic algorithms for dermatoscopy use pattern analysis to some extent. Different algorithms may be better suited to dermatologists at different levels of training. In a clinical setting, using the simple and practical approach may be most appropriate for dermatologists with less experience in dermatoscopy. This method involves the identification of pattern analysis features of known benign and malignant patterns, and the biopsy of otherwise unknown patterns. With this principle in mind, less experienced dermatoscopists should maintain a high index of suspicion. By performing a biopsy on every lesion that has an unknown dermatoscopic pattern, the goal is to avoid missing any malignant lesions. As the level of the dermatologist's experience with dermatoscopy and its patterns increases, the level of unknown features decreases, which improves the diagnostic accuracy of dermatoscopy over time.

There are limitations in the use of dermatoscopy. However, understanding some of the dermatoscopic patterns of featureless melanoma and the use of digital dermatoscopy imaging may help dermatologists avoid missing these lesions. The optimal diagnostic approach to melanoma and pigmented lesions includes a multimodal system approach that combines clinical history and examination with different imaging technologies.

REFERENCES

1. U.S. Cancer Statistics Working Group. United States cancer statistics: 1999–2007 incidence and mortality Web-based report. Atlanta (GA): US Department of Health and Human Services, Centers for Disease Control and Prevention and National Cancer Institute; 2010. Available at: http://www.cdc.gov/uscs. Accessed November 18, 2011.
2. Rivers JK, Wulkan S. The case for early detection of melanoma. J Cutan Med Surg 2010;14:24–9.
3. Campos-do-Carmo G, Ramos-e-Silva M. Dermoscopy: basic concepts. Int J Dermatol 2008;47:712–9.
4. Pehamberger H, Steiner A, Wolff K. In vivo epiluminescence microscopy of pigmented skin lesions. I. Pattern analysis of pigmented skin lesions. J Am Acad Dermatol 1987;17:571–83.

5. Soyer H, Smolle J, Hödl S, et al. Surface microscopy. A new approach to diagnosis of cutaneous pigment tumors. Am J Dermatopathol 1989;11:1–10.

6. Bahmer FA, Fritsch P, Kreusch J, et al. Terminology in surface microscopy. Consensus meeting of the Committee on Analytical Morphology of the Arbeitsgemeinschaft Dermatologische Forschung, Hamburg, Federal Republic of Germany, Nov 17, 1989. J Am Acad Dermatol 1990;23:1159–62.

7. Tasli L, Kaçar N, Argenziano G. A scientometric analysis of dermoscopy literature over the past 25 years. J Eur Acad Dermatol Venereol 2011. DOI:10.1111/j.1468-3083.2011.04262.x. [Epub ahead of print].

8. Benvenuto-Andrade C, Dusza SW, Agero AL, et al. Differences between polarized light dermoscopy and immersion contact dermoscopy for the evaluation of skin lesions. Arch Dermatol 2007;143(3): 329–38.

9. Charles CA, Yee VS, Dusza SW, et al. Variation in the diagnosis, treatment, and management of melanoma in situ: a survey of US dermatologists. Arch Dermatol 2005;141(6):723–9.

10. Nehal KS, Oliveria SA, Marghoob AA, et al. Use of and beliefs about dermoscopy in the management of patients with pigmented lesions: a survey of dermatology residency programmes in the United States. Melanoma Res 2002;12:601–5.

11. Terushkin V, Oliveria SA, Marghoob AA, et al. Use of and beliefs about total body photography and dermatoscopy among US dermatology training programs: an update. J Am Acad Dermatol 2010; 62:794–803.

12. Noor O 2nd, Nanda A, Rao BK. A dermoscopy survey to assess who is using it and why it is or is not being used. Int J Dermatol 2009;48:951–2.

13. Venugopal SS, Soyer HP, Menzies SW. Results of a nationwide dermoscopy survey investigating the prevalence, advantages and disadvantages of dermoscopy use among Australian dermatologists. Australas J Dermatol 2011;52:14–8.

14. van der Leest RJ, de Vries E, Bulliard JL, et al. The Euro-melanoma skin cancer prevention campaign in Europe: characteristics and results of 2009 and 2010. J Eur Acad Dermatol Venereol 2011;25:1455–65.

15. Argenziano G, Soyer HP, Chimenti S, et al. Dermoscopy of pigmented skin lesions: results of a consensus meeting via the Internet. J Am Acad Dermatol 2003;48:679–93.

16. Henning JS, Dusza SW, Wang SQ, et al. The CASH (color, architecture, symmetry, and homogeneity) algorithm for dermoscopy. J Am Acad Dermatol 2007;56:45–52.

17. Johr RH. Dermoscopy: alternative melanocytic algorithms—the ABCD rule of dermatoscopy, Menzies scoring method, and 7-point checklist. Clin Dermatol 2002;20:240–7.

18. Blum A, Rassner G, Garbe C. Modified ABC-point list of dermoscopy: a simplified and highly accurate dermoscopic algorithm for the diagnosis of doubtful melanocytic lesions. J Am Acad Dermatol 2003;48: 672–8.

19. MacKie RM, Fleming C, McMahon AD, et al. The use of the dermoscope to identify early melanoma using the three-colour test. Br J Dermatol 2002; 146:481–4.

20. Blum A, Clemens J, Argenziano G. Three-colour test in dermoscopy: a re-evaluation. Br J Dermatol 2004; 150:1040.

21. Binder M, Kittler H, Steiner A, et al. Reevaluation of the ABCD rule for epiluminescence microscopy. J Am Acad Dermatol 1999;40:171–6.

22. Dolianitis C, Kelly J, Wolfe R, et al. Comparative performance of 4 dermoscopic algorithms by nonexperts for the diagnosis of melanocytic lesions. Arch Dermatol 2005;141:1008–14.

23. Henning JS, Stein JA, Yeung J, et al. CASH algorithm for dermoscopy revisited. Arch Dermatol 2008;144:554–5.

24. Carli P, De Giorgi V, Massi D, et al. The role of pattern analysis and the ABCD rule of dermoscopy in the detection of histological atypia in melanocytic naevi. Br J Dermatol 2000;143:290–7.

25. Carli P, Quercioli E, Sestini S, et al. Pattern analysis, not simplified algorithms, is the most reliable method for teaching dermoscopy for melanoma diagnosis to residents in dermatology. Br J Dermatol 2003;148: 981–4.

26. Argenziano G, Soyer HP, Chimenti S, et al. Impact of dermoscopy on the clinical management of pigmented skin lesions. Clin Dermatol 2002;20:200–2.

27. Haenssle HA, Korpas B, Hansen-Hagge C, et al. Seven-point checklist for dermatoscopy: performance during 10 years of prospective surveillance of patients at increased melanoma risk. J Am Acad Dermatol 2010;62:785–93.

28. Argenziano G, Fabbrocini G, Carli P, et al. Epiluminescence microscopy for the diagnosis of doubtful melanocytic skin lesions. Comparison of the ABCD rule of dermatoscopy and a new 7-point checklist based on pattern analysis. Arch Dermatol 1998; 134:1563–70.

29. Carli P, de Giorgi V, Chiarugi A, et al. Addition of dermoscopy to conventional naked-eye examination in melanoma screening: a randomized study. J Am Acad Dermatol 2004;50:683–9.

30. van der Rhee JI, Bergman W, Kukutsch NA. The impact of dermoscopy on the management of pigmented lesions in everyday clinical practice of general dermatologists: a prospective study. Br J Dermatol 2010;162:563–7.

31. Mayer J. Systematic review of the diagnostic accuracy of dermatoscopy in detecting malignant melanoma. Med J Aust 1997;167:206–10.

32. Menzies SW, Zalaudek I. Why perform dermoscopy? The evidence for its role in the routine management of pigmented skin lesions. Arch Dermatol 2006;142:1211–2.

33. De Giorgi V, Grazzini M, Rossari S, et al. Adding dermatoscopy to naked eye examination of equivocal melanocytic skin lesions: effect on intention to excise by general dermatologists. Clin Exp Dermatol 2011;36:255–9.

34. Vestergaard ME, Macaskill P, Holt PE, et al. Dermoscopy compared with naked eye examination for the diagnosis of primary melanoma: a meta-analysis of studies performed in a clinical setting. Br J Dermatol 2008;159:669–76.

35. van der Rhee JI, Bergman W, Kukutsch NA. Impact of dermoscopy on the management of high-risk patients from melanoma families: a prospective study. Acta Derm Venereol 2011;91:428–31.

36. Argenziano G, Catricalà C, Ardigo M, et al. Dermoscopy of patients with multiple nevi: improved management recommendations using a comparative diagnostic approach. Arch Dermatol 2011;147:46–9.

37. Rosendahl C, Tschandl P, Cameron A, et al. Diagnostic accuracy of dermatoscopy for melanocytic and nonmelanocytic pigmented lesions. J Am Acad Dermatol 2011;64:1068–73.

38. Binder M, Schwarz M, Winkler A, et al. Epiluminescence microscopy: a useful tool for the diagnosis of pigmented skin lesions for formally trained dermatologists. Arch Dermatol 1995;131:286–91.

39. Kittler H, Pehamberger H, Wolff K, et al. Diagnostic accuracy of dermoscopy. Lancet Oncol 2002;3:159–65.

40. Piccolo D, Ferrari A, Peris K, et al. Dermoscopic diagnosis by a trained clinician vs. a clinician with minimal dermoscopy training vs. computer-aided diagnosis of 341 pigmented skin lesions: a comparative study. Br J Dermatol 2002;147:481–6.

41. Bafounta ML, Beauchet A, Aegerter P, et al. Is dermoscopy (epiluminescence microscopy) useful for the diagnosis of melanoma? Results of a meta-analysis using techniques adapted to the evaluation of diagnostic tests. Arch Dermatol 2001; 137:1343–50.

42. Tan E, Levell NJ. Regular clinical dermatoscope use with training improves melanoma diagnosis by dermatologists. Clin Exp Dermatol 2009;34:876–8.

43. Troyanova P. A beneficial effect of a short-term formal training course in epiluminescence microscopy on the diagnostic performance of dermatologists about cutaneous malignant melanoma. Skin Res Technol 2003;9:269–73.

44. Pagnanelli G, Soyer HP, Argenziano G, et al. Diagnosis of pigmented skin lesions by dermoscopy: web-based training improves diagnostic performance of non-experts. Br J Dermatol 2003;148:698–702.

45. Skvara H, Teban L, Fiebiger M, et al. Limitations of dermoscopy in the recognition of melanoma. Arch Dermatol 2005;141:155–60.

46. Neila J, Soyer HP. Key points in dermoscopy for diagnosis of melanomas, including difficult to diagnose melanomas, on the trunk and extremities. J Dermatol 2011;38:3–9.

47. Pizzichetta MA, Canzonieri V, Massarut S, et al. Pitfalls in the dermoscopic diagnosis of amelanotic melanoma. J Am Acad Dermatol 2010;62:893–4.

48. Puig S, Argenziano G, Zalaudek I, et al. Melanomas that failed dermoscopic detection: a combined clinicodermoscopic approach for not missing melanoma. Dermatol Surg 2007;33:1262–73.

49. Menzies SW, Kreusch J, Byth K, et al. Dermoscopic evaluation of amelanotic and hypomelanotic melanoma. Arch Dermatol 2008;144:1120–7.

50. Altamura D, Avramidis M, Menzies SW. Assessment of the optimal interval for and sensitivity of short-term sequential digital dermoscopy monitoring for the diagnosis of melanoma. Arch Dermatol 2008;144: 502–6.

51. Kittler H, Guitera P, Riedl E, et al. Identification of clinically featureless incipient melanoma using sequential dermoscopy imaging. Arch Dermatol 2006;142:1113–9.

52. Argenziano G, Zalaudek I, Ferrara G, et al. Dermoscopy features of melanoma incognito: indications for biopsy. J Am Acad Dermatol 2007;56: 508–13.

53. Marghoob AA, Changchien L, Defazio J, et al. The most common challenges in melanoma diagnosis and how to avoid them. Australas J Dermatol 2009; 50:1–13.

54. Weinstock MA. Cutaneous melanoma: public health approach to early detection. Dermatol Ther 2006;19: 26–31.

55. Resneck JS Jr, Lipton S, Pletcher MJ. Short wait times for patients seeking cosmetic botulinum toxin appointments with dermatologists. J Am Acad Dermatol 2007;57:985–9.

56. Griffiths WA. Improving melanoma diagnosis in primary care–a tele-dermatoscopy project. J Telemed Telecare 2010;16(4):185–6.

57. Carli P, Chiarugi A, De Giorgi V. Examination of lesions (including dermoscopy) without contact with the patient is associated with improper management in about 30% of equivocal melanomas. Dermatol Surg 2005;31:169–72.

58. Warshaw EM, Lederle FA, Grill JP, et al. Accuracy of teledermatology for pigmented neoplasms. J Am Acad Dermatol 2009;61:753–65.

59. Segura S, Pellacani G, Puig S, et al. In vivo microscopic features of nodular melanomas: dermoscopy, confocal microscopy, and histopathologic correlates. Arch Dermatol 2008;144:1311–20.

60. Carli P, De Giorgi V, Crocetti E, et al. Improvement of malignant/benign ratio in excised melanocytic lesions in the 'dermoscopy era': a retrospective study 1997-2001. Br J Dermatol 2004;150:687–92.

Biopsy of the Pigmented Lesions

David Silverstein, MD[a], Kavita Mariwalla, MD[a,b],*

KEYWORDS

- Skin biopsy • Pigmented lesions • Shave biopsy • Punch biopsy • Incisional biopsy
- Excisional biopsy

KEY POINTS

- The skin biopsy is the fundamental procedure all dermatologists should be familiar with when approaching patients with pigmented lesions.
- When deciding to perform a skin biopsy of a pigmented lesion it is important to decide which type of biopsy is appropriate: shave, incisional or excisional.
- Determining which type of biopsy to perform should be guided by clinical suspicion and informed by area on the body.
- For pigmented lesions, partial biopsies are not recommended.
- While complete excision of a pigmented lesion allows the pathologist to fully evaluate the depth and margins of a suspicious lesion, this may not always be practical. In such cases, the dermatologist must always remember that a biopsy is a diagnostic tool and additional tissue can always be taken at a later time if needed.

INTRODUCTION

The rate of melanoma has increased significantly in the last several decades.[1] It is not clear whether this is a true increase in the incidence of the biologic process or a function of improved diagnostic acumen amongst dermatologists and dermatopathologists. Early-stage lesions comprise most newly diagnosed melanomas, suggesting that the increase may be because of an uptick in biopsy rates. However, given that melanoma continues to claim several thousand lives annually, an argument can be made that melanocytic lesions are still not biopsied enough. Although new technologies are becoming available to aid in diagnosis, the skin biopsy continues to be the fundamental tool of the dermatologist to evaluate the nature of a pigmented lesion.

When a decision to biopsy is made, the method by which to do it can represent a challenging dilemma. There are 3 major techniques for the biopsy of a pigmented lesion: shave biopsy, punch/incisional biopsy, and excisional biopsy. Each has its advantages and drawbacks and which the clinician chooses is based on many factors, including, but not limited to, the morphologic characteristics and anatomic site of the pigmented lesion, the clinician's level of suspicion regarding the aggressiveness of the lesion, the clinician's level of comfort with each technique under varying circumstances, and the cosmesis of the resultant defect.

This article discusses when to biopsy a pigmented lesion and reviews the different biopsy techniques. Specific clinical scenarios are discussed. When approaching a pigmented lesion, the most important end point is realizing that a biopsy is needed and then choosing the technique that provides an accurate diagnosis.

LESION EVALUATION

Before performing a biopsy, the first step for the clinician is determining whether a pigmented

a State University of New York at Stony Brook, East Setauket, NY, USA; b Columbia University, New York, NY, USA
* Corresponding author. 181 N. Belle Meade Road, Suite 5, East Setauket, NY 11733.
E-mail address: kavita.mariwalla@yale.edu

Dermatol Clin 30 (2012) 435–443
doi:10.1016/j.det.2012.04.013
0733-8635/12/$ – see front matter © 2012 Published by Elsevier Inc.

derm.theclinics.com

lesion is suspicious enough to warrant removal. There are multiple factors that influence the clinician's decision regarding the biologic behavior of a pigmented lesion. The most widely known are probably best encapsulated by the ABCDE criteria.[2] Lesions that are asymmetric (A) warrant a heightened level of suspicion, as do lesions with irregular borders (B), multiple colors (C), or a diameter (D) greater than 6 mm. The evolution of the lesion (E), or how it is changing, is one of the newly added criteria, although it can lead to diagnostic challenges, especially in children whose nevi are often growing as they are.[3]

In general, the dermatologist has few tools other than their clinical experience to evaluate the malignant potential of a pigmented lesion in vivo. The most widely used is dermoscopy, which has gained significant traction in recent years. As a technique, it requires a hand-held device that allows for closer inspection of the structural pattern of a lesion. Although there are multiple published criteria and methods for evaluation of pigmented lesions with dermoscopy, many of the criteria are still in flux[4] and subject to interpreter variability. Another tool used at some academic medical centers for diagnosis of melanoma is confocal microscopy.[5] However, the science is still in its early stages; it is time-consuming, the machinery is expensive, and few operators are trained on its interpretation. MelaFind (Mela Sciences, Irvington, NY, USA) is a new technology that received approval by the United States Food and Drug Administration in 2011. The device evaluates a pigmented lesion and uses a series of algorithms to guide the dermatologist in the decision to perform a biopsy. It is used as an adjunct in the overall clinical picture because it is still at the discretion of the physician to biopsy MelaFind-negative and nonevaluable lesions. Thus, in general, the decision to biopsy a pigmented lesion rests principally on the clinician's experience.

When deciding whether to biopsy, Bolognia[6] has said that the first step is visualizing the gross configuration of the tumor as well as a cross-section of the skin that contains the tumor cells. Thus, an important part of the physical examination is palpation of the suspicious lesion. Because a melanoma with invasion feels thicker than a melanoma in situ, palpation can aid in the selection of the biopsy method. For example, a pigmented nodule is not appropriately sampled by means of a simple shave biopsy, in which the lesion is removed at a level even with the skin; this misses the depth of a melanoma and results in inappropriate management of the patient.

Patients with numerous nevi are especially challenging for the clinician. In this scenario, it is important to assess whether the patient has a signature nevus, which can range from nevi that present as couplets to darkly pigmented nevi that are otherwise benign.[7] For these patients, or patients with greater than 50 nevi (and thus an increased risk for melanoma), regular total body skin examinations with biopsy of the most unusual appearing nevus on an annual basis should be considered.

ANESTHESIA

Depending on the biopsy method, the tools for biopsy vary slightly. However, universal to all biopsies is the selection of anesthesia. Typically, 1% lidocaine with epinephrine at 1:100,000 is used to achieve local anesthesia.[8] However, it is possible to use concentrations as dilute as 1:500,000. The epinephrine provides for vasoconstriction, thereby minimizing the risk of bleeding, although it takes 7 to 10 minutes to achieve its full effect. The duration of action is 1 to 2 hours. Some patients report an allergy to lidocaine, although this is usually more likely a reflection of the sympathomimetic effects of epinephrine, leading to tachycardia. If there is a true allergy to lidocaine (and thus other amide anesthetics), an ester anesthetic such as procainamide can be used. Depending on the size of the lesion to be biopsied, it is also possible to use saline alone for anesthesia.

The area to be biopsied should be injected using a 30-gauge, 1.27-cm (half-inch) needle and infiltrated with the anesthetic until a raised bleb is visible on the skin surface. When infiltrating the skin with anesthesia, it is preferable to insert the needle adjacent to the lesion so as not to disrupt the epidermis of the pigmented lesion itself. If the lesion is greater than 1.0 cm, a ring block technique can be used. In this method, anesthesia is placed peripherally and allowed to diffuse to the center of the lesion. Techniques for minimizing discomfort include warming the anesthetic, injecting slowly, alkalinizing the lidocaine with sodium bicarbonate, and inserting the needle in areas already anesthetized to minimize the number of needlesticks the patient feels.

In children, it is advisable to pretreat the area with topical anesthetic such as eutectic mixture of local anesthetics (EMLA) or a 4 or 5% lidocaine cream for 45 minutes under occlusion with either a bandage or Tegaderm clear dressing. Doing so prevents the patient from feeling the needlestick for additional anesthesia. Depending on the age of the child and their weight, the patient can be placed in a papoose or the parent can hold the child in their lap. It is critical when performing biopsies on children that arms and legs are immobilized as well as the head, if needed. It is important to discuss the biopsy at length with the parent because children often react at the sight of a needle regardless of the amount of pain felt, which can be difficult for a parent to witness. Other modes of pretreating a biopsy area before injection include ice packs, cryogen (which should be sprayed at a distance), or Medi-First cold spray.

In pregnant women, biopsies should be performed without epinephrine. In the first trimester, total amount of lidocaine should be minimized and should not exceed 10 mL. If an excision is performed, patients should be alerted that the scar may spread (depending on the area) because of stretch and that healing time is slightly prolonged.

EQUIPMENT

The tools required for the biopsy of a pigmented lesion depend, in part, on the method chosen (see later discussion). However, most tools are present in the dermatologist's outpatient office. The most commonly used pieces of equipment include a disposable scalpel with a number 15 blade, Webster needle holder, Adson type forceps, Iris scissor, skin hook, Dermablade, punch biopsy tool, suture, aluminum chloride, electrocautery, gauze, and a cotton-tipped applicator. We do not recommend the use of an iron-based solution (eg, Monsel) for coagulation after biopsy of a pigmented lesion because the solution can leave residual pigment (the so-called "Monsel tattoo") in the area. Thus, if a second biopsy or additional tissue is required, light-brown exogenous pigment is seen on permanent section of the tissue, which could make evaluation difficult.

HOW TO BIOPSY: THE GUIDELINES

Many different national organizations have issued guidelines on the biopsy of a suspicious pigmented lesion. In 2002, the British Association of Dermatologists issued their evidence-based guidelines for the management of cutaneous melanoma, and this was updated in 2010.[9] Their guidelines indicate that excisional biopsy of clinically suspicious lesions is almost always preferable to any other technique. However, they note that their guidelines are just that, and each clinical scenario relies on decision making that takes into account many factors. Similarly, the American Academy of Dermatology has recently issued a position statement on the management of melanoma, recommending that a narrow excisional biopsy with 1-mm to 3-mm margins is required to clear the subclinical component of most

atypical melanocytic lesions and is therefore preferable in almost all scenarios.[10]

BIOPSY TECHNIQUES
Shave Biopsy (Saucerization Technique)

Method
The shave biopsy technique is the most commonly performed to evaluate pigmented lesions. The equipment needed is shown in **Fig. 1**. First, the border of the lesion is clearly delineated. A woods lamp (365 nm) can be useful in finely demarcating the lesion; pigment is visualized as a darker area when compared with normal, unaffected background skin. The area is then anesthetized with lidocaine and epinephrine. A disposable scalpel with a number 15 blade or flexible razor blade is then used to remove the lesion, usually with a 1-mm margin of normal surrounding skin.

The advantage of the flexible razor blade over a number 15 scalpel blade is that the diameter of the biopsy can be altered by curving the blade; a greater curvature decreases the diameter of the sampling. Ideally, the lesion should be completely removed so that the depth can be evaluated. This strategy can be accomplished by angling the blade deeper toward the subcutis. If residual pigment remains in the dermis and it is appreciated immediately after performing the biopsy, the lesion should be either reshaved to make sure all the pigment is removed or completely excised. A razor blade is best used in areas of thick skin such as the back or nonfacial areas. A disadvantage of this blade is that it can leave a depressed scar if angled too much and the scar can be hypopigmented after biopsy.

A disposable scalpel with a number 15 blade is helpful when cosmesis is an issue because the scalpel can be used to remove a lesion at the level of the skin. In this scenario, the tip of the needle used for injection can be placed into the lesion and

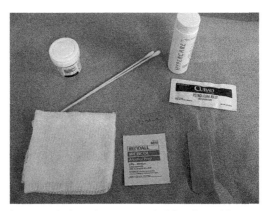

Fig. 1. Typical equipment needed for shave biopsy.

pulled upwards; this holds the lesion in place and provides for countertraction while the scalpel is used to remove the suspicious area. A scalpel with a number 15 blade is ideal to use on the face, the ears, and areas of thin skin such as the dorsal hand.

When performing a shave biopsy of a pigmented lesion, it is best to remove the diameter of the lesion completely, otherwise the biopsy is considered a partial biopsy and the true nature of the lesion cannot be ascertained with accuracy by the examining pathologist. If a lesion is large and biopsy of the entire area would leave a significant scar, it is best to biopsy the darkest or most unusual part of the lesion and note that the biopsy is partial for the dermatopathologist. If the lesion is benign, the area not biopsied should continue to be monitored on a regular basis.

After biopsy, hemostasis is usually achieved using 35% to 50% aluminum chloride, which deposits small crystal plugs into blood vessels. The area is then allowed to heal by secondary intention. Patients are instructed to keep the area moist and coated with Vaseline daily and then covered with a bandage. We do not recommend the use of antibiotic ointments, because there is significant risk for allergic contact dermatitis and the potential for wound infection is low given that the dermis is usually not broken. In addition, recent studies suggest a selection bias toward methicillin-resistant *Staphylococcus aureus* by these antibiotic ointments.[11]

Patients should be advised that the biopsy site looks red initially followed by the appearance of yellow fibrinous tissue, which is normal and not a sign of infection. In addition, patients should be informed that biopsies on the lower extremities may take up to 1 month or longer to heal completely because of the poor circulation in the area. This situation is especially true in obese and vasculopathic patients. We also instruct patients to allow shower water to flow over the wound gently rather than allowing it to hit the area directly because water leaving most shower heads does so at a force of 5.6 kilograms per square centimeter and can slow wound healing. Patients are instructed to use mild soap to clean the area and refrain from swimming in chlorinated pools while the biopsy site is healing. We also advise against the use of hydrogen peroxide on biopsy sites because this too impedes healing.

Given that this method is usually selected for small lesions, it tends to provide good cosmetic outcome, especially if used off the face. The defect created is usually circular in shape and shallow so that a significant scar is not evident if the procedure is performed well. Also, because scars contract as they fibrose, the patient can be reassured from the outset that the cosmetic defect will likely be smaller than the pigmented lesion with respect to size.

Controversies

This method of sampling pigmented lesions offers many benefits but also has some disadvantages. In terms of advantages, the procedure is quick. Typically, this procedure can be performed within a few minutes, thus allowing for little patient anxiety and good in-office flow. The training to adequately perform this procedure is not unduly burdensome, and most dermatology residents are proficient early in their careers. The procedure may even be learned using common household fruits instead of human skin.[12] It is also inexpensive to perform because sutures are not required. Nondermatologists are capable of performing this procedure accurately, which is especially important in areas in which primary care physicians provide most of the dermatologic care without training in skin surgery. In addition, in a patient who has multiple suspicious melanocytic lesions, the shave biopsy might be preferable because performing multiple excisional biopsies can become laborious for both provider and patient. Finally, most providers cannot interrupt their clinic to perform a surgery and must reschedule the patient. There is a significant potential of loss to follow-up in such a scenario. The patient may be too fearful to undertake a cutaneous surgery or scheduling difficulties may not allow for a return visit in the immediate future. In such cases, the saucerization method might at least allow for immediate diagnostic testing.

The biggest problem with this technique arises when the procedure is inadequately selected or the operator is inexperienced. For example, larger lesions are more difficult to completely sample and may best be sampled by other means (see later discussion). Lesions with deep pigment are also difficult to completely evaluate, and a major criticism of this technique has been the potential for transection at the base of the specimen, thereby losing the ability to accurately evaluate the depth of the lesion. A retrospective study of 223 patients showed that shave biopsy specimens left a positive deep margin in 22 patients.[13] This problem becomes especially important when the depth of the lesion affects prognosis and additional intervention (ie, what margins to undertake with a wide excision or whether a sentinel node biopsy is needed). In this regard, a recent retrospective study of 139 patients with melanoma showed that 18 patients had a thicker Breslow depth as determined by excision compared with initial shave biopsy of the lesion. Seven of these patients required additional surgery after the initial wide local excision because of the discrepancy.[14] A more recent study, with a bigger sample size of 600 patients, noted that the initial shave biopsy accurately predicted the lesion depth and thus the correct treatment strategy in 97% of patients.[15] Thus, when properly performed in the right setting, the shave technique may yield the accurate melanoma depth in 97% of patients, but it may be incorrect in as much as 10%. The most worrisome scenario could occur if a biopsy is performed too superficially and the pathologist notes that there are atypical features but does not interpret them as a melanoma. Here, it is possible that the deeper portions of the specimen would have resulted in pathologic interpretation as melanoma and the lesion is being undercalled without this additional tissue. Thus, if the pathologist notes that a lesion has significant atypia and it extends to the base of the specimen, it is advisable to have it definitively sampled.

Incisional or Punch Biopsy

Technique

There are several settings in which an incisional biopsy may be useful. For example, as congenital nevi age, there are often areas that become cobblestoned, bleed from irritation, or become darker. An incisional biopsy using a punch biopsy tool is helpful to sample a portion of the larger lesion. Similarly, in a nevus spilus, areas of hyperpigmentation can become darker and may require sampling. Incisional biopsies have been recommended in other circumstances, including extensive or large pigmented lesions with unclear margins, extensive facial lentigo maligna, pigmented lesions in acral areas, and pigmented lesions in mucosal areas.[16]

The tools needed to complete a punch biopsy are shown in **Fig. 2**. As with the shave biopsy,

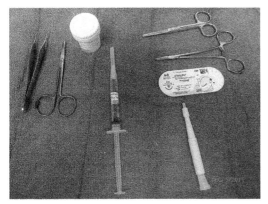

Fig. 2. Typical example of equipment needed for a punch biopsy.

the portion of the lesion to be biopsied is clearly marked. We recommend the use of a camera to photograph exactly where in the lesion the biopsy is taken from. Anesthesia is again provided with 1% lidocaine with epinephrine.

The biopsy can be performed using a punch tool, which is placed over the area and rotated in one direction while consistent pressure is applied in a downward fashion. The skin should be held taught in the direction of the relaxed skin tension lines so that the punch creates a small ellipse rather than a perfect circle. Depending on the area, the rotation should continue until the hub of the punch is at the surface of the skin. If working in an area of thin skin, the punch should be rotated until the level of the fat is reached. The punch tool is then removed and an Adson forceps is used to gently raise the specimen, and tissue cutting scissors are used to transect the specimen at the deep fat. Care should be taken not to crush the specimen with the forceps. In pigmented lesions, the size of the punch should be no smaller than 3 mm to be sectioned and processed appropriately. A hemostatic foam or gauze can be used to pack the biopsy site if it is 3 mm. For larger punch sizes, we recommend the use of a simple, interrupted stitch using nonabsorbable suture such as ethilon. If there is concern that the patient cannot return for a suture removal visit, then an absorbable suture can be used with cyanoacrylate or liquid adhesive and Steri-Strips for epidermal approximation.

If the lesion is larger than a punch tool, a scalpel with a number 15 blade can be used. An ellipse in the direction of skin tension lines is made over the area to be biopsied and removed by cutting down to the layer of the fat. Closure is then performed using dermal and epidermal sutures as needed.

Controversies

Historically, there have been 2 major issues with incisional biopsy. One is whether putting a defect in the middle of the tumor allows for further spread or seeding of the tumor. This theory has largely been debunked and, if it occurs at all, is not considered clinically relevant.[16,17] The more important and clinically relevant issue relates to diagnosis and evaluation of depth. Similar to shave or saucerization biopsies, there is potential for misinterpretation of tumor depth with the incisional technique. Unlike the saucerization biopsy, which is usually selected with intent to remove the entire lesion, the incisional biopsy is intended to remove only a portion of the lesion. Some have argued that the most worrisome portion of the lesion, as determined clinically and dermascopically, should thus be sampled. However, Somach and colleagues[18] found through a survey that there are differences amongst clinicians as to what might represent the most worrisome area of a suspected lentigo maligna lesion. Although there are no studies comparing the clinician's greatest area of concern before biopsy within a lesion with tumor depth on histology, Somach and colleagues' study found a diagnostic discordance between incisional and excisional biopsy by as much as 40% in lesions evaluated by the clinicians they surveyed. This finding indicates that the portion of the lesion most worrisome to a clinician may not correspond to the most histologically aggressive portion of a melanocytic lesion. Although this observation may be true, once a diagnosis is made, most patients subsequently undergo complete excisions of melanoma, with full interpretation of disease and treatment modification if necessary. Studies have therefore not documented negative implications for patient outcome overall, even although this technique may end up subjecting the patient to additional procedures. Pflugfelder and colleagues[16] reviewed 9 such studies, which were mainly retrospective, and overall found no difference in patient outcomes when comparing incisional with excisional samples. However, similar to concerns with the shave biopsy, if a lesion is interpreted as melanoma in 1 region but not another, and the nonmelanoma portion of it is sampled, the pathologist's interpretation may be undercalling the true nature of the lesion and the diagnosis missed. Thus, if the pathologist notes that there is atypia with extension to peripheral margins when performing an incisional biopsy, consideration should be given to complete excision of the pigmented lesion.

Conversely, a major disadvantage of the incisional biopsy technique is overcalling the lesion as a melanoma when it is not (ie, a false-positive result). Evaluation of the symmetry and borders of the lesion is important for the pathologist when interpreting specimens; when an incisional biopsy is performed the area of interest always extends to the periphery of a sample, thereby making a proper diagnosis difficult to render.[19] This situation can be especially confusing with histologic melanoma mimickers such as Spitz nevi or deep penetrating nevi. In addition, a particularly problematic scenario could arise when evaluating recurrent nevi by partial biopsy, because recurrent nevi can share features of melanoma with regression.[20] Because many recurrent nevi occur on the back, this could be further confusing because it may be difficult for patients, especially those with many moles, to know which lesion is being questioned because they cannot easily monitor this area of the body.

Excisional Biopsy

Technique

Excisional biopsy is considered the gold standard for melanoma diagnosis. This technique allows for the entire lesion to be examined, thereby giving the dermatopathologist optimal opportunity to evaluate the margins, depth, and cellular behavior of the pigmented lesion. Excisional biopsy should be performed on any lesion that is highly suspicious for melanoma.

First, the margins of the melanocytic lesion are clearly determined; as in the techniques mentioned earlier; a Wood's lamp can be helpful to detect subclinical pigmentation. Then a 2-mm to 3-mm margin of skin is outlined around the lesion and the lesion is anesthetized with lidocaine and epinephrine as described earlier. A scalpel with a number 15 blade is used to remove the specimen in an elliptical fashion down to the layer of the fat. The orientation is along the relaxed skin tension lines and the draining lymphatics from the site. This orientation theoretically allows for a more accurate sentinel lymph node biopsy if it is later needed. On the extremities, it is preferable to orient such excisions vertically rather than horizontally to better preserve lymphatic architecture. Deep absorbable subcutaneous sutures can be placed if wound strength is needed followed by nonabsorbing epidermal sutures.

Controversies

There has been discussion regarding the accuracy of sentinel lymph node biopsy when performed as a separate procedure after wide local excision (ie, definitive treatment) of melanoma. It has generally been accepted that, if there is not significant tissue rearrangement after defect closure, the accuracy of sentinel lymph node biopsy is still good, although sentinel lymph node biopsy at the time of wide local excision is most preferred.[21,22] Few studies have attempted to address specifically whether an initial diagnostic excisional biopsy affects the subsequent accuracy of sentinel lymph node biopsy. One small study of 60 patients found no difference in lymphatic flow between groups who had previously had diagnostic excision of melanoma with less than 10-mm margins and those whose melanoma was still present after biopsy.[23] Although no studies specifically compare the accuracy of sentinel lymph node biopsy with skin biopsy technique (ie, shave vs incisional vs excisional), it is generally accepted that narrow excisional biopsy does not alter the subsequent accuracy of a sentinel lymph node biopsy and therefore does not change patient prognosis. Further, if wide local excision, which has been studied, does not appreciably alter the accuracy of sentinel lymph node biopsy, neither does the initial biopsy with narrow margins.[24]

SPECIAL SITUATIONS
Evaluation of Melanonychia

The evaluation of longitudinal melanonychia remains difficult, and there are competing methods for biopsy. The evaluation of melanonychia and biopsy techniques has been reviewed by Jellinek.[25] When the decision to biopsy is made, there are 3 main methods to do so, although the most widely accepted is a longitudinal full-thickness excisional procedure, given that shave biopsies fail to evaluate the thickness of the lesion.[26] Many investigators have suggested that, before obtaining a biopsy, the nail plate is viewed end-on with dermoscopy, because lesions that are present in the dorsal nail plate reflect a melanocytic origin at the proximal nail matrix, whereas lesions present in the ventral nail plate correspond to origin at the distal nail matrix.[27] Regardless of which technique is chosen, the procedure is best performed with a digital block using lidocaine and a tourniquet. There has been much controversy over the years regarding the use of epinephrine, although it is generally now accepted that it can be used safely in small quantities to ensure hemostasis.[28] We find the use of epinephrine helpful but recommend not exceeding a total volume of 3 mL of anesthesia for a single digit. Similarly, tourniquet time should be recorded in the patient record and should not exceed 20 minutes.

Shave biopsy of the nail matrix
After achieving adequate anesthesia, tangential incisions are made at the junction of the proximal and lateral nail folds. The skin can be undermined with use of a Freer elevator, and the proximal nail fold is reflected proximally, thereby exposing the proximal nail plate and underlying matrix. The proximal nail plate is then reflected laterally through use of an English anvil-action nail splitter. This procedure allows full exposure of the proximal nail bed and matrix. The matrix is then inspected to fully visualize pigment. The origin of the band is identified and then scored with 1-mm to 2-mm margins with a scalpel blade, which is then turned horizontally to shave the specimen. The laterally reflected nail plate is trimmed longitudinally at its lateral free edge and returned to its original position. The proximal nail fold is released and returned to its normal position. The skin is then sutured at each tangential incision.

Punch biopsy of the nail matrix
As with the shave biopsy, anesthesia is achieved and the proximal nail fold is reflected. The nail plate is left intact because it may serve to help visualize the origin of the pigment. A punch-biopsy tool is used to score the overlying plate above the origin of melanonychia and carried down through matrix to bone. Fine-tipped scissors are used to snip the specimen at the level of the periosteum. Given that the underlying nail plate is secure, suturing is not necessary after realigning the proximal nail fold, and a simple pressure dressing may suffice for wound healing.

Lateral longitudinal excision
A scalpel blade is inserted halfway between the cuticle and distal interphalangeal crease, 1 to 2 mm medial to the pigmented band. Incision is made through skin and soft tissue to the level of bone, extending distally through the nail plate to the hyponychium, to a level 3 to 4 mm distally onto the digital tip. The blade is then reinserted proximally at the same starting point and moved laterally, coursing around the entire matrix horn, so that a final elliptical shape is achieved, with a thin margin around the entire pigmented band. Repair is performed using a single suture that realigns the proximal nail fold to the lateral nail fold, a suture at the proximal nail fold, and a distal suture at the hyponychium. This technique can also be used for larger lesions in the middle of the nail when shave or punch biopsies are deemed inadequate.

Evaluation of Scalp Nevi in Children

Scalp nevi remain a difficult diagnostic dilemma, especially given that they frequently undergo change and may manifest unusual morphologic characteristics.[29] However, most scalp nevi in children are benign, and most investigators recommend conservative observation instead of biopsy unless the lesion becomes clinically suspicious. Further adding difficulty to this scenario, some scalp nevi, although considered benign, manifest histology that has been shown to be unusual,[30] thus making even their pathologic evaluation complicated. Thus, some investigators have recommended excision with conservative margins for these children.[31] When evaluating pigmented lesions of the scalp with biopsy, a full-thickness sampling with excisional biopsy is therefore best, because it allows the dermatopathologist the most tissue to evaluate these sometimes unusual lesions.

Labial Melanotic Macules

Melanotic macules on the lips can have several causes, including medications, physiologic pigmentation, carcinoma, and syndromes such as Laugier-Hunziker or Peutz-Jegher disease. Biopsy is often indicated, and the technique used depends on where on the lip the lesion is located. On the cutaneous lip, a shave biopsy is acceptable if the lesion does not cross the vermilion border. The area can be left to heal by secondary intention and does well with minimal scarring if the area is kept moist. On the mucosal lip, a punch biopsy is preferred, with closure using silk suture and removal at 5 days. If the pigmented lesion crosses the vermilion border, a punch biopsy should be performed, with orientation vertically. The border of the lip should be marked with a gentian violet marking pen so that when the suture is placed to close the defect, the border can be aligned precisely.

Genital Melanotic Macules

Nevi in the genital region should be monitored and photographed to assess for change. If biopsy is required, a punch biopsy using a silk suture for closure is the preferred method. Sutures should be removed at 5 days and patients should be prescribed Bactroban to place over the area twice daily. Although shave biopsies heal well, patients often complain of stinging and irritation in the area while healing takes place.

CONSIDERATIONS IN THE EVALUATION OF PIGMENTED LESIONS ON SUN-DAMAGED SKIN

The histopathologic evaluation of melanocytic lesions on sun-damaged skin has historically been replete with difficulties because multiple studies have shown that chronically sun-damaged skin often has features that are indistinguishable from lentigo maligna.[32,33] Thus, even with an adequately sampled specimen, dermatopathologists may have difficulty in the interpretation of a clinically suspicious pigmented lesion. To that end, some have argued for the simultaneous biopsy of a negative control when biopsying clinically suspicious pigmented lesions on sun-damaged skin to aid in diagnosis. Bowen and colleagues[34] have suggested that a small fusiform excision (12 × 3 mm) be performed on an equivalent site of sun damage to act as a negative control,

thereby allowing for direct comparison of the suspicious lesion with the patient's own sun-damaged skin.

SUMMARY

The technique by which a pigmented lesion is biopsied is influenced by many factors. In general, the preferred method by site can be found in **Table 1**, but the clinician's suspicion, the patient's comfort, and many other circumstances play a role in which technique is chosen. Full excision with complete evaluation of the depth and margins always yields the most data and therefore allows for the most accurate diagnosis, but this is not always practical. Therefore, the clinician must remember to interpret the pathologist's report in the entire clinical context. For example, a lesion in which the clinician is strongly suspicious for melanoma but biopsies only a portion of the neoplasm could be undercalled; it is therefore essential that the clinician question the diagnosis or take additional tissue for pathologic examination. On the other hand, a lesion that was biopsied in the past but repigments could be overcalled. In this case, it would be important for the pathologist to know that a lesion had previously been biopsied. It is the responsibility of the dermatologist to best protect patients by keeping accurate records, including photographs, and to choose the best method for biopsy given the clinical scenario and to adequately communicate this with the pathologist.

REFERENCES

1. Welch HG, Woloshin S, Schwartz LM. Skin biopsy rates and incidence of melanoma: population based ecological study. BMJ 2005;331(7515):481.
2. Rigel DS, Friedman RJ, Kopf AW, et al. ABCDE–an evolving concept in the early detection of melanoma. Arch Dermatol 2005;141(8):1032–4.
3. Grichnik JM. Age-dependent differences in growth curves for distinct melanocytic nevus subsets. Arch Dermatol 2011;147(6):731–2.
4. Marghoob AA, Braun R. Proposal for a revised 2-step algorithm for the classification of lesions of the skin using dermoscopy. Arch Dermatol 2010; 146(4):426–8.
5. Nobre Moura F, Dalle S, Depaepe L, et al. Melanoma: early diagnosis using in vivo reflectance confocal microscopy. Clin Exp Dermatol 2011; 36(2):209–11.
6. Bolognia JL. I. Biopsy techniques for pigmented lesions. Dermatol Surg 2000;26(1):89–90.
7. Suh KY, Bolognia JL. Signature nevi. J Am Acad Dermatol 2009;60(3):508–14.

Table 1 Biopsy recommendations by site	
Site	Technique
Scalp	Excision
Nail	Excision, shave, or punch
Lip	Shave (external) or punch (mucosal)
Genital	Punch

8. Norris RL Jr. Local anesthetics. Emerg Med Clin North Am 1992;10(4):707–18.

9. Marsden JR, Newton-Bishop JA, Burrows L, et al. Revised UK guidelines for the management of cutaneous melanoma 2010. J Plast Reconstr Aesthet Surg 2010;63(9):1401–19.

10. Bichakjian CK, Halpern AC, Johnson TM, et al. Guidelines of care for the management of primary cutaneous melanoma. J Am Acad Dermatol 2011; 65(5):1032–47.

11. Suzuki M, Kazuhiro Y, Nagao M, et al. Antimicrobial ointments and methicillin-resistant *Staphylococcus aureus* USA300. Emerg Infect Dis 2011;17(10): 1917–20.

12. Chen TM, Mellette JR. Surgical pearl: tomato–an alternative model for shave biopsy training. J Am Acad Dermatol 2006;54(3):517–8.

13. Stell VH, Norton HJ, Smith KS, et al. Method of biopsy and incidence of positive margins in primary melanoma. Ann Surg Oncol 2007;14(2):893–8.

14. Moore P, Hundley J, Hundley J, et al. Does shave biopsy accurately predict the final breslow depth of primary cutaneous melanoma? Am Surg 2009; 75(5):369–73 [discussion: 374].

15. Zager JS, Hochwald SN, Marzban SS, et al. Shave biopsy is a safe and accurate method for the initial evaluation of melanoma. J Am Coll Surg 2011; 212(4):454–60 [discussion: 460–2].

16. Pflugfelder A, Weide B, Eigentler TK, et al. Incisional biopsy and melanoma prognosis: facts and controversies. Clin Dermatol 2010;28(3):316–8.

17. Sober AJ, Balch CM. Method of biopsy and incidence of positive margins in primary melanoma. Ann Surg Oncol 2007;14(2):274–5.

18. Somach SC, Taira JW, Pitha JV, et al. Pigmented lesions in actinically damaged skin. Histopathologic comparison of biopsy and excisional specimens. Arch Dermatol 1996;132(11):1297–302.

19. Elenitsas R, Schuchter LM. The role of the pathologist in the diagnosis of melanoma. Curr Opin Oncol 1998;10(2):162–9.

20. King R, Hayzen BA, Page RN, et al. Recurrent nevus phenomenon: a clinicopathologic study of 357 cases and histologic comparison with melanoma with regression. Mod Pathol 2009;22(5):611–7.

21. Gannon CJ, Rousseau DL Jr, Ross MI, et al. Accuracy of lymphatic mapping and sentinel lymph node biopsy after previous wide local excision in patients with primary melanoma. Cancer 2006; 107(11):2647–52.

22. Evans HL, Krag DN, Teates CD, et al. Lymphoscintigraphy and sentinel node biopsy accurately stage melanoma in patients presenting after wide local excision. Ann Surg Oncol 2003;10(4):416–25.

23. Koller J, Rettenbacher L. The influence of diagnostic biopsies on the sentinel lymph node detection in cutaneous melanoma. Arch Dermatol 2000;136(9):1176.

24. Morton DL, Thompson JF, Essner R, et al. Validation of the accuracy of intraoperative lymphatic mapping and sentinel lymphadenectomy for early-stage melanoma: a multicenter trial. Multicenter Selective Lymphadenectomy Trial Group. Ann Surg 1999;230(4): 453–63 [discussion: 463–5].

25. Jellinek N. Nail matrix biopsy of longitudinal melanonychia: diagnostic algorithm including the matrix shave biopsy. J Am Acad Dermatol 2007;56(5): 803–10.

26. O'Connor EA, Dzwierzynski W. Longitudinal melonychia: clinical evaluation and biopsy technique. J Hand Surg Am 2011;36(11):1852–4.

27. Tran KT, Wright NA, Cockerell CJ. Biopsy of the pigmented lesion–when and how. J Am Acad Dermatol 2008;59(5):852–71.

28. Chowdhry S, Seidenstricker L, Cooney DS, et al. Do not use epinephrine in digital blocks: myth or truth? Part II. A retrospective review of 1111 cases. Plast Reconstr Surg 2010;126(6):2031–4.

29. Gupta M, Berk DR, Gray C, et al. Morphologic features and natural history of scalp nevi in children. Arch Dermatol 2010;146(5):506–11.

30. Mason AR, Mohr MR, Koch LH, et al. Nevi of special sites. Clin Lab Med 2011;31(2):229–42.

31. Fabrizi G, Pagliarello C, Parente P, et al. Atypical nevi of the scalp in adolescents. J Cutan Pathol 2007;34(5):365–9.

32. Hendi A, Brodland DG, Zitelli JA. Melanocytes in long-standing sun-exposed skin: quantitative analysis using the MART-1 immunostain. Arch Dermatol 2006;142(7):871–6.

33. Barlow JO, Maize J Sr, Lang PG. The density and distribution of melanocytes adjacent to melanoma and nonmelanoma skin cancers. Dermatol Surg 2007;33(2):199–207.

34. Bowen GM, Bowen AR, Florell SR. Lentigo maligna: one size does not fit all. Arch Dermatol 2011; 147(10):1211–3.

The Pathology of Melanoma

Clay J. Cockerell, MD[a,b],*

KEYWORDS

- Melanoma • Skin cancer • Cutaneous melanoma • Pathology

KEY POINTS

- Although melanoma represents only 10% of all skin cancer diagnoses, it accounts for at least 65% of all skin cancer-related deaths.
- The most important point in melanoma management is its early recognition by a clinician or patients themselves by using ABCDE melanoma mnemonic.
- The use of an adequate biopsy technique that will provide the entire lesion for microscopic evaluation is essential to ensure the correct diagnosis.
- The most important stain in microscopic evaluation of melanocytic lesions remains hematoxylin and eosin with special stains used only if melanocytic differentiation is not readily apparent.
- The depth of melanoma remains the most important prognostic factor.

INTRODUCTION

Although melanoma represents only 10% of all skin cancer diagnoses, it accounts for at least 65% of all skin cancer–related deaths.[1] The number of new cutaneous melanoma cases projected during 2010 was 68,000—a 23% increase from the 2004 prediction of 55,100 cases.[2,3] In 2015, the lifetime risk of developing melanoma is estimated to increase to 1 in 50. As the incidence of melanoma continues to rise, now more than ever, clinicians and histopathologists must have familiarity with the various clinical and pathologic features of cutaneous melanoma.

CLINICAL FEATURES OF MELANOMA

Cutaneous melanoma may present with many different clinical appearances and histopathologic correlates. Most early lesions of melanoma demonstrate the ABCDE features physicians and some patients are now aware of; however, rare cases of melanoma may demonstrate only some or none of these features. Morphologically, most melanomas appear as patches, plaques, nodules, or tumors; however, rarely, melanomas may be polypoidal with a stalk.[4] Usually, lesions measure greater than 6 mm in diameter at diagnosis but smaller lesions are well recognized.

The most common and well-known types of melanoma include superficial spreading melanoma, nodular melanoma, lentigo maligna, and acral lentiginous melanoma. Rare variants of melanoma include desmoplastic melanoma (DM), amelanotic melanoma, verrucous melanoma, follicular melanoma, and melanomas arising from or mimicking blue nevi. Due to a lack of familiarity, these rare variants pose a greater diagnostic challenge to clinicians and histopathologists. DMs present subtly as an indurated patch, plaque, or papule that is either skin colored or pigmented. These lesions are notoriously difficult to diagnose, appear on sun-exposed skin, and clinically resemble a fibroma or scar.

Amelanotic melanomas, which account for 2% to 8% of all melanomas,[5] contain little or no pigment and are the most difficult variant of melanoma to diagnose.[6] Fortunately, truly amelanotic

[a] Department of Dermatology, UT Southwestern Medical Center, 5323 Harry Hines Boulevard, Dallas, TX 75390, USA; [b] Department of Pathology, UT Southwestern Medical Center, 5323 Harry Hines Boulevard, Dallas, TX 75390, USA
* Department of Dermatology, UT Southwestern Medical Center, 5323 Harry Hines Boulevard, Dallas, TX 75390.
E-mail address: ccockerell@skincancer.com

Dermatol Clin 30 (2012) 445–468
doi:10.1016/j.det.2012.04.007
0733-8635/12/$ – see front matter © 2012 Published by Elsevier Inc.

melanomas completely devoid of pigment are rare and account for less than 2% of all melanomas.[6] These lesions present as pink or skin-colored patches, plaques, or nodules that may ulcerate. Clinicians commonly mistake these for pyogenic granulomas, basal cell carcinomas, nevi, seborrheic keratoses, or fibromas. A potential clue to the correct diagnosis is recognition of faint pigmentation at the periphery of the lesion, which may be easier with dermascopy.[7] Dermascopy may also show small red dots evenly distributed or grouped on a whitish or pink-red background,[7] regression structures, irregular dots/globules, or a blue-whitish veil.[5]

Verrucous melanoma, first described in 1967,[8] presents as hyperkeratotic pigmented lesions commonly on the extremities (71%).[9] Clinically, they mimic benign lesions, including seborrheic keratoses, verrucae, nevi, and Spitz nevi.[10–12]

Follicular melanoma, first described in 2004, represents a rare form of melanoma that presents as a perifollicular, darkly pigmented papule measuring less than 5 mm.[13] It commonly occurs on the face or neck of older patients (46–82 years of age)[13,14] with sun-damaged skin. Clinically, it more closely resembles a comedo or pigmented cyst than a melanoma.[13]

Occasionally, melanomas arise in association with blue nevi or arise de novo but clinically resemble blue nevi.[15] This type of melanoma favors the head and neck and may affect children, adults, or the elderly.[15] These lesions tend to evade detection, which leads to a poor prognosis, because they typically grow slowly and predominantly involve the deep dermis.[15] The clinicopathologic correlations of all melanomas remain critical in the effective management of melanoma.

HISTOLOGIC DIAGNOSIS OF MELANOMA

Although the pathogenesis of melanoma remains unsettled, the most valid and currently accepted pathway was proposed by Ackerman and colleagues in the 1980s.[16,17] According to their hypothesis, a de novo melanoma arises when an oncogenic stimulus, usually chronic ultraviolet radiation, acts on one or more melanoctyes in the epidermis at the dermoepidermal (DE) junction. These mutated melanoctyes then proliferate at the junction as solitary units that appear histologically as scattered, single hyperchromatic cells with a cleft or halo surrounding them. At this stage clinically, the lesion may appear as nothing or a light tan macule (**Fig. 1**). With time, these melanocytes multiply and coalesce to form small nests that remain confined to the DE junction. Adnexal involvement, including acrotrichia and acrosyringia, may also occur. At this point clinically, a small tan or brown macule (3–4 mm in diameter) that lacks significant atypia (**Fig. 2**) can be appreciated.

As the tumor progresses, more nests of atypical melanocytes accumulate at the DE junction. Eventually, spread throughout the epidermis occurs and both singular atypical melanocytes and nests of atypical melanocytes extending into the upper layers of the epidermis are seen.[18] Clinically, this manifests as tan lesions ranging in size from 3 mm to greater than 6 mm in diameter, which contain foci of dark brown or black pigment (**Fig. 3**).

Dark brown or black coloration reflects the presence of melanin in the upper levels of the epidermis, including the cornified layer. At this point, lesions manifest noticeable abnormalities, including asymmetry, color variation, and irregular borders, which should prompt a biopsy.

With further progression, the epidermis and adnexal structures becomes more involved and occupied with atypical melanocytes arranged either in nests or singularly. For the first time, melanocytes invade the papillary dermis, initially as small foci of neoplastic melanocytes. Eventually, the papillary dermis becomes filled with neoplastic melanocytes and expands. Clinically, these lesions are macular or slightly elevated, greater than 6 mm in diameter, and demonstrate the ABCDEs

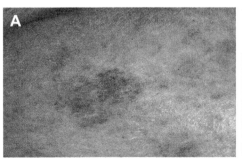
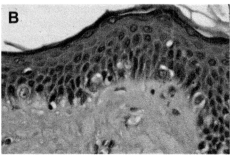

Fig. 1. (A) Early evolving melanoma manifested by pigment alteration inside a faint macule on sun damage skin. (B) Single proliferation of hyperchromatic cells with surrounding halo located on the basement membrane.

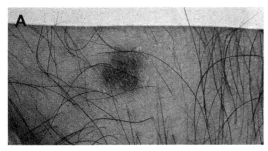
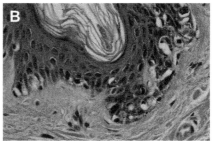

Fig. 2. (A) In time, melanocytes begin to coalesce into nests producing aggregates of darker pigment evident in this 4-mm brown tan macule with irregular border and mild erythema. (B) Histologically single proliferation melanocytes along with nests can be seen at the dermal epidermal junction and along adnexal structures.

characteristic of most melanomas. Skin markings are typically obliterated at this point (Fig. 4).

With even further progression, neoplastic melanocytes spread to involve deeper structures, such as the reticular dermis and subcutaneous fat. At this point, ulceration, nodule formation, and the emergence of colors, including red, blue, and white, may occur. The appearance of white, a poor prognostic sign, indicates regression has occurred (Fig. 5). All of these findings (ulceration, nodule formation, and regression) signify more advanced lesions and a poorer prognosis.[19]

The final stage of progression in melanomas, like many other cancers, is metastasis. The primary metastasis in two-thirds of patients is classified as locoregional metastasis, which comprises satellite, in-transit, and regional lymph node metastasis.[20] Regional lymph node metastasis accounts for one-half of all melanoma metastases.[20] Satellite metastasis is defined as the formation of metastatic nodules within 2 cm of the primary tumor. In-transit metastasis develops in the metastatic drainage area en route to the first regional lymph node. The remaining one-third of metastases in melanoma present primarily as distant metastases to virtually any organ.[20]

Metastatic melanoma presents with different clinical and histologic manifestations depending on which site in the body is involved. In cutaneous metastasis, histology reveals aggregates of atypical neoplastic melanocytes in the dermis often without contiguity with the epidermis. These atypical melanocytes may be arranged in nodular aggregates or cords of cells between and among dermal collagen bundles. The superficial papillary dermis may also be involved in so-called epidermotropic metastases. Blood vessels, lymphatics, and nerves may contain neoplastic cells. Clinically, cutaneous metastases of melanoma present as intracutaneous or subcutaneous nodules, ranging in color from that of normal skin to jet-black. Lymph node involvement usually manifests as one or more firm nodules in a lymph node chain that may be fixed to underlying structures. Histologically, the normal lymph node architecture is replaced by atypical neoplastic melanocytes.

The pathway, described previously, applies to melanomas that arise de novo. Approximately 25% of melanomas develop in association with nevi, however. Clark and colleagues[21] recognized this and proposed a pathway to melanoma that begins with precursor lesions, which are nevi containing dysplastic melanocytes. All melanocytic nevi, especially giant congenital nevi, must be monitored regularly for changes signaling the development of melanoma.

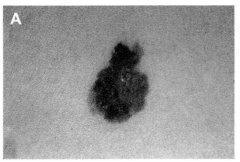
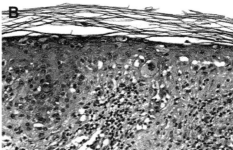

Fig. 3. (A) Clinically asymmetry, irregular color, and shape indicate neoplastic growth. (B) Nests and single atypical melanocytes accumulate and coalesce at the DE junction.

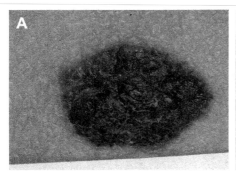
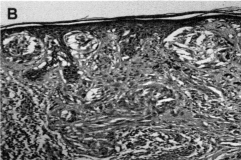

Fig. 4. (A) Morphologic change occurs from a macule to a papule when the papillary dermis is occupied by proliferating melanocytes. (B) Atypical melanocytes occupying the papillary dermis and adnexal structures.

Clark and colleagues described a model for the progression of melanoma that involves 2 separate and distinct growth phases: the radial phase followed by the vertical phase.[21,22] The radial growth phase, which lacks metastatic potential, is characterized by expansion of malignant melanocytes throughout the epidermis and papillary dermis at the periphery of the lesion. Cells in this stage show limited capacity for growth in cell culture[23,24] and are considered less biologically aggressive than cells in the vertical growth phase, which have the capacity for immortality in cell culture.[24] As the name suggests, melanomas in the vertical phase expand vertically to involve deeper layers of the skin and are more likely to metastasize. Significant exceptions to this model of melanoma progression exist, however. Nodular melanomas have only a short or no radial growth phase,[21,25] and thin melanomas may metastasize without a vertical growth phase. In addition, acrolentiginous melanoma demonstrates genotypic features of metastatic melanoma while confined to the epidermis. These findings led some to question the validity of assigning a radial and vertical growth phase to melanomas.

Molecular studies suggest some dysplastic nevi (DN) might represent intermediate lesions in a multistep melanoma tumorigenesis pathway.[26]

Studies have found common genetic alterations between DN and melanoma, including loss of identical tumor suppressor genes, the presence of similar microsatellite instability patterns, and reduced mismatch repair enzyme activity.[27] Many experts do not consider dysplastic nevi to represent precursors of melanoma but rather markers. A recent study has produced evidence that tends to corroborate this position.[28]

BIOPSY TECHNIQUE FOR MELANOMA

The accurate histologic diagnosis of melanoma requires a biopsy that appropriately represents the lesion in question. The biopsy must achieve adequate depth, symmetry, and circumscription to allow for microscopic evaluation of as many diagnostic criteria as possible. Obtaining adequate depth and breadth is especially important to ensure capture of the entire process. Once obtained, specimens must remain intact and receive appropriate processing. Fragmented, deteriorated, or damaged specimens are often not interpretable and may lead to misdiagnosis. Additionally, because several entities mimic melanoma both clinically and histologically, truly representative and pristine biopsies are critical for accurate diagnosis.

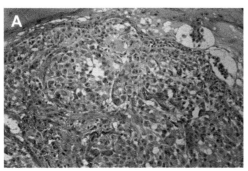
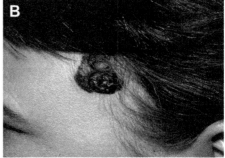

Fig. 5. (A) Atypical melanocytic proliferation involving the deeper structures of the dermis. (B) Nodular growth and ulceration as well as regression (*white color*) are signs of advanced disease.

Biopsy can remove part of the lesion (incisional) or the entire lesion (excisional). Incisional biopsy techniques include superficial shave biopsy, saucerization, and punch biopsy. Superficial shave biopsy should never be used for suspected melanomas because this technique does not sample deeply enough. Excisional biopsy is the preferred method because it encompasses the entire breadth of the lesion as judged clinically.[26]

The most important prognostic factor for melanoma remains the thickness of the lesion (Breslow depth). A nonrepresentative biopsy may provide inaccurate information concerning the true depth of the lesion as well as other important prognostic factors and lead to mismanagement. A retrospective review of 145 cutaneous melanomas compared the accuracy at which saucerization, punch biopsy, or excisional biopsy estimated the Breslow depth found at subsequent therapeutic excision. Saucerization outperformed punch biopsies that were less than 5 mm in diameter for thin melanomas (≤1 mm). Excisional biopsy was found the most accurate method of biopsy.[27] Hsu and Cockerell showed similar results when they reviewed 1123 histologically proved cutaneous melanomas to compare Breslow depth determined from saucerization, punch biopsy, or excisional biopsy to the Breslow depth at re-excision. They found significant diagnostic discrepancy between the re-excision specimens and the initial punch biopsies (86.5% accurate), whereas both excisional biopsy and saucerization demonstrated near 100% accuracy. (Hsu M, Cockerell CJ. Punch biopsy of melanocytic neoplasms: a poorly recognized pitfall in the diagnosis of cutaneous malignant melanoma. Submitted for publication, 2012.) Karimipour and colleagues[29] examined 253 patients with suspected melanoma who underwent subtotal incisional biopsy with retainment of a significant portion of the initial lesion (≥50%). They found a statistically significant ($P = .001$) and substantial discrepancy between the initial Breslow depth (mean of 0.66 mm) and the final depth (mean of 1.07 mm) after re-excision. After complete excision, 21% of these patients were upstaged and 10% became eligible for sentinel lymph node (SLN) biopsy. This study underscores the importance of obtaining representative specimens to ensure patients are managed properly.

The American Academy of Dermatology published updated guidelines for the management of primary cutaneous melanoma in 2011.[30] For the biopsy of lesions suspicious for melanoma, they endorse narrow excisional biopsy that encompasses the entire breadth of the lesion with clinically negative margins to a depth sufficient to ensure the lesion is not transected.[27,29–39] Obtaining clinical margins of 1 mm to 3 mm during the excisional biopsy is recommended.[26,30] This can be accomplished using an elliptical or punch excision (with sutures) or saucerization. Saucerization is commonly used when the suspicion for melanoma is low, when the lesion lends itself to complete removal by this technique, or in the setting of suspected lentigo maligna.[27,30,33] Incisional biopsy of the most atypical portion is acceptable in lesions that are large, have a low clinical suspicion for melanoma, or have on a facial or acral location.[30] Incisional biopsies, however, can potentially underestimate the true depth of the lesion.[29]

HISTOPATHOLOGIC CRITERIA FOR MELANOMA

Ackerman and colleagues proposed a unifying concept regarding the histologic classification of melanoma based on both architectural and cytologic features. Architectural characteristics of melanoma include asymmetry, poor circumscription, and the presence of irregularly distributed melanocytes, arranged singly or in nests, occupying the epidermis (pagetoid spread), adnexa, and dermis. Melanocytes exist above the DE junction and sometimes form irregular nests, which may become confluent (**Fig. 6**). The nests and individual melanocytes lack maturation with progressive descent into the dermis. Additionally, melanin is irregularly distributed in the lesion within the epidermis, dermis, and adnexa. Cytologic characteristics include the presence of atypical melanocytes, necrotic melanocytes, and melanocytes undergoing mitosis.[40]

PATHOLOGIC FEATURES OF DIFFERENT CLINICAL FORMS OF CUTANEOUS MELANOMA
Superficial Spreading Melanoma

Superficial spreading melanoma commonly demonstrates the characteristic features described previously. In addition, it typically demonstrates prominent spread of large atypical melanocytes with abundant pale cytoplasm throughout the epidermis.

Melanoma in Situ

Virtually all forms of melanoma possess a stage in which the neoplasm is confined to the epidermis. Lentigo maligna refers to a subtype typically affecting older individuals with sun-damaged skin. (Note: Not all is Lentigo Maligna—Melanoma in Situ on Acral Skin would not be called that.) Histologically,

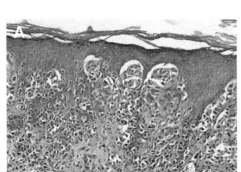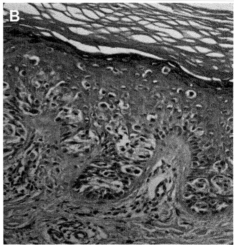

Fig. 6. (A) Asymmetric atypical melanocytic proliferation involving the epidermis, dermis, and adnexal structures. (B) The ascent of atypical melanocytes in the epidermis is characteristic of pagetoid spread in melanoma.

atypical melanocytes, arranged singly and in nests, are distributed irregularly at and above the DE junction. These atypical melanocytes are often present within hair follicles and appendageal structures. The epidermis is commonly thin and atrophic with loss of retia. Solar elastosis is usually abundant on lesions that develop on sun-damaged skin. The superficial dermis might contain a lichenoid infiltrate of lymphocytes and mimic benign lichenoid keratosis on low-magnification evaluation.

The histologic evaluation of margin involvement in melanoma in situ on sun-damaged skin may be difficult because of diffuse melanoctyic proliferation caused by longstanding sun damage.[41] As a general guide, diffuse melanocytic proliferation caused by sun damage contains fewer melanocytes per unit area and typically lacks nests of melanocytes. Clinical correlation may be needed if the pathology is equivocal.

Nodular Melanoma

Virtually all melanomas, if left untreated, may eventually progress to involve the dermis and form papules or nodules clinically. Nodular melanoma, however, tends to involve the dermis at an early point in time in contrast to others that tend to remain confined to the epidermis. Nevertheless, some investigators contend that a nodule appearing in a melanoma is a sign of metastatic potential rather than a distinct subtype of melanoma.[40,42,43]

Acrolentiginous Melanoma

Relative to the other forms of melanoma, acrolentiginous melanoma predominantly affects the palms and soles and contains a greater number of dendritic melanocytes with dendrites extending into the upper layers of the epidermis. Initially, the degree of cytologic atypia may be minimal. With time, melanocytes become more spindle shaped in appearance and display prominent pleomorphism and pagetoid spread. Eventually, involvement of the dermis and deeper structures occurs.

Desmoplastic Melanoma

DM is notoriously difficult to diagnose clinically, so dermatopathologists must have a high index of suspicion for this lesion. Unfortunately, most lesions present at an advanced stage. Several histologic variants of DM exist. In one form, melanocytes appear delicate and spindle shaped and are arranged in fascicles in the upper dermis. These cells may demonstrate minimal atypia and simulate a neural neoplasm, such as neurofibroma. A myxoid stroma is usually present. A second variant demonstrates prominent collagen in the dermis with admixed spindle cells and, occasionally, epitheliod cells; this lesion resembles a scar or fibroma. Many of these lesions have been previously biopsied and may contain scar tissue admixed with neoplasm. A third variant is compromised of numerous markedly atypical spindle and/or epitheliod cells arranged in sheets or fascicles. This variant contains abundant pleomorphic cells with hyperchromatic and bizarre nuclei.[44] The majority of DM lesions (80%) have a component of melanoma in situ in the overlying dermis. They arise either in association with a preexisting melanoma of another type or de novo. They commonly contain nodular aggregates of lymphocytes scattered throughout the dermis.

Perineural invasion, which can cause recurrence and allow spread along nerves, is more common in DM compared with the other types of melanoma. Immunohistochemsitry is often needed to diagnose DM. Most DM lesions are positive for S-100 protein, p75 neurotrophin receptor, and vimentin.[45] Smooth muscle actin may be positive, whereas HMB-45 and Melan-A are inconsistent.[45]

Verrucous Melanoma

Many investigators consider verrucous melanoma a variant of superficial spreading melanoma. Verrucous melanoma is characterized by an exophytic papilliferous growth pattern.[11] Prominent features include pseudoepitheliomatous hyperplasia and overlying hyperkeratosis. These findings may obscure the underlying melanoma cells that exhibit varying degrees of cellular pleomorphism at the DE junction and beneath it.[12] Blessing and colleagues[12] reviewed 20 cases of verrucous melanoma and found 10% of patients initially received benign histologic diagnoses. Furthermore, greater than 50% of patients were given benign clinical diagnoses before biopsy. The investigators also reported difficulty in assigning Breslow depth given the papilliferous architecture of these lesions. Unfortunately, 8 of the 20 patients developed metastases and 7 died of their disease. This study underscores the difficulty clinicians and pathologists face when encountering verrucous melanoma.

Animal Melanoma

Animal melanoma is a rare dermal-based melanocytic neoplasm comprised of sheets of heavily pigmented epithelioid or spindle cells with numerous melanophages. Epidermal hyperplasia is common[46] and mitoses are infrequent.[47] Abundant pigment makes the cytology difficult to evaluate. Animal melanoma may be confused with heavily pigmented blue nevi although diffuse architecture and deep extension are features of animal melanoma that are consistent with this diagnosis.

Nevoid Melanoma

At scanning magnification, these lesions resemble ordinary compound or dermal nevi. In the past, some investigators favored calling these lesions "minimal deviation melanoma" or "borderline melanoma" because they contain only subtle deviations from a nevus. These terms have fallen out of favor, however, and are no longer used. With close inspection, these lesions contain sufficiently distinct characteristics that portray a malignant nature.[48] Clues to the malignant nature of these lesions include pleomorphism, impaired maturation, asymmetry, and mitoses.[49] In addition, the junctional component may contain melanoma in situ, which is a good clue to the diagnosis.[48] Another characteristic of this variant is the presence of irregularly sized and shaped dermal melanocytic nests. Also commonly seen in these lesions is pseudomaturation, which mimics true maturation. True maturation demonstrates progressive smaller melanocytes and cytoplasmic volume at increased depths of the lesion. Pseudomaturation, like true maturation, exhibits a decrease in cytoplasmic volume with increasing depth; however, nuclear size does not follow this trend and are larger than immature nuclei. Finally, unlike most other types of melanomas, inflammatory cell infiltrates are typically absent in this variant. Pathologists should recognize this entity because although they may appear benign, these lesions are no less aggressive than conventional melanomas.[49,50]

Malignant Blue Nevus

Malignant blue nevus, a misnomer, refers to either de novo melanoma that simulates a cellular blue nevus or melanoma that arises in association with a blue nevus. Histologically, these lesions resemble animal melanoma in that they are characterized by large, deep proliferations of melanocytes with sheet-like growth patterns. Individual cells are epithelioid or spindle shaped and demonstrate mitoses, necrosis, nuclear atypia, pleomorphism, hyperchromasia, and prominent nucleoli. Pigmented dendritic cells exist in virtually all lesions.[15] Three histologic patterns are recognized.[45] The first is a lesion with an overtly malignant component adjacent to a benign blue nevus component. The second resembles a subtle sarcoma-like presentation (without florid benign and malignant components), which initially suggests a cellular blue nevus. These lesions, however, exhibit large densely cellular fascicles or nodules of spindle cells that on closer inspection express adequate atypia for malignancy. The third pattern also suggests a benign cellular blue nevus but contains atypical features, including large diameter, asymmetry, prominent cellular density, nuclear pleomorphism, and some mitotic activity. This pattern, not as obviously malignant as the first two patterns, is termed *biologically indeterminate*.[45]

Balloon Cell Melanoma

Balloon cell melanoma is a rare variant of melanoma characterized by the presence of balloon cells, which are epithelioid cells containing abundant eosinophilic or foamy cytoplasm.[51] These balloon cells may present either focally or diffusely throughout the lesion. These lesions typically stain for the usual melanoma markers, including S-100, HMB-45, and Melan-A. Additionally, balloon cell melanoma may simulate benign balloon nevus cells by exhibiting similar cytoplasmic features. The presence of nuclear pleomorphism, atypia, and mitoses and the absence of intervening stroma help distinguish balloon cell melanoma from a balloon cell nevus.[51]

Clear Cell Saoft Part Sarcoma

Clear cell sarcoma (CCS), also called melanoma of soft parts, is a rare variant of a soft tissue sarcoma showing melanocytic differentiation.[52] These deep lesions primarily affect soft tissues in the foot and ankle of young adults.[52] Genetically, these malignant cells express a characteristic translocation of t(12;22)(q13;q12) involving EWS and ATF-1 genes.[53,54] Histologically, they are characterized by a diffuse neoplasm of atypical, pleomorphic, clear-staining cells arranged in sheets and focally in nests. The absence of a direct connection to the epidermis is a useful feature in distinguishing CCS and melanoma.[52] The presence of melanin pigment is occasionally seen in scattered cells. Neoplastic cells demonstrate immunoreactivity for S-100 protein (100%), HMB-45 antigen (97%), Melan-A (71%), and microphthalmia-associated transcription factor (MITF) (81%).[55] The clinical course of CCS is usually protracted with multiple local recurrences and late metastases.[52]

Spitzoid Melanoma

Spitz nevus and melanoma histologically simulate one another and are sometimes impossible to differentiate. Features that favor the diagnosis of melanoma over Spitz nevus include asymmetry, prominent confluence, high cellular density of melanoctyes, failure of maturation, deep invasion, increased mitotic rate, deep mitoses, lack of Kamino (dull-pink) bodies, and necrosis en masse.[45] In adults, a low threshold should exist to diagnose melanoma if any of these features are present. The reverse is true of similar lesions in children (especially prepubertal children).

Sarcomatoid Melanoma

Sarcomatoid melanomas are rare melanomas with features that simulate a spindle cell or epithelioid cell sarcoma.[56] Sarcomatoid melanoma lesions are extremely poorly differentiated and exhibit diffuse sheets of anaplastic cells with ulceration and necrosis en masse. Because these lesions are poorly differentiated, immunoperoxidase stains are necessary to render an accurate diagnosis.

Spindle Cell Melanoma

Spindle cell melanomas are characterized by a proliferation of spindle-shaped melanocytes arranged in fascicles and sheets. Unlike sarcomatoid and DM variants, these lesions do not demonstrate diffuse and deep involvement. Features that suggest melanoma include involvement of the epidermis, pagetoid spread of melanocytes, nesting, and the presence of melanin pigment. Because these lesions are poorly differentiated, they must be distinguished from other malignant neoplasms of the skin that may demonstrate a spindle cell morphology, including spindle cell squamous carcinoma and atypical fibroxanthoma. As with sarcomatoid melanoma and other poorly differentiated variants of melanoma, immunoperoxidase stains are required to render a precise diagnosis.

Follicular Melanoma

Follicular melanoma, a rare and newly reported variant, involves hair follicles. Atypical melanocytes, arranged in nests or singly, may involve the entire length of the hair follicle, including the sebaceous duct, with extension into the adjacent papillary dermis.[14]

Melanoma in Children

Cutaneous melanoma is rare in childhood, particularly before puberty. Clinically, as with adults, melanoma in children mainly affects the white population. There likely exists a minor female predominance with slightly worse males prognoses[57]; however, some studies report equal gender distributions and prognoses.[58] Similar to adults, clinical characteristics concerning for melanoma in children include rapid size increase, bleeding, color change, itch, lymph node enlargement, subcutaneous mass, pain, and distant metastases.[59,60] The most common primary tumor sites are the extremities, followed by the trunk.[58] Most melanomas in children arise from large or giant congenital nevi. Histologic features of melanomas in children and adults are identical, including asymmetry, atypical melanocytes, mitoses, pagetoid spread, irregular epidermal nest formation, and failure of maturation with progressive depth.[57] The diagnosis is difficult when the lesions demonstrate spitzoid morphology because most such lesions represent Spitz nevi. When spitzoid lesions in children exhibit poor maturation and contain deep mitoses near their bases, the diagnosis of melanoma should be strongly considered. In questionable cases, err on the cautious side by performing excision with appropriate margins, and if necessary, also perform SLN excision. The 10-year cause-specific survival rate in children with melanoma is 89.4%.[61]

SPECIAL PROBLEMS IN THE HISTOLOGIC DIAGNOSIS OF CUTANEOUS MELANOMA

There are several problems clinicians and pathologists must be aware of that can create difficulty in the diagnosis of melanoma other than those described previously. Some of these represent mimics of melanoma whereas others involve certain settings in which melanoma may develop or be altered by other factors.

Dyplastic Nevi

DN are associated with an increased risk of melanoma (up to a 10-fold increased risk) when present in an individual with a personal or family history of melanoma.[62] Melanoma risk increases as the number of DN increases. DN have been reported in up to 34% to 56% of melanoma cases although these findings are somewhat controversial because the criteria used to distinguish between DN and malignant melanoma (MM) as well as DN and other forms of nevi are somewhat subjective.[63] Several studies have investigated the ability of pathologists to distinguish melanoma from DN. Concordance rates in these studies have ranged from 49% to 76%,[64–67] which illustrates the diagnostic challenge melanocytic lesions present to pathologists.

Criteria for the histologic diagnosis of DN include both architectural and cytologic features. Architectural features include poor circumscription, lentiginous melanocytic hyperplasia, subepidermal fibroplasia, and variable degrees of associated dermal lymphohistiocytic infiltrate. Cytologic features include the presence of random cytologic atypia and small dermal melanocytes with at least some maturation with dermal descent. In the past, some investigators have proposed classifying the cytology of DN as mild, moderate, or severe.[68] Due to difficulty in distinguishing between mild and moderate dysplasia, however, a simplified classification scheme using low-grade and high-grade dysplasia was proposed.[69] Nevertheless, none of the proposed classification schemes have proved to provide guidelines for the consistent diagnosis or classification of DN.

Nevi on Special Sites

Certain body sites show a tendency to express melanocytic nevi in a way that may closely simulate melanoma. These sites include the breast, scalp, ear, umbilicus, perineal area, genital area, and flexural sites, such as the axilla, neck, popliteal, and antecubital fossa (**Fig. 7**). Clinicians and pathologists must recognize the potential for mimicry at these sites to avoid overdiagnosing melanoma. Histologic features that may cause benign nevi to simulate melanoma include large size of individual melanocytes, large nests of melanocytes, and slight pagetoid spread of melanocytes in the epidermis. An especially confusing situation arises in nevi that develop on genital areas affected by lichen sclerosus et atrophicus. These nevi, like melanoma, may demonstrate prominent pagetoid spread and atypia but in actuality are benign.

Congenital Nevi Biopsied in Neonates

Congenital nevi biopsied shortly after birth and rarely up to 2 to 3 years may simulate melanoma by exhibiting pagetoid spread of large melanocytes with abundant cytoplasm throughout the epidermis. This is believed to result from migration of evolving nevus cells (melanoblasts) through the epidermis. As congenital nevi mature, the single melanocytes in the epidermis congregate in nests that then become positioned at the DE junction and in the dermis. In addition to prominent intraepidermal melanoctyic proliferation, there exists concurrent expression of nests of typical-appearing melanocytes in the dermis situated between and among collagen bundles and around adnexal structures. The presence of these benign nests is characteristic of a congenital nevus. Clinical correlation, including the location of the lesion, size of the lesion (large congenital melanoctyic nevi carry a 2.5%–5% risk of developing into melanoma),[70] and presence of evolution in the lesion, remains valuable in making an accurate diagnosis.

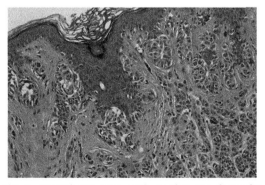

Fig. 7. Special site nevi, such as this one from the pubic area, can closely simulate melanoma with large nests of melanocytes and slight pagetoid spread.

Congenital Melanoblastic Proliferation

Occasionally seen in congenital nevi are large nodular aggregates of small hyperchromatic melanocytes. Pleomorphism and mitoses may occur in these lesions simulating melanoma. Distinguishing histologic features indicating a benign nature include symmetry, good circumscription, and evidence of maturation. Furthermore, this lesion is almost always present at birth, matures with age, and may undergo complete regression.

Persistent (Recurrent) Nevi

Nevi that have been previously biopsied or damaged by trauma, such as shaving, may develop histologic features that simulate melanoma. In these situations, melanocytes in the epidermis may be large and can coalesce with involvement at all levels of the epidermis, including the granular and cornified layers. In addition, scattered mitotic figures may be present. Characteristic of these lesions is confinement of atypical changes in the area of epidermis directly above the scar tissue in the dermis (**Fig. 8**). If the melanocytic proliferation extends beyond the margin of the scar, diagnosis of melanoma should be considered. Clinical correlation, as well as review of any available histologic sections from prior biopsies at that site, may be helpful. If doubt exists, conservative re-excision would be a reasonable action.

Single Cell Melanocytic Proliferations

In some instances, a benign proliferation of single melanocytes in the epidermis may occur and simulate melanoma in situ, which begins in a similar fashion. This may occur in many different settings, including in the presence of an underlying congenital nevus on sun-damaged skin, on the eyelid, in the epidermis overlying fibrous papules, within solar lentigines, and on mucocutaneous sites, such as the nail unit. Benign features include a lower density of melanocytes compared with melanoma in situ as well as a lack of nests. The presence of an obvious underlying congenital nevus in the dermis beneath the epidermal proliferation allows the diagnosis to be made with certainty. Clinical correlation may be valuable because most of these lesions do not demonstrate visible pigment. This is particularly important when dealing with excision margins of melanoma.

Regressed Melanoma

After regression, melanomas exhibit a characteristic pattern of dermal fibrosis in the upper dermis along with telangiectasias, lymphocytes, and abundant melanophages. The fibromucinous stroma differs from fibroplasias seen in scars. In regression, fibrosis occurs broadly and mirrors the position of the original melanoma that was present previously. Residual scattered single melanocytes may remain in the epidermis along with a few nests of atypical melanocytes in the fibrotic dermis.

Metastatic Melanoma

Cutaneous metastases of melanoma are typically characterized by atypical melanocytes in the deep dermis or subcutis arranged in either nodules or diffusely in cords and strands. Occasionally, involvement of the superficial dermis and epidermis occurs. Generally, these lesions are as deep as they are broad and contain atypical melanocytes with mitoses throughout. These lesions can be small, however, which further complicates diagnosis.

A distinct form of metastatic melanoma expresses atypical but delicate pigmented spindle or dendritic melanocytes in the dermis. These lesions may simulate blue nevi; however, this variant of metastatic melanoma usually develops rapidly and demonstrates at least some atypia with occasional mitoses, allowing the diagnosis to be made.

Artifact from Monsel Solution

Dermatologists commonly use Monsel solution (ferrous subsulfate) to control bleeding after a biopsy. This solution contains iron that, when applied to the skin, is engulfed by histiocytes. The iron-containing histiocytes appear brown and may simulate atypical melanocytes or melanoma.[71] Careful inspection reveals a refractile quality of the pigment similar to the appearance of hemosiderin. In addition, the cells themselves in this instance are not significantly pleomorphic or atypical.

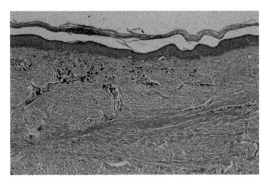

Fig. 8. Atypical-appearing melanocytes and melanophages in an area directly above scar tissue.

TECHNIQUES TO IMPROVE ACCURACY OF HISTOPATHOLOGIC DIAGNOSIS OF MELANOMA

Special Stains and Immunohistochemical Stains

As discussed previously, melanoma may present with a wide spectrum of histologic features that mimic epithelial, hematologic, mesenchymal, and neural tumors.[72] For poorly differentiated tumors or amelanotic melanomas, chemical and immunohistochemical stains are often necessary for correct diagnosis. A commonly used silver stain, which stains melanin, is the Fontana-Masson stain. Immunohistochemical stains directed against S-100 protein remain the most sensitive marker for melanocytic lesions (sensitivity for melanoma is 97%–100%).[72] The name S-100 is derived from the observation that this 21-kDa calcium-binding protein is soluble in 100% saturated ammonium sulfate solution.[73] Unfortunately, S-100 stain lacks specificity, because the protein is also expressed in nerve sheath cells, myoepithelial cells, adiopocytes, chondrocytes, Langerhans cells, and all tumors derived from these cells.[72]

Most spindle or desmoplastic lesions only express S-100 positivity, which gives the other available stains little value in these cases. Particularly challenging is differentiating DM, which can appear scar-like, from actual scar tissue, because both lesions stain positive for S-100. Chorny and Barr[74] found the spindle cell component from previously biopsied nonmelanocytic neoplasms showed S-100 positivity in 90% of cases. In addition, they found 100% S-100 positivity in re-excision scars from previously biopsied nevomelanocytic lesions. They concluded the presence of S-100 positive spindle cells in scars may create a diagnostic pitfall, particularly in the evaluation of re-excision specimens of DM.[74] To further exacerbate this potential pitfall, the vast majority of desmoplastic lesions only express S-100, rendering the remaining arsenal of melanoma stains useless.

A more specific, albeit less sensitive, marker for melanoma, is HMB-45. This marker stains the cytoplasmic premelanosomal glycoprotein, gp100. Reported sensitivities for melanoma range from 69% to 93%; sensitivity for primary melanomas is greater than metastatic melanoma.[72] HMB-45 is specific for melanocytic differentiation and was reported to be absent 100% of the time in nonmelanocytic tumors in several studies.[75–78] HMB-45 is also expressed, however, in tumors other than melanoma, including PEComas, sweat gland tumors, meningeal melanocytomas, CCS of the tendons, and aponeuroses as well as certain ovarian steroid cell, breast, and renal cell carcinoma tumors.[72] Fortunately, most of these tumors are histologically distinct from melanomas.

A cocktail that stains for HMB45, Mart-1, and tyrosinase exhibits a high sensitivity for all forms of melanoma and is a complementary marker to polyclonal S-100 protein.[79] Additional stains that are available clinically include MITF, NKI/C3, CD10 antigen, and vimentin. MITF has good sensitivity (81%–100%) and specificity (88%–100%) for melanoma but is less specific for spindle cell lesions and stains tumors of many other lineages.[72] NKI/C3 is not widely used due to poor specificity and high cost. CD10 antigen, a neutral endopeptidase expressed by a variety of mesenchymal tumors, is significantly up-regulated during the process of metastasis in melanoma and may help distinguish between primary versus metastatic melanoma.[80] Vimentin exhibits good sensitivity (96%) and if negative can be used to rule out melanoma.[72] Newer markers for melanoctyic differentiation that are being investigated but are not yet widely used clinically, include MUM-1, melanocortin 1, SM5-1, PNL2, and TRP-1/TRP-2.[72]

Cytogenetics

Understanding of the genetics of melanoma has greatly improved in recent years. Melanoma is recognized as a heterogenous tumor characterized, in part, by DNA mutations that lead to either a loss of function of tumor suppressor genes or activation of oncogenes.[79] Different subtypes of melanoma express characteristic mutational and karyotypic profiles.[81–83] Two important and well studied pathways are implicated in the pathogenesis of melanoma: the mitogen-activated protein kinase (MAPK) (or RAS-[B]RAF-MEK-ERK) pathway, which contributes to the regulation of cell growth, and the phosphatidylinositol-3-kinase-PTEN (PI3K/AKT/PTEN/mTOR) pathway, which is involved in the regulation of cell death.[79] In melanoma, the MAPK and PTEN/AKT pathways may become activated aberrantly by one of several activating oncogenic mutations. Known mutations involve BRAF, NRAS, and HRAS.[79]

The activating BRAF V600E mutation was found in 60% of melanomas in one study.[84] These melanomas, however, are the type that arises in association with intense intermittent sun exposure.[79] Some melanoctyic nevi, however, contain activating BRAF mutations that play a role in melanocytic growth arrest: stimulating oncogene-induced senescence. In these lesions, the progression to melanoma might occur after the loss of cell cycle regulators, such as p16.

Many studies have looked at genetic mutations in specific variants of melanoma, particularly those variants where distinction between benign and malignant is challenging. A few studies looking at BRAF and NRAS have shown these mutations are common in spitzoid melanomas but absent in Spitz nevi.[85–87] Other studies, however, have disputed this claim.[88] HRAS mutations seem limited to Spitz nevi, so detection of this mutation favors the diagnosis of Spitz nevus over spitzoid melanoma.[89] Congenital nevi tend to have NRAS mutations, not BRAF mutations. Blue nevi are characterized by GNAQ mutations. In the hereditary melanoma syndrome, germline mutations in the cyclin-dependent kinase inhibitor 2A (CDKN2A) encoding p16 tumor suppressor proteins is frequently mutated.[90] Further studies are needed to assess the potential diagnostic value of these mutations.

Array Comparative Genomic Hybridization

Array comparative genomic hybridization (CGH) is a powerful technique that can assess the entire genome for genetic aberrations. A landmark study by Bastian and colleagues[91] in 2003 used CGH to evaluate genetic aberrations in melanocytic lesions. They found multiple genetic aberrations in 96% of melanomas whereas nevi only rarely exhibited mutations. The only nevi to express mutations were Spitz nevi, where a specific single gain on the short arm of chromosome 11 was found. This mutation seen in Spitz nevi was not appreciated in any of the melanomas studied. Subsequent studies evaluating array CGH in congenital nevi showed no aberrations whereas melanomas arising in congenital nevi showed aberrations typical of de novo cutaneous melanoma.[79] Additionally, proliferative nodules seen in congenital pattern nevi have genetic aberrations but these differ from those seen in melanoma.[92] Ultimately, the use of array CGH will likely be limited to research because of its high cost, time-consuming nature, need for special equipment/expertise, and the requirement of a significant amount of relatively pure (primarily tumor) tissue.

Fluorsescence in Situ Hybridation

Fluorescence in situ hybridization (FISH) technique has emerged as the preferred molecular technique to interrogate chromosomal abnormalities because of its low cost compared with CGH, efficacy with use of archival tissue, and increasing availability in pathology laboratories.[93] This technique is limited in the sense it can only investigate a maximum of 4 genetic aberrations per experiment.

Currently, a 4-probe melanoma FISH test targeting chromosomes 6 (6p25, 6q23, and centromere) and 11 (11q13) is commercially available. A validation study of this test revealed a sensitivity of 87% and specificity of 95%.[94] Subsequent studies have found similar results. The majority of these investigations, however, have only studied the performance of the 4-probe melanoma FISH test in unequivocal cases. This test would not be ordered in cases where the diagnosis of a melanocytic lesion is certain. Thus, if FISH proves to have diagnostic value, it will be in ambiguous cases. Gerami and colleagues[94] evaluated the performance of the 4-probe FISH test in 27 cases of ambiguous melanocytic lesions. After 5+ years of follow-up, 6 cases developed macroscopic metastatic disease whereas 21 cases remained disease-free. Of the 6 patients who went on to develop metastatic disease, all 6 of them had a positive FISH test. Six of the 21 disease-free patients, however, were FISH positive as well. A limitation of this investigation is that follow-up can only prove malignancy of the lesion. Follow-up cannot differentiate benign lesions from malignant lesions that were cured with removal.[89] Nevertheless, mounting numbers of cases with long-term event-free follow-up and negative FISH tests increases confidence in the ability of this test to identify benign lesions.

The efficacy of FISH has been explored in several other settings. One study found FISH can be used to help distinguish benign intranodal nevi from metastatic melanoma.[95] In a study of lentiginous junctional melanomas of the elderly, 84% of cases tested positive using FISH.[96] FISH might also be helpful in distinguishing between epithelioid blue nevi and blue nevus-like metastatic melanomas based on a small study that showed excellent sensitivity (90%) and specificity (100%).[97] Similarly, another small study used FISH to distinguish nevoid melanomas from mitotically active nevi. They found the 4-probe melanoma FISH test performed perfectly in this setting (100% sensitive and specific).[98]

Several problems with FISH exist in addition to a paucity of data evaluating FISH in equivocal cases. For one, the currently widely available 4-probe test is not sufficiently sensitive or specific to accurately diagnose melanoma by itself. The results of this test must be interpreted in conjunction with histologic and clinical information. Also, FISH requires 20 to 30 well-visualized cells to get an accurate count of fluorescent signals, so small melanoctyic lesions may not have sufficient cells for FISH analysis.[89] Additionally, FISH relies on mathematic algorithms to define positive and negative results. If rigid standards of technique and assessment are not followed, diagnostic discrepancy and uncertainty increase and limit the diagnostic value of FISH.[89] One study investigated intraobserver variation in FISH and found that 3 pathologists, evaluating the same data, failed to reach agreement in 32% of cases.[99] This study calls into question the reproducibility of FISH tests. For FISH tests to be of any diagnostic use, it is important that pathologists adhere to stringent standards at every step of the testing process.

Pathologists face a difficult situation when deciding when to order a FISH test. Gerami and Zembowicz advocate using this test as an adjunctive test to routine pathologic examination and clinical correlation in borderline cases.[93] Other investigators advocate using FISH in challenging cases where no consensus diagnosis is reached, particularly in those cases where clinical consequences are substantial.[89] Further studies are needed to clarify the diagnostic value of FISH.

Proliferation Markers

Many malignancies exhibit identifiable proliferation markers that can aid in both diagnosis and prognosis. Ki-67, a nuclear antigen present in all active phases of cell cycle proliferation, is the most widely used proliferation marker in pathology. This antigen is not expressed during nonproliferative stages of the cell cycle (G0 and early G1). Antibodies to Ki-67 can be used to label melanocytes in an effort to correlate the rate of melanocyte proliferation with histologic malignancy.

Smolle and colleagues[100] were the first group to investigate the proliferative potential of melanoctyic lesions by staining for Ki-67. They examined 25 melanocytic skin tumors using antibodies to Ki-67 on fresh frozen tissue. Using the parameter of growth fraction (percentage of positively stained nuclei to total nuclei), they found statistically significant differences between nevi, primary melanomas, and MMs. Similarly, Boni and colleagues[101] successfully used MIB1, another antibody to Ki-67, to stain Ki-67 on formalin-fixed, paraffin-embedded specimens. This discovery permitted Ki-67 staining of archival tissues. Since the work of Smolle and colleagues, several studies looking at Ki-67 as a proliferation marker in melanoma have found similar results. Benign nevi typically express Ki-67 positivity in less than 5% of tumor cells, although some reports have shown up to 15% positivity in Spitz nevi and DN.[72] Conversely, melanoma lesions stain positive for Ki-67 in 13% to 30% of cells.[72] Spitz neoplasms also typically demonstrate increased Ki-67 staining. There are conflicting data concerning whether Ki67 is an independent risk factor for adverse outcome in melanoma.[72]

Another marker of cellular proliferation is proliferating cell nuclear antigen (PCNA). There is increased expression of this marker in MM compared with benign nevi; however, Spitz nevi also show increased expression of PNCA.[72,102–104] Like Ki-67, the prognostic implication of PCNA remains subject to debate.

Cyclins (A, B, D1, D3, and E), another class of proliferation marker, bind and activate cyclin-dependent kinases causing the cell to progress through the cell cycle. Cyclin A, rarely expressed in benign nevi, is expressed in 42% to 99% of melanomas.[105] Florenes and colleagues[105] reported an inverse correlation between cyclin A staining and disease-free survival in superficial melanoma but not in nodular melanoma. Similarly, cyclin B is rarely expressed in benign nevi but is expressed in approximately 50% of melanomas.[106,107] The prognostic implication of cyclin B has not been adequately studied. Cyclins D1 and D3 are rarely expressed in benign nevi and commonly expressed in melanoma.[107,108] No prognostic significance was seen in cyclin D1, whereas increased cyclin D3 staining was associated with early relapse and decreased survival in superficial melanomas only.[108]

Other markers of proliferation under investigation include p16, p21, p27, p53, HDM2, and GADD proteins.[72] HDM2 and GADD proteins possess promise as prognostic markers in melanoma; however to this point, none of the proliferation markers has been definitely shown to have independent prognostic value.[72]

STAGING AND PROGNOSIS: AMERICAN JOINT COMMITTEE ON CANCER MELANOMA STAGING GUIDELINES

In 2009, the American Joint Committee on Cancer (AJCC) revised the staging system for cutaneous melanoma for the 2010 edition of AJCC melanoma guidelines on the basis of data from the AJCC melanoma staging database: 30,946 patients with stage I, II, and III and 7972 patients with stage IV melanoma.[109] Findings and changes in the 2010 AJCC guidelines include the following: (1) in patients with localized melanoma, tumor thickness, mitotic rate and ulceration were the most dominant prognostic factors; (2) mitotic rate replaces level of invasion (Clark level) as a primary criterion from defining T1b melanomas; (3) among the 3307 patients with regional metastases, components that defined the N category were the number of metastatic nodes, tumor burden, and ulceration of the primary melanoma; (4) for staging purposes, all patients with microscopic nodal metastases, regardless of extent or tumor burden, are classified as stage III; micrometastases detected by immunohistochemistry are specifically included; and (5) on the basis of a multivariate analysis of patients with distant metastases, the 2 dominant components in defining the M category continue to be the site of distant metastases (nonvisceral vs lung vs all other visceral metastatic sites) and an elevated serum lactate dehydrogenase.[109]

HISTOLOGIC FEATURES RELATED TO PROGNOSIS
Breslow Depth

In 1970, Alexander Breslow evaluated the relationship between histologic depth and prognosis. He looked at melanoma excision specimens from 98 patients and followed them over a 5-year period. After 5 years, 71 of the patients remained disease-free whereas 27 patients developed either recurrent or metastatic disease. Using an ocular micrometer, Breslow measured the distance from the skin surface to the deepest level of extension of the tumor. In patients whose lesions measured less than 0.76 mm in depth (n = 38), there were no reports of metastasis or recurrence.[110] Breslow thickness, defined as the distance from the granular layer to the deepest level of neoplasm, remains the most important prognostic indicator of survival in primary cutaneous melanomas.[19,111]

There exist special situations where the Breslow depth is measured slightly differently. For example, if ulceration exists within the lesion, measurement should be from the top-most viable melanoma cell to the deepest dermal tumor. In the case of a polypoid primary melanoma, report the largest measurement perpendicular to the surface epidermis. In all primary melanomas, avoid including the measurement tumor cells within the adventitial dermis, perineural space, or blood vessels.[112]

There are, however, several limitations when relying on Breslow depth to determine prognosis. Certain areas of the body contain either very thick or very thin skin. The volar areas (palms and soles) contain a very thick epidermis, which contributes significantly to the Breslow depth and may artificially inflate this number. Conversely, the skin covering the eyelid is very thin, and lesions extending into the deep dermis or subcutis may exhibit smaller Breslow depths that underestimate the severity of the lesion. Additionally, thickness measurements may vary depending on the histopathologist, microscope, biopsy technique, and cuts chosen. Remember that re-excision specimens may reveal areas that are deeper than the original biopsy specimen. Thus, whereas thickness measurements no doubt provide valuable prognostic information, their absolute value should not be overemphasized.

Mitotic Rate

The mitotic rate, reported as the mitotic index, is the number of mitoses per square millimeter. The maximum number found in the tumor is reported as the mitotic index. The AJCC melanoma staging committee recommends using the hot spot approach to determine the mitotic index.[112] In this method, the hematoxylin-eosin–stained tissue sections of the primary melanoma are reviewed for the region with the greatest number of mitotic figures—the hot spot. From this region, the mitotic index is determined. If only a single mitosis is found after examining all tissue sections, the mitotic index should be reported as $1/mm^2$ (rather than reporting this as $<1\ mm^2$).[112]

A seminal study assessing the prognostic value of mitotic rate was conducted by Azzola and colleagues[113] using the Sydney Melanoma Unit database. This study, which examined 3661 patients with melanoma, showed patients with a mitotic index of 0 mitoses/mm^2 had a significantly improved survival compared with those with 1 or more mitoses. A similar study showed mitotic rate is a predictor of SLN positivity in patients with thin melanomas.[114] Data from the AJCC melanoma staging database showed the most significant correlation between mitotic rate and survival exists at threshold of at least $1/mm^2$. In a multifactorial analysis of 10,233 patients with clinically localized melanoma, mitotic rate was the second most powerful predictor of survival, after tumor thickness.[109]

Unfortunately, there remain several important unanswered questions regarding the utility of counting mitoses in melanomas not addressed before the new AJCC recommendations were issued. First, the studies performed were all retrospective in nature and there was minimal to no interobserver evaluation of histology because all cases were reviewed by pathologists from the same groups. Determination of whether a cell is in mitosis may be difficult and subjective and also would skew data and determination between 0 and 1 and 1 and 2 mitoses per 5 fields may be difficult to assess.

Many biopsies had been performed on lesions not thought to be melanoma clinically and may be superficial and not representative of the entire lesion, which could easily compromise evaluation. Furthermore, some lesions with no mitoses could have been nevi and not melanoma, which would have skewed the data. In contrast, occasionally very thick melanomas present with no or few mitoses, the significance of which was not evaluated. No comment was made about traumatized lesions, which may lead to mitoses not only in melanocytes but also in keratinocytes and fibroblasts, all of which would lead to erroneous interpretation.

No consideration as to the type of melanoma was noted, which is even more important now that MM has been shown to differ genetically, such as in BRAF+ and BRAF− lesions. DM is also known to represent a different subset of MM, one in which sentinel LN biopsy is not recommended, yet this was not accounted for. Furthermore, no description of the morphology of mitoses was evaluated (ie, whether a mitosis was bipolar or multipolar), no assessment of the location of the mitoses was made (ie, whether near the surface as opposed to the deep part of lesion), and no segregation was made between lesions that were very thin, Clark level 2 versus thin but Clark level 3 lesions, which contain a greater number of neoplastic cells per unit area. In addition, some melanomas have a significant number of intraepidermal mitoses, another important variable that was not evaluated.

To address some of these questions, especially the utility of counting mitoses in thin MM less than or equal to 1 mm in thickness, the authors evaluated 100 melanomas sequentially in prospective fashion to determine the number of mitoses in these lesions.[115] Of these, 9 melanomas were found to have epidermal mitoses only (9%), 14 had dermal mitoses (1 in 12; 2 in 2), and 77 had no mitoses (77%). Four MMs of 100 MMs demonstrated multiple mitoses: 2 with 2 dermal mitoses/mm^2 and 2 with multiple epidermal mitoses—1 with 3 and the other with 15, without dermal mitoses. The authors also demonstrated a significant difference between the number of mitoses in very thin, Clark level 2 lesions versus Clark level 3 lesions. Thus, the authors concluded that the number of thin melanomas with greater than 1 mitosis/mm^2 is low and even lower in exceedingly thin Clark level 2 lesions. The importance of reporting mitoses in thin melanomas is likely overemphasized and probably of limited significance and calls into question whether it is truly worth the time or the unnecessary anxiety conveyed to patients and families and the utility of performing sentinel lymphadenectomy in all melanoma patients with even 1 dermal mitosis.

Because melanoma grows by hyperplasia and not hypertrophy, theoretically there should be mitoses in every melanoma. The number of mitoses is probably most important when they are multiple and easily identifiable, which is usually seen in thick lesions with other poor prognostic features.

Ulceration

Ulceration is defined histologically as total loss of the epidermis and some of the dermis. In 1980, Balch and colleagues[116] evaluated the prognostic significance of melanoma ulceration on 5-year survival. Stage I melanoma with ulceration had a decreased survival compared with those without ulceration (55% vs 80%).[116] Stage II melanomas exhibited a similar trend (12%–53%). These trends remained even when corrected for thickness. The width but not the depth of ulceration significantly correlated with survival.[116] Balch later evaluated 5-year survival in 17,600 melanoma patients.[19] Using Cox regression analysis, he showed ulceration and thickness the most powerful predictors of survival. Because of these findings, ulceration was added to the revised 2002 AJCC melanoma staging system. In this system, the presence of ulceration upstages the melanoma to the next worst prognostic level.[117] The 2010 AJCC guidelines for ulceration are unchanged from 2002 because ulceration remains a major predictor of survival in patients with melanoma.[112]

Although ulceration is a valuable prognostic indicator, it is not without problems. The definition of ulceration as applied to melanoma is highly subjective. In addition, it did not define the extent of ulceration or differentiate between lesions that may have been previously traumatized or biopsied. Recently, the definition was expanded to include the presence of reactive changes, such as nuclear debris, inflammatory infiltrate, and fibrin deposition, as well as the absence of history of trauma or prior surgery at the site.[118] Application of these additional criteria will hopefully reduce overcalling ulceration that occurs due to prior biopsy and in cases where epithelium is lost due to processing artifact.[112]

As with mitoses, the significance of ulceration in thin lesions is likely overemphasized. In a study by Googe and colleagues,[119] which was a retrospective review of invasive melanomas with ulceration between 1998 and 2007, 156 of 2752 (5.7%) melanomas were found to have ulceration. Virtually all of these were in the "vertical growth phase." Only 16 were less than or equal to 1 mm in thickness and only 2 had ulceration greater 3 mm across the lesion. Three of 1493 (0.2%) Clark level II melanomas had ulceration. Furthermore, there was no discussion about whether or not the ulceration could have been traumatic. Thus, thin melanomas rarely ulcerate and, as with mitoses, ulcerated melanomas are almost always thick and associated with other poor prognostic variables.

Clark Levels

In 1969, Clark and colleagues[120] proposed a schema to describe melanomas by their anatomic depth of involvement. Clark levels are as follows:

I—Confined to the epidermis (in situ)
II—Neoplasm to the papillary dermis but not filling the papillary dermis
III—Neoplasm present to level of the junction between the papillary and reticular dermis (filling the papillary dermis)
IV—Neoplasm extending into the reticular dermis
V—Neoplasm extending into the subcutaneous fat.

In relation to prognosis, Clark level derives most of its prognostic value from a secondary correlation with tumor thickness.[121] In a large study of 17,600 primary melanomas,[19] Clark level was found to hold prognostic significance within the subgroup of patients with melanomas less than 1 mm. In these thin tumors, Clark level IV or V invasion significantly predicted survival.[19,122] The 2002 AJCC staging system included Clark level for thin melanomas only.[19] In 2010, however, the AJCC replaced Clark level in favor of mitotic index for thin melanomas. Mitotic index, although still codependent on tumor thickness, was shown to have more independent prognostic significance than Clark level.[112] In spite of the AJCC recommendations, many dermatopathologists continue to report Clark levels because they can be an important check to ensure that the report is accurate. A lesion reported as Clark level 2 but 1.75 mm in thickness is likely erroneous.

Tumor-Infiltrating Lymphocytes

In 1989, Clark and coworkers[123] demonstrated tumor-infiltrating lymphocytes were independent predictors of 8-year survival. The patterns for infiltrating lymphoctyes are described as "brisk, nonbrisk or absent." A brisk pattern, defined as a dense infiltrate of lymphocytes present in both the substance of neoplasm as well as its periphery, was associated with improved prognosis.[123] A total of 9 studies have looked into tumor-infiltrating lymphocytes as a prognostic indicator in primary melanoma. Five of the 9 studies support the prognostic significance of a brisk response, whereas 4 of the 9 did not.[124] In 3 of the 4 studies that found no prognostic significance of a brisk response, they did show that the absence of tumor-infiltrating lymphocytes predicted the presence of nodal metastasis, which is itself an important predictor of decreased survival.[124]

Burton and colleagues[125] conducted a large randomized controlled trial of 515 cutaneous melanomas with Breslow depth greater than or equal to 1 mm. They demonstrated that nonbrisk response is a significant predictor of SLN positivity. Using multivariate analysis, however, they concluded tumor-infiltrating lymphocyte response is not a significant independent factor predicting disease-free survival or overall survival.

Regression

Regression is defined histologically as destruction of melanoma cells with replacement by fibrous tissue. Also seen are melanophages, varying degrees of inflammation, and increased vascularity. Between 10% and 35% of melanomas show histologic regression.[126] Clinically, this may appear as depigmented areas within or around the melanoma; white, red, blue, or gray colors may be present.[127] Regression almost exclusively accompanies thin melanomas and is rare in nodular melanomas. Some speculate regression may cause thinning of tumors, which were previously deeper, hence creating a misleading association between regression and thin melanomas.[128]

Conflicting reports exist surrounding the prognostic implications of regression. Traditionally, the presence of regression portended a poor prognosis. Many hospitals carry out sentinel node biopsy if regression is found, regardless of Breslow depth.[127] A recent article by Requena and colleagues[127] in 2009 reviewed the medical literature to assess the prognostic significance of regression. They found numerous contradictory studies; some studies show regression portended poorer prognoses whereas others show no association or oven improved prognoses in patients with regression. They concluded that the prognostic significance of regression remains unclear. Further studies are needed to address the creation of accurate and consistent criteria for regression as well as studies that separate the early (inflammatory) and late (fibrotic) phases of regression when assessing prognosis.

Histologic Satellite Metastases

Day and coworkers[129] defined microscopic satellites as discrete tumor nests greater than 0.05 mm in diameter that are separated from the main body of the melanoma by normal reticular dermal collagen or subcutaneous fat. In 1981 they published a seminal study that looked at histologic sections of 596 patients with stage 1 melanoma.[129] There found a dramatic difference in the 5-year disease-free survival for patients with microscopic satellites compared with those without: 36% versus 89%. Supporting these data, several subsequent studies found an association between microsatellites and increased regional recurrences as well as decreased disease-free survival.[130–134] Based on these studies, the 2002 AJCC melanoma staging guidelines included microscopic satellites under the N2 category, indicating stage IIIB disease.[109]

Sentinel Node Biopsy

In the 1970s, many investigators favored elective lymph node dissection at the time of wide resection in cutaneous melanoma because consensus held that this led to improved outcomes. This belief was based on the clinical observation that lymph node metastasis usually precedes more widespread metastatic disease; thus, if caught early enough, systemic metastases may be prevented by removing metastatic lymph nodes. When Cascinelli and colleagues[135] reviewed long-term results from several World Health Organization studies (conducted between 1967 and 1989) investigating this practice, no survival benefit was found in the groups of patients who underwent elective lymphadenectomy.

Another investigation performed by Cascinelli and colleagues[136] did reveal that immediate regional lymph node dissection provides valuable prognostic information. In this study, 240 melanoma patients with lesions on the trunk deeper than 1.5 mm were followed after receiving either immediate or delayed regional lymphadenectomy. Again, no overall survival benefit was shown in the group that received immediate elective regional lymphadenectomy. It did show, however, regional lymph node positivity is a strong indicator of worsened prognosis. Moreover, in patients with occult metastasis limited to lymph nodes, prognosis improved with immediate regional lymphadenectomy.

The idea of SLN biopsy was first advocated by Cochran and colleagues[137] in 1992. This technique offers a less-invasive method to detect occult lymph node metastasis in clinical stage I and II melanoma by excising only the primary draining lymph nodes of that region of skin—the SLNs.[137] Numerous data show the sentinel node is the most likely site of initial metastasis, and if the sentinel node is histologically negative, the remaining nodes are unlikely to contain disease.[138–140] The goals of SLN biopsy include accurate nodal staging, enhanced regional disease control, and improved survival.[141] In short, the test is designed to detect occult nodal disease in patients with nonpalpable lymph nodes and improve outcomes in those patients by preventing the development of

clinically detectable regional lymph node metastasis. Additionally, it identifies patients without nodal metastasis for whom additional treatment may not be indicated.[141]

The current technique of SLN biopsy relies on a dual modality approach, owing to the use of both a radionuclide tracer and dye, to localize SLNs. The radionuclide tracer used in the United States is a technetium 99m–labeled sulfur colloid. This tracer serves two purposes. First, either the day before surgery, or just before surgery, the radionuclide is injected at the site of the primary melanoma for lymphoscintigraphy. Lymphoscintigraphy establishes a preoperative road map of nodal basins that are at risk for metastasis. If lymphoscintigraphy is performed the day before surgery as opposed to just before surgery, the radionuclide must be reinjected 1 to 2 hours before surgery. The second role of the technetium 99m is to allow intraoperative localization of sentinel nodes through the use of a handheld scanner with a gamma sensor probe. Using the lymphoscintogram as a guide to initially direct the scanner, an incision is made around the region of skin with the highest gamma emission and thus the highest localization of technetium 99m.

The second lymph node tag used in the dual modality approach is isosulfan blue dye. Injected just before surgery, it stains any draining nodes blue and allows the surgeon to locate them for excision amidst surrounding nonlymphatic tissue.[141]

After excision, detailed examination of the sentinel nodes is performed by histopathologists using both hematoxylin-eosin and immunohistochemical stains. The sensitivity of melanoma detection in formalin-fixed tissue (postoperative) was found superior to frozen tissue (intraoperative); thus, intraoperative evaluation of SLNs is not recommended.[142]

The first study to look at the prognostic significance of SLN status was published by Gershenwald and colleagues in 1999.[143] They looked at 612 stage I or II melanoma patients who underwent lymphatic mapping and SLN biopsy. In the 580 patients who experienced successful lymphatic mapping and SLN biopsy, SLN was positive by conventional histology in 85 patients (15%) and negative in 495 patients (85%). The 3-year disease-specific survival for negative SLN was 96.8% compared with only 69.9% for those patients with a positive SLN. Analysis of 3-year disease-free survival showed a similar trend (88.5% for negative SLN vs 55.8% for positive SLN). Using univariate and multiple covariate analyses, they determined SLN status was the most significant prognostic factor with respect to disease-free and disease-specific survival. Additionally, they found tumor thickness and ulceration provided important prognostic implications in SLN-negative patients but provided no additional prognostic information in SLN-positive patients. Subsequent studies corroborated the prognostic significance of the sentinel node biopsy.[144,145]

One small study (n = 46) evaluated SLN biopsy in patients with thin melanomas (≤1 mm).[146] Three patients (7%) had a positive SLN or micrometastatic disease. Clark level in these 3 patients was III or higher; therefore, these investigators recommend SLN biopsy for melanomas less than 1 mm if Clark level is III or higher. Other investigators have advocated pursuing sentinel node biopsy in thin melanomas if Clark level is IV or greater.[141] The latest AJCC analysis, however, failed to confirm the usefulness of Clark level as an independent predictor of prognosis.[109] Due to conflicting data on this matter, the debate continues surrounding whether SLN biopsy should be performed based on Clark level in thin melanomas.

The AJCC included the powerful prognostic significance of the sentinel node in their revised 2002 staging guidelines. The 2010 AJCC staging guidelines support the use of sentinel node biopsy for patients who have T2, T3, and T4 melanomas and clinically uninvolved regional lymph nodes.[109] SLN biopsy should be used selectively in patients with T1B melanomas (depth <1 mm with either ulceration or mitosis ≥1/mm^2).

With respect to the histologic evaluation of the sentinel node, the 2010 AJCC staging guidelines require the detection of only a single melanoma cell to confer N+ status and assign that patient to clinical stage III.[112] The immunohistochemical detection of tumor in conjunction with cytologically malignant features is considered sufficient for the identification of nodal metastasis, even if hematoxylin-eosin evaluation is negative.[112]

To date, the only randomized trial to investigate the potential survival benefit of sentinel-lymph biopsy is the Multicenter Selective Lymphadenectomy Trial I.[147] In this trial, 1269 patients with a primary melanoma greater than or equal to 1 mm in depth were randomly assigned to sentinel node biopsy or nodal observation. In the SLN biopsy group, complete nodal dissection was performed if the SLN was positive. In the nodal observation group, complete nodal dissection was performed if the patient developed clinically detectable (palpable) nodes. At the 5-year point, there was no significant difference in melanoma-specific survival between the two groups.[147] Patients in the observation group, however, who went on to develop clinical nodal involvement

(and who, therefore, underwent delayed lymphadenectomy) had significantly poorer survival at 5 years compared with patients who had positive SLNs and underwent immediate lymphadenectomy (52% vs 72%).[147] The significance of this comparison rests on the assumption that all micrometastases seen on examination of the SNL would have progressed to palpable disease if left untreated, and some evidence exists that suggests this is true.[141,148,149]

Other Prognostic Markers

Other potential markers that have shown prognostic value were compiled in a review article by Tejera-Vaquerizo and colleagues in 2011.[150] These prognostic markers include the presence of tumor lymphangiogenesis,[150,151] paratumoral epidermal hyperplasia,[152] vascular invasion,[153,154] neurotropism,[155,156] cellular atypia,[157,158] and the presence of an associated melanocytic nevus.[159–162] Whether or not any of these markers becomes incorporated into future AJCC staging guidelines or contribute to the management of melanoma remains to be seen.

Future Outlook

Despite tremendous advancement in recent years, the histologic diagnosis of melanoma remains a challenge. In the future, biometric techniques may be available that allow the quick and accurate diagnosis of melanoma. In addition to providing diagnostic certainty, these new techniques might improve estimates of prognosis and metastatic potential. Even more exciting is the prospect that improved melanoma treatments will soon be individualized based on the genetic profile of each melanoma—as is occurring in metastatic melanoma patients with BRAF V600E mutations treated with vemurafenib.

REFERENCES

1. Linos E, Swetter SM, Clarke CA, et al. Increasing burden of melanoma in the United States. J Invest Dermatol 2009;129:1666–74.
2. Jemal A, Tiwari RC, Ward E, et al. Cancer statistics, 2004. CA Cancer J Clin 2004;54:8–29.
3. Jemal A, Siegel R, Xu J, et al. Cancer statistics, 2010. CA Cancer J Clin 2010;60:277–300.
4. Plotnick H, Rachmaninoff N, VandenBerg HJ Jr. Polypoid melanoma: a virulent variant of nodular melanoma. Report of three cases and literature review. J Am Acad Dermatol 1990;23:880–4.
5. Pizzichetta MA, Talamini R, Argenziano G, et al. Amelanotic/hypomelanotic melanoma: clinical and

dermoscopic features. Br J Dermatol 2004;150: 1117–24.

6. Giuliano AE, Cochran AJ, Morton DL. Melanoma from unknown primary site and amelanotic melanoma. Semin Oncol 1982;9:442–7.

7. Bono A, Maurichi A, Lualdi M, et al. Clinical and dermatoscopic diagnosis of early amelanotic melanoma. Melanoma Res 2001;11:491–4.

8. Montgomery RM. Differential diagnosis and treatment of warts. West Med Med J West 1967;1:34–6.

9. Kuehnl-Petzoldt C, Berger H, Wiebelt H. Verrucous-keratotic variations of malignant melanoma: a clinicopathological study. Am J Dermatopathol 1982;4:403–10.

10. Suster S, Ronnen M, Bubis JJ. Verrucous pseudonevoid melanoma. J Surg Oncol 1987;36: 134–7.

11. Steiner A, Konrad K, Wolff K, et al. Verrucous malignant melanoma. Arch Dermatol 1988;124: 1534–7.

12. Blessing K, Evans AT, al-Nafussi A. Verrucous naevoid and keratotic malignant melanoma: a clinicopathological study of 20 cases. Histopathology 1993;23:453–8.

13. Hantschke M, Mentzel T, Kutzner H. Follicular malignant melanoma: a variant of melanoma to be distinguished from lentigo maligna melanoma. Am J Dermatopathol 2004;26:359–63.

14. Hu SW, Tahan SR, Kim CC. Follicular malignant melanoma: a case report of a metastatic variant and review of the literature. J Am Acad Dermatol 2011;64:1007–10.

15. Granter SR, McKee PH, Busam K, et al. Melanoma associated with blue nevus and melanoma mimicking cellular blue nevus: a clinicopathologic study of 10 cases on the spectrum of so-called 'malignant blue nevus'. Am J Surg Pathol 2001; 25:316–23.

16. Ackerman AB. Malignant melanoma: a unifying concept. Hum Pathol 1980;11:591–5.

17. Ackerman AB, David KM. A unifying concept of malignant melanoma: biologic aspects. Hum Pathol 1986;17:438–40.

18. Bono A, Bartoli C, Grassi G, et al. Small melanomas: a clinical study on 270 consecutive cases of cutaneous melanoma. Melanoma Res 1999;9: 583–6.

19. Balch CM, Soong SJ, Cascinelli N, et al. Prognostic factors analysis of 17,600 melanoma patients: validation of the American Joint Committee on Cancer melanoma staging system. J Clin Oncol 2001;19:3622–34.

20. Leiter U, Meier F, Garbe C, et al. The natural course of cutaneous melanoma. J Surg Oncol 2004;86: 172–8.

21. Clark WH Jr, Elder DE, Van Horn M, et al. A study of tumor progression: the precursor lesions of superficial spreading and nodular melanoma. Hum Pathol 1984;15:1147–65.

22. Clark WH Jr, Elder DE, Van Horn M. The biologic forms of malignant melanoma. Hum Pathol 1986; 17:443–50.

23. Elder DE, Guerry DT, Van Horn M, et al. Invasive malignant melanomas lacking competence for metastasis. Am J Dermatopathol 1984;6:55–61.

24. Herlyn M, Clark WH, Koprowski H, et al. Biology of tumor progression in human melanocytes. Lab Invest 1987;56:461–74.

25. Barnhill RL, Mihm MC Jr. The histopathology of cutaneous malignant melanoma. Semin Diagn Pathol 1993;10:47–75.

26. Coit DG, Andtbacka R, Guild V, et al. Melanoma. J Natl Compr Canc Netw 2009;7:250–75.

27. Ng PC, Barzilai DA, Gilliam AC, et al. Evaluating invasive cutaneous melanoma: is the initial biopsy representative of the final depth? J Am Acad Dermatol 2003;48:420–4.

28. Decarlo K, Yang S, Mahalingam M, et al. Oncogenic BRAF-positive dysplastic nevi and the tumor suppressor IGFBP7—challenging the concept of dysplastic nevi as precursor lesions? Hum Pathol 2010;41:886–94.

29. Karimipour DJ, Schwartz JL, King AL, et al. Microstaging accuracy after subtotal incisional biopsy of cutaneous melanoma. J Am Acad Dermatol 2005; 52:798–802.

30. Bichakjian CK, Halpern AC, Swetter SM, et al. Guidelines of care for the management of primary cutaneous melanoma. J Am Acad Dermatol 2011; 65:1032–47.

31. Stell VH, Norton HJ, White RL Jr, et al. Method of biopsy and incidence of positive margins in primary melanoma. Ann Surg Oncol 2007;14: 893–8.

32. Austin JR, Byers RM, Wolf P, et al. Influence of biopsy on the prognosis of cutaneous melanoma of the head and neck. Head Neck 1996;18:107–17.

33. Ng JC, Swain S, Kelly JW, et al. The impact of partial biopsy on histopathologic diagnosis of cutaneous melanoma: experience of an Australian tertiary referral service. Arch Dermatol 2010;146: 234–9.

34. Pariser RJ, Divers A, Nassar A. The relationship between biopsy technique and uncertainty in the histopathologic diagnosis of melanoma. Dermatol Online J 1999;5:4.

35. Armour K, Mann S, Lee S. Dysplastic naevi: to shave, or not to shave? A retrospective study of the use of the shave biopsy technique in the initial management of dysplastic naevi. Australas J Dermatol 2005;46:70–5.

36. Bong JL, Herd RM, Hunter JA. Incisional biopsy and melanoma prognosis. J Am Acad Dermatol 2002;46:690–4.

37. Lederman JS, Sober AJ. Does biopsy type influence survival in clinical stage I cutaneous melanoma? J Am Acad Dermatol 1985;13:983–7.

38. Lees VC, Briggs JC. Effect of initial biopsy procedure on prognosis in Stage 1 invasive cutaneous malignant melanoma: review of 1086 patients. Br J Surg 1991;78:1108–10.

39. Martin RC 2nd, Scoggins CR, Edwards MJ, et al. Is incisional biopsy of melanoma harmful? Am J Surg 2005;190:913–7.

40. Ackerman AB. Malignant melanoma. A unifying concept. Am J Dermatopathol 1980;2:309–13.

41. Florell SR, Boucher KM, Malone JC, et al. Histopathologic recognition of involved margins of lentigo maligna excised by staged excision: an interobserver comparison study. Arch Dermatol 2003;139:595–604.

42. Heenan PJ. Nodular melanoma is not a distinct entity. Arch Dermatol 2003;139:387 [author reply: 388].

43. Chamberlain AJ, Fritschi L, Kelly JW, et al. Nodular type and older age as the most significant associations of thick melanoma in Victoria, Australia. Arch Dermatol 2002;138:609–14.

44. From L, Hanna W, Baumal R, et al. Origin of the desmoplasia in desmoplastic malignant melanoma. Hum Pathol 1983;14:1072–80.

45. Barnhill RL, Gupta K. Unusual variants of malignant melanoma. Clin Dermatol 2009;27:564–87.

46. Antony FC, Sanclemente G, Calonje E, et al. Pigment synthesizing melanoma (so-called animal type melanoma): a clinicopathological study of 14 cases of a poorly known distinctive variant of melanoma. Histopathology 2006;48:754–62.

47. Crowson AN, Magro CM, Mihm MC Jr. Malignant melanoma with prominent pigment synthesis: "animal type" melanoma–a clinical and histological study of six cases with a consideration of other melanocytic neoplasms with prominent pigment synthesis. Hum Pathol 1999;30:543–50.

48. Diwan AH, Lazar AJ. Nevoid melanoma. Clin Lab Med 2011;31:243–53.

49. Zembowicz A, McCusker M, Calonje E, et al. Morphological analysis of nevoid melanoma: a study of 20 cases with a review of the literature. Am J Dermatopathol 2001;23:167–75.

50. Schmoeckel C, Castro CE, Braun-Falco O. Nevoid malignant melanoma. Arch Dermatol Res 1985; 277:362–9.

51. Kao GF, Helwig EB, Graham JH. Balloon cell malignant melanoma of the skin. A clinicopathologic study of 34 cases with histochemical, immunohistochemical, and ultrastructural observations. Cancer 1992;69:2942–52.

52. Kosemehmetoglu K, Folpe AL. Clear cell sarcoma of tendons and aponeuroses, and osteoclast-rich tumour of the gastrointestinal tract with features

resembling clear cell sarcoma of soft parts: a review and update. J Clin Pathol 2010;63:416–23.

53. Langezaal SM, Graadt van Roggen JF, Hogendoorn PC, et al. Malignant melanoma is genetically distinct from clear cell sarcoma of tendons and aponeurosis (malignant melanoma of soft parts). Br J Cancer 2001;84:535–8.

54. Panagopoulos I, Mertens F, Kardas I, et al. Molecular genetic characterization of the EWS/ATF1 fusion gene in clear cell sarcoma of tendons and aponeuroses. Int J Cancer 2002;99:560–7.

55. Hisaoka M, Ishida T, Nishida K, et al. Clear cell sarcoma of soft tissue: a clinicopathologic, immunohistochemical, and molecular analysis of 33 cases. Am J Surg Pathol 2008;32:452–60.

56. Wick MR, Fitzgibbon J, Swanson PE. Cutaneous sarcomas and sarcomatoid neoplasms of the skin. Semin Diagn Pathol 1993;10(2):148–58.

57. Paradela S, Fonseca E, Prieto VG. Melanoma in children. Arch Pathol Lab Med 2011;135:307–16.

58. Paradela S, Fonseca E, Herzog C, et al. Prognostic factors for melanoma in children and adolescents: a clinicopathologic, single-center study of 137 Patients. Cancer 2010;116:4334–44.

59. Ruiz-Maldonado R, Orozco-Covarrubias ML. Malignant melanoma in children. A review. Arch Dermatol 1997;133:363–71.

60. Fishman C, Mihm MC Jr, Sober AJ. Diagnosis and management of nevi and cutaneous melanoma in infants and children. Clin Dermatol 2002; 20:44–50.

61. Livestro DP, Kaine EM, Muzikansky A, et al. Melanoma in the young: differences and similarities with adult melanoma: a case-matched controlled analysis. Cancer 2007;110:614–24.

62. Gandini S, Sera F, Masini C, et al. Meta-analysis of risk factors for cutaneous melanoma: III. Family history, actinic damage and phenotypic factors. Eur J Cancer 2005;41:2040–59.

63. Tucker MA. Melanoma epidemiology. Hematol Oncol Clin North Am 2009;23:383–95.

64. Farmer ER, Gonin R, Hanna MP. Discordance in the histopathologic diagnosis of melanoma and melanocytic nevi between expert pathologists. Hum Pathol 1996;27:528–31.

65. Corona R, Mele A, Piccardi P, et al. Interobserver variability on the histopathologic diagnosis of cutaneous melanoma and other pigmented skin lesions. J Clin Oncol 1996;14:1218–23.

66. Urso C, Rongioletti F, Chimenti S, et al. Interobserver reproducibility of histological features in cutaneous malignant melanoma. J Clin Pathol 2005;58:1194–8.

67. Cerroni L, Kerl H. Tutorial on melanocytic lesions. Am J Dermatopathol 2001;23:237–41.

68. Shea CR, Vollmer RT, Prieto VG. Correlating architectural disorder and cytologic atypia in Clark

(dysplastic) melanocytic nevi. Hum Pathol 1999;30: 500–5.

69. Pozo L, Naase M, Diaz-Cano SJ, et al. Critical analysis of histologic criteria for grading atypical (dysplastic) melanocytic nevi. Am J Clin Pathol 2001;115:194–204.

70. Shah KN. The risk of melanoma and neurocutaneous melanosis associated with congenital melanocytic nevi. Semin Cutan Med Surg 2010; 29:159–64.

71. Duray PH, Livolsi VA. Recurrent dysplastic nevus following shave excision. J Dermatol Surg Oncol 1984;10:811–5.

72. Ohsie SJ, Sarantopoulos GP, Binder SW, et al. Immunohistochemical characteristics of melanoma. J Cutan Pathol 2008;35:433–44.

73. Cochran AJ, Wen DR. S-100 protein as a marker for melanocytic and other tumours. Pathology 1985; 17:340–5.

74. Chorny JA, Barr RJ. S100-positive spindle cells in scars: a diagnostic pitfall in the re-excision of desmoplastic melanoma. Am J Dermatopathol 2002; 24:309–12.

75. Kaufmann O, Koch S, Dietel M, et al. Tyrosinase, melan-A, and KBA62 as markers for the immunohistochemical identification of metastatic amelanotic melanomas on paraffin sections. Mod Pathol 1998;11:740–6.

76. Ordonez NG, Ji XL, Hickey RC. Comparison of HMB-45 monoclonal antibody and S-100 protein in the immunohistochemical diagnosis of melanoma. Am J Clin Pathol 1988;90:385–90.

77. Trefzer U, Rietz N, Siegel P, et al. SM5-1: a new monoclonal antibody which is highly sensitive and specific for melanocytic lesions. Arch Dermatol Res 2000;292:583–9.

78. Wick MR, Swanson PE, Rocamora A. Recognition of malignant melanoma by monoclonal antibody HMB-45. An immunohistochemical study of 200 paraffin-embedded cutaneous tumors. J Cutan Pathol 1988;15:201–7.

79. Junkins-Hopkins JM. Malignant melanoma: molecular cytogenetics and their implications in clinical medicine. J Am Acad Dermatol 2010;63: 329–32.

80. Kanitakis J, Narvaez D, Claudy A. Differential expression of the CD10 antigen (neutral endopeptidase) in primary versus metastatic malignant melanomas of the skin. Melanoma Res 2002;12: 241–4.

81. Curtin JA, Fridlyand J, Kutzner H, et al. Distinct sets of genetic alterations in melanoma. N Engl J Med 2005;353:2135–47.

82. Pleasance ED, Cheetham RK, Greenman CD, et al. A comprehensive catalogue of somatic mutations from a human cancer genome. Nature 2010;463: 191–6.

83. Blokx WA, van Dijk MC, Ruiter DJ. Molecular cytogenetics of cutaneous melanocytic lesions - diagnostic, prognostic and therapeutic aspects. Histopathology 2010;56:121–32.

84. Smalley KS. Understanding melanoma signaling networks as the basis for molecular targeted therapy. J Invest Dermatol 2010;130:28–37.

85. van Dijk MC, Bernsen MR, Ruiter DJ. Analysis of mutations in B-RAF, N-RAS, and H-RAS genes in the differential diagnosis of Spitz nevus and spitzoid melanoma. Am J Surg Pathol 2005;29: 1145–51.

86. Yazdi AS, Palmedo G, Rutten A, et al. Mutations of the BRAF gene in benign and malignant melanocytic lesions. J Invest Dermatol 2003;121: 1160–2.

87. Da Forno PD, Pringle JH, Potter L, et al. BRAF, NRAS and HRAS mutations in spitzoid tumours and their possible pathogenetic significance. Br J Dermatol 2009;161:364–72.

88. Fullen DR, Poynter JN, Nair RP, et al. BRAF and NRAS mutations in spitzoid melanocytic lesions. Mod Pathol 2006;19:1324–32.

89. Song J, Mooi WJ, Krausz T, et al. Nevus versus melanoma: to FISH, or not to FISH. Adv Anat Pathol 2011;18:229–34.

90. Hornyak TJ. Future advances in melanoma research. Clin Plast Surg 2010;37:169–76.

91. Bastian BC, Olshen AB, Pinkel D, et al. Classifying melanocytic tumors based on DNA copy number changes. Am J Pathol 2003;163:1765–70.

92. Bastian BC, Xiong J, Busam K, et al. Genetic changes in neoplasms arising in congenital melanocytic nevi: differences between nodular proliferations and melanomas. Am J Pathol 2002;161: 1163–9.

93. Gerami P, Zembowicz A. Update on fluorescence in situ hybridization in melanoma: state of the art. Arch Pathol Lab Med 2011;135: 830–7.

94. Gerami P, Jewell SS, Ruffalo T, et al. Fluorescence in situ hybridization (FISH) as an ancillary diagnostic tool in the diagnosis of melanoma. Am J Surg Pathol 2009;33:1146–56.

95. Dalton SR, Gerami P, LeBoit PE, et al. Use of fluorescence in situ hybridization (FISH) to distinguish intranodal nevus from metastatic melanoma. Am J Surg Pathol 2010;34:231–7.

96. Newman MD, Mirzabeigi M, Gerami P. Chromosomal copy number changes supporting the classification of lentiginous junctional melanoma of the elderly as a subtype of melanoma. Mod Pathol 2009;22:1258–62.

97. Pouryazdanparast P, Newman M, Gerami P, et al. Distinguishing epithelioid blue nevus from blue nevus-like cutaneous melanoma metastasis using

fluorescence in situ hybridization. Am J Surg Pathol 2009;33:1396–400.

98. Gerami P, Wass A, Busam KJ, et al. Fluorescence in situ hybridization for distinguishing nevoid melanomas from mitotically active nevi. Am J Surg Pathol 2009;33:1783–8.

99. Gaiser T, Kutzner H, Bruckner T, et al. Classifying ambiguous melanocytic lesions with FISH and correlation with clinical long-term follow up. Mod Pathol 2010;23:413–9.

100. Smolle J, Soyer HP, Kerl H. Proliferative activity of cutaneous melanocytic tumors defined by Ki-67 monoclonal antibody. A quantitative immunohistochemical study. Am J Dermatopathol 1989;11:301–7.

101. Boni R, Doguoglu A, Dummer R, et al. MIB-1 immunoreactivity correlates with metastatic dissemination in primary thick cutaneous melanoma. J Am Acad Dermatol 1996;35:416–8.

102. Rieger E, Hofmann-Wellenhof R, Smolle J, et al. Comparison of proliferative activity as assessed by proliferating cell nuclear antigen (PCNA) and Ki-67 monoclonal antibodies in melanocytic skin lesions. A quantitative immunohistochemical study. J Cutan Pathol 1993;20:229–36.

103. Kanoko M, Ueda M, Ichihashi M. PCNA expression and nucleolar organizer regions in malignant melanoma and nevus cell nevus. Kobe J Med Sci 1994;40:107–23.

104. Niemann TH, Argenyi ZB. Immunohistochemical study of Spitz nevi and malignant melanoma with use of antibody to proliferating cell nuclear antigen. Am J Dermatopathol 1993;15:441–5.

105. Florenes VA, Maelandsmo GM, Holm R, et al. Cyclin A expression in superficial spreading malignant melanomas correlates with clinical outcome. J Pathol 2001;195:530–6.

106. Tran TA, Ross JS, Mihm MC Jr, et al. Mitotic cyclins and cyclin-dependent kinases in melanocytic lesions. Hum Pathol 1998;29:1085–90.

107. Alonso SR, Ortiz P, Acuna MJ, et al. Progression in cutaneous malignant melanoma is associated with distinct expression profiles: a tissue microarray-based study. Am J Pathol 2004;164:193–203.

108. Florenes VA, Faye RS, Holm R, et al. Levels of cyclin D1 and D3 in malignant melanoma: deregulated cyclin D3 expression is associated with poor clinical outcome in superficial melanoma. Clin Cancer Res 2000;6:3614–20.

109. Balch CM, Gershenwald JE, Byrd DR, et al. Final version of 2009 AJCC melanoma staging and classification. J Clin Oncol 2009;27:6199–206.

110. Breslow A. Thickness, cross-sectional areas and depth of invasion in the prognosis of cutaneous melanoma. Ann Surg 1970;172:902–8.

111. Barnhill RL, Fine JA, Berwick M, et al. Predicting five-year outcome for patients with cutaneous melanoma in a population-based study. Cancer 1996;78:427–32.

112. Piris A, Mihm MC Jr, Duncan LM. AJCC melanoma staging update: impact on dermatopathology practice and patient management. J Cutan Pathol 2011;38:394–400.

113. Azzola MF, Shaw HM, Watson GF, et al. Tumor mitotic rate is a more powerful prognostic indicator than ulceration in patients with primary cutaneous melanoma: an analysis of 3661 patients from a single center. Cancer 2003;97:1488–98.

114. Kesmodel SB, Karakousis GC, Wahl PM, et al. Mitotic rate as a predictor of sentinel lymph node positivity in patients with thin melanomas. Ann Surg Oncol 2005;12:449–58.

115. Litzner B, EE, Cockerell CJ. Tumor mitotic index in melanomas less than or equal to 1 mm in thickness: a Proscpective Study. Am J Dermatopathol, in press.

116. Balch CM, Wilkerson JA, Maddox WA, et al. The prognostic significance of ulceration of cutaneous melanoma. Cancer 1980;45:3012–7.

117. Kanzler MH, Swetter SM. Malignant melanoma. J Am Acad Dermatol 2003;48:780–3.

118. Piris A, Mihm MC Jr. Progress in melanoma histopathology and diagnosis. Hematol Oncol Clin North Am 2009;23:467–80.

119. Googe P, King R, Page R, et al. Ulceration in thin melanoma. J Cut Pathol 2011;38(1):112–3.

120. Clark WH Jr, From L, Mihm MC, et al. The histogenesis and biologic behavior of primary human malignant melanomas of the skin. Cancer Res 1969;29:705–27.

121. Maize JC. Primary cutaneous malignant melanoma. J Am Acad Dermatol 1983;8:857–63.

122. Zettersten E, Shaikh L, Kashani-Sabet M, et al. Prognostic factors in primary cutaneous melanoma. Surg Clin North Am 2003;83:61–75.

123. Clark WH Jr, Elder DE, Schultz D, et al. Model predicting survival in stage I melanoma based on tumor progression. J Natl Cancer Inst 1989;81:1893–904.

124. Cipponi A, Wieers G, Coulie PG, et al. Tumor-infiltrating lymphocytes: apparently good for melanoma patients. But why? Cancer Immunol Immunother 2011;60:1153–60.

125. Burton AL, Roach BA, Vierling AM, et al. Prognostic significance of tumor infiltrating lymphocytes in melanoma. Am Surg 2011;77:188–92.

126. Blessing K, McLaren KM. Histological regression in primary cutaneous melanoma: recognition, prevalence and significance. Histopathology 1992;20:315–22.

127. Requena C, Botella-Estrada R, Guillen C, et al. Problems in defining melanoma regression and prognostic implication. Actas Dermosifiliogr 2009;100:759–66 [in Spanish].

128. Olah J, Gyulai R, Dobozy A, et al. Tumour regression predicts higher risk of sentinel node involvement in thin cutaneous melanomas. Br J Dermatol 2003;149:662–3.

129. Day CL Jr, Harrist TJ, Friedman RJ, et al. Malignant melanoma. Prognostic significance of "microscopic satellites" in the reticular dermis and subcutaneous fat. Ann Surg 1981;194:108–12.

130. Harrist TJ, Rigel DS, Rhodes AR, et al. "Microscopic satellites" are more highly associated with regional lymph node metastases than is primary melanoma thickness. Cancer 1984;53:2183–7.

131. Leon P, Daly JM, Synnestvedt M, et al. The prognostic implications of microscopic satellites in patients with clinical stage I melanoma. Arch Surg 1991;126:1461–8.

132. Rao UN, Ibrahim J, Kirkwood JM, et al. Implications of microscopic satellites of the primary and extracapsular lymph node spread in patients with high-risk melanoma: pathologic corollary of Eastern Cooperative Oncology Group Trial E1690. J Clin Oncol 2002;20:2053–7.

133. Shaikh L, Sagebiel RW, Kashani-Sabet M, et al. The role of microsatellites as a prognostic factor in primary malignant melanoma. Arch Dermatol 2005;141:739–42.

134. Nagore E, Oliver V, Fortea JM, et al. Prognostic factors in localized invasive cutaneous melanoma: high value of mitotic rate, vascular invasion and microscopic satellitosis. Melanoma Res 2005;15: 169–77.

135. Cascinelli N, Santinami M, Pennacchioli E, et al. World Health Organization experience in the treatment of melanoma. Surg Clin North Am 2003;83: 405–16.

136. Cascinelli N, Morabito A, Belli F, et al. Immediate or delayed dissection of regional nodes in patients with melanoma of the trunk: a randomised trial. WHO Melanoma Programme. Lancet 1998;351: 793–6.

137. Cochran AJ, Wen DR, Morton DL. Management of the regional lymph nodes in patients with cutaneous malignant melanoma. World J Surg 1992;16:214–21.

138. Ross MI, Reintgen D, Balch CM. Selective lymphadenectomy: emerging role for lymphatic mapping and sentinel node biopsy in the management of early stage melanoma. Semin Surg Oncol 1993;9:219–23.

139. Reintgen D, Cruse CW, Glass F, et al. The orderly progression of melanoma nodal metastases. Ann Surg 1994;220:759–67.

140. Thompson JF, McCarthy WH, Paramaesvaran S, et al. Sentinel lymph node status as an indicator of the presence of metastatic melanoma in regional lymph nodes. Melanoma Res 1995;5:255–60.

141. Gershenwald JE, Ross MI. Sentinel-lymph-node biopsy for cutaneous melanoma. N Engl J Med 2011;364:1738–45.

142. Scolyer RA, Thompson JF, Cochran AJ, et al. Intraoperative frozen-section evaluation can reduce accuracy of pathologic assessment of sentinel nodes in melanoma patients. J Am Coll Surg 2005; 201:821–3 [author reply: 823–4].

143. Gershenwald JE, Thompson W, Tseng CH, et al. Multi-institutional melanoma lymphatic mapping experience: the prognostic value of sentinel lymph node status in 612 stage I or II melanoma patients. J Clin Oncol 1999;17:976–83.

144. Statius Muller MG, van Leeuwen PA, Ferwerda CC, et al. The sentinel lymph node status is an important factor for predicting clinical outcome in patients with Stage I or II cutaneous melanoma. Cancer 2001;91:2401–8.

145. Vuylsteke RJ, van Leeuwen PA, Meijer S, et al. Clinical outcome of stage I/II melanoma patients after selective sentinel lymph node dissection: long-term follow-up results. J Clin Oncol 2003;21: 1057–65.

146. Lowe JB, Hurst E, Cornelius LA, et al. Sentinel lymph node biopsy in patients with thin melanoma. Arch Dermatol 2003;139:617–21.

147. Morton DL, Thompson JF, Essner R, et al. Sentinel-node biopsy or nodal observation in melanoma. N Engl J Med 2006;355:1307–17.

148. Morton DL, Cochran AJ, Thompson JF. The rationale for sentinel-node biopsy in primary melanoma. Nat Clin Pract Oncol 2008;5:510–1.

149. Kanzler MH, Levitt L, Lin A. Sentinel-node biopsy in melanoma. N Engl J Med 2007;356:419 [author reply: 21].

150. Tejera-Vaquerizo A, Solis-Garcia E, Moreno-Ramirez D, et al. Primary cutaneous melanoma: prognostic factors not included in the classification of the American Joint Committee on Cancer. Actas Dermosifiliogr 2011;102:255–63.

151. Dadras SS, Lange-Asschenfeldt B, Muzikansky A, et al. Tumor lymphangiogenesis predicts melanoma metastasis to sentinel lymph nodes. Mod Pathol 2005;18:1232–42.

152. Drunkenmolle E, Marsch W, Helmbold P, et al. Paratumoral epidermal hyperplasia: a novel prognostic factor in thick primary melanoma of the skin? Am J Dermatopathol 2005;27: 482–8.

153. Kashani-Sabet M, Sagebiel RW, Miller JR 3rd, et al. Vascular involvement in the prognosis of primary cutaneous melanoma. Arch Dermatol 2001;137: 1169–73.

154. Straume O, Akslen LA. Independent prognostic importance of vascular invasion in nodular melanomas. Cancer 1996;78:1211–9.

155. Quinn MJ, Crotty KA, McCarthy WH, et al. Desmoplastic and desmoplastic neurotropic melanoma: experience with 280 patients. Cancer 1998;83: 1128–35.

156. Chen JY, Hruby G, Fitzgerald P, et al. Desmoplastic neurotropic melanoma: a clinicopathologic analysis of 128 cases. Cancer 2008;113: 2770–8.

157. Larsen TE, Grude TH. A retrospective histological study of 669 cases of primary cutaneous malignant melanoma in clinical stage I. 3. The relation between the tumour-associated lymphocyte infiltration and age and sex, tumour cell type, pigmentation, cellular atypia, mitotic count, depth of invasion, ulceration, tumour type and prognosis. Acta Pathol Microbiol Scand A 1978;86:523–30.

158. Schmoeckel C, Bockelbrink A, Braun-Falco O, et al. Low- and high-risk malignant melanoma–III. Prognostic significance of the resection margin. Eur J Cancer Clin Oncol 1983;19:245–9.

159. Friedman RJ, Rigel DS, Harris MN, et al. Favorable prognosis for malignant melanomas associated with acquired melanocytic nevi. Arch Dermatol 1983;119:455–62.

160. Masback A, Olsson H, Jonsson N, et al. Prognostic factors in invasive cutaneous malignant melanoma: a population-based study and review. Melanoma Res 2001;11:435–45.

161. MacKie RM, Aitchison T, Watt DC, et al. Prognostic models for subgroups of melanoma patients from the Scottish Melanoma Group database 1979-86, and their subsequent validation. Br J Cancer 1995;71:173–6.

162. Kaddu S, Smolle J, Kerl H, et al. Melanoma with benign melanocytic naevus components: reappraisal of clinicopathological features and prognosis. Melanoma Res 2002;12:271–8.

Prognostic Factors for Melanoma

Oliver J. Wisco, DO[a,b,*], Arthur J. Sober, MD[c]

KEYWORDS

• Melanoma • Prognosis • Histology • Biomarkers • Survival

KEY POINTS

- The AJCC melanoma staging system defines prognosis based on the standard TNM (tumor, regional nodes, distant metastasis) classification to create 4 (I–IV) clinical and pathologic stages.
- The tumor thickness serves as the main prognostic factor, with the mitotic rate and ulceration further subcategorizing the Breslow thickness to increase its prognostic accuracy.
- For advanced disease, the determination of lymph node involvement is the first step in evaluating for systemic involvement and predicting survivability.
- The AJCC has created an online melanoma prediction tool (www.melanomaprognosis.org) to more accurately determine melanoma prognosis for localized and regional disease.
- Research into identifying the major genetic pathways that contribute to the development of melanoma has created a new model to determine prognosis and develop new therapeutic options.

INTRODUCTION

The pioneering work by Drs Wallace H. Clark, Jr and Alexander Breslow established the framework for today's melanoma prognosis models.[1,2] Following the establishment of the Clark levels of invasion and the Breslow thickness in 1969 and 1970, respectively, Clark and colleagues,[3] in 1989, described 6 independently predictive factors (mitotic rate, tumor-infiltrating lymphocytes, tumor thickness, anatomic site, patient sex, and histologic regression) that, when analyzed with tumor thickness, became the standard melanoma prognostic model. Today, the American Joint Committee on Cancer (AJCC) serves as the dominant staging system for melanoma, with the Breslow thickness being the principle component in determining outcomes.[4] As medical science evolves into a genetic approach to understanding the balance between disease and health, research on genetic biomarkers has introduced an additional factor that influences prognosis.[5] This article summarizes the current melanoma AJCC staging system and predictive model, discusses the more recent larger clinical studies and current reviews on common prognostic factors, and summarizes recent genetic biomarker development to understand the current staging system and future implications.

2009 AJCC MELANOMA STAGING AND CLASSIFICATION

The AJCC melanoma staging system defines prognosis based on the standard TNM (tumor, regional nodes, distant metastasis) classification to create 4 (I–IV) clinical and pathologic stages (**Tables 1** and **2**). This classification system is pivotal because it unifies the staging nomenclature to predict the prognosis and determine the appropriate treatment.[6]

The T classification describes the state of the primary tumor by the thickness, presence of

[a] Dermatology Clinic, 81st Medical Group, 81 MDOS/SGOMD, 301 Fisher Street STE 1F-136, Keesler AFB, MS 39534, USA; [b] Massachusetts General Hospital's Wellman Center for Photobiology Research, 40 Blossom Street, Boston, MA 02114, USA; [c] Department of Dermatology, Massachusetts General Hospital, Harvard Medical School, Bartlett Hall, Room 622, 40 Blossom Street, Boston, MA 02114, USA
* Corresponding author. 81 MDOS/SGOMD, 301 Fisher Street, Suite 1F-136, Keesler AFB, MS 39534.
E-mail address: wiscooj@gmail.com

Dermatol Clin 30 (2012) 469–485
doi:10.1016/j.det.2012.04.008
0733-8635/12/$ – see front matter Published by Elsevier Inc.

derm.theclinics.com

Table 1
TNM melanoma classification

Classification	Thickness (mm)	Ulceration Status/Mitoses
T		
Tis	NA	NA
T1	≤ 1.00	a: Without ulceration and mitosis <1/mm^2 b: With ulceration or mitoses $\geq$1/mm^2
T2	1.01–2.00	a: Without ulceration b: With ulceration
T3	2.01–4.00	a: Without ulceration b: With ulceration
T4	>4.00	a: Without ulceration b: With ulceration
N	**Number of Metastatic Nodes**	**Nodal Metastatic Burden**
N0	0	NA
N1	1	a: Micrometastasis[a] b: Macrometastasis[b]
N2	2–3	a: Micrometastasis[a] b: Macrometastasis[b] c: In-transit metastases/satellites without metastatic nodes
N3	4+ metastatic nodes, or matted nodes, or in-transit metastases/satellites with metastatic nodes	
M	**Site**	**Serum LDH**
M0	No distant metastases	NA
M1a	Distant skin, subcutaneous, of nodal metastases	Normal
M1b	Lung metastases	Normal
M1c	All other visceral metastases	Normal
	Any distant metastasis	Elevated

Abbreviations: NA, not applicable; LDH, lactate dehydrogenase.
[a] Micrometastases are diagnosed after sentinel lymph node biopsy.
[b] Macrometastases are defined as clinically detectable nodal metastases confirmed pathologically.
Adapted from Balch CM, Gershenwald JE, Soong SJ, et al. Final version of 2009 AJCC melanoma staging and classification. J Clin Oncol 2009;27:6199–206; with permission.

ulceration, and mitotic rate. The N designation signifies the degree of regional lymph node involvement subcategorized by microscopic and macroscopic disease, and the M category defines the presence and location of distant metastatic disease. The current melanoma TNM classification system is predominantly an anatomic and pathologic staging system; the Breslow thickness continues to be the main prognostic factor.[4] The 2009 classification introduced a few significant modifications to the 2002 classification (**Table 3**). The mitotic rate in the T category replaces the Clark level of invasion in the 2009 staging system and the integration of immunohistochemical tumor detection with no lower tumor threshold in the N category has also been added.[4,7] The AJCC's prognosis determinations were based on a multivariate analysis, using the Cox proportional hazards model, of prospective data on 30,946 patients with stages I, II, and III melanoma and 7972 patients with stage IV disease in the AJCC melanoma staging database. Survival curves were created through the Kaplan-Meier product-limit method and compared using the log-rank test.[4]

T Primary Tumor Classification

The AJCC uses tumor thickness, mitotic rate, and ulceration as the primary independent prognostic factors to define the local tumor burden (see **Tables 1** and **2**). The T classification is labeled as T1 to 4 based on increasing tumor thickness (≤1.00 mm, 1.01–2.00 mm, 2.01–4.00, >4.00), with survivability decreasing as the depth increases.[2,8]

Table 2
TNM melanoma staging

	Clinical Staging[a]				Pathologic Stagingt[b]		
	T	N	M		T	N	M
0	Tis	N0	M0	0	Tis	N0	M0
IA	T1a	N0	M0	IA	T1a	N0	M0
IB	T1b	N0	M0	IB	T1b	N0	M0
	T2a	N0	M0		T2a	N0	M0
IIA	T2b	N0	M0	IIA	T2b	N0	M0
	T3a	N0	M0		T3a	N0	M0
IIB	T3b	N0	M0	IIB	T3b	N0	M0
	T4a	N0	M0		T4a	N0	M0
IIC	T4b	N0	M0	IIC	T4b	N0	M0
III	Any T	N > N0	M0	IIIA	T14a	N1a	M0
					T14a	N2a	M0
				IIIB	T14b	N1a	M0
					T14b	N2a	M0
					T14a	N1b	M0
					T1-4a	N2b	M0
					T14a	N2c	M0
				IIIC	T1-4b	N1b	M0
					T14b	N2b	M0
					T14b	N2c	M0
					Any T	N3	M0
IV	Any T	Any N	M1	IV	Any T	Any N	M1

[a] Clinical staging includes microstaging of the primary melanoma and clinical/radiologic evaluation for metastases. By convention, it should be used after complete excision of the primary melanoma with clinical assessment for regional and distant metastases.

[b] Pathologic staging includes microstaging of the primary melanoma and pathologic information about the regional lymph nodes after partial (ie, sentinel lode biopsy) or complete lymphadenectomy. Pathologic stage 0 or stage IA patients are the exception; they do not require pathologic evaluation of their lymph nodes.

Adapted from Balch CM, Gershenwald JE, Soong SJ, et al. Final version of 2009 AJCC melanoma staging and classification. J Clin Oncol 2009;27:6199–206; with permission.

Although the tumor thickness serves as the main prognostic factor, the mitotic rate and the ulceration further subcategorize the Breslow thickness to increase its prognostic accuracy (**Table 4**). Subcategorization with the designation of *a* indicates no ulceration or less than $1/mm^2$ mitoses in tumors in the T1 category. The designation of *b* indicates the presence of ulceration in all T categories or greater than or equal to $1/mm^2$ mitoses in tumors in the T1 category. Clark level of invasion is still occasionally used for staging purposes in T1 tumors when the mitotic rate cannot be evaluated or has not been reported. Clark levels are defined by the presence of tumor cells within the various anatomic layers of the skin (**Table 5**).[1] The presence of a Clark level of 4 or 5 will upstage a tumor less than 1.00 mm from T1a to T1b in the absence of a mitotic rate determination.

As defined by Dr Alexander Breslow, the Breslow thickness, or the tumor thickness, is a measure of the melanoma from the top of the granular layer down to the lowest tumor cell.[2]

Numerous studies have validated the clinical significance of the Breslow thickness as an independent prognostic factor, with the 2008 AJCC melanoma staging database verifying its prognostic power.[6] Tumor thickness is the most powerful prognostic indicator for localized cutaneous melanoma ($\chi^2 = 84.6$, $P<.0001$, see **Table 4**); as thickness increases, there is a significant decline in 5- and 10-year survival ($P<.0001$). A 10-year 96% survival is found in patients with 0.01- to 0.5-mm thick localized cutaneous melanomas, whereas a 10-year 42% survival is found in localized melanomas greater than 6.00 mm thick.[6]

Mitotic rate was added to the seventh edition staging system, replacing the Clark level of invasion in the T1 category because the Clark level was not found to add clinical significance ($\chi^2 = 1.9$, $P = .17$) in the multivariate analysis when tumor thickness, mitotic rate, and ulceration are included (**Table 6**).[4,7] The mitotic rate is determined by first identifying the area in the dermis with the highest number of mitotic figures, which is called the hot

Table 3
Differences between the sixth edition (2002) and the seventh edition (2009) of the melanoma staging system

Factor	Sixth Edition Criteria	Recommended Seventh Edition Criteria	Comments
Thickness	Primary determinant of T staging	Same	Thresholds of 1.0, 2.0, and 4.0 mm
Level of invasion	Used only for defining T1 melanomas	Same	Used as a default criterion only if mitotic rate cannot be determined
Ulceration	Included as a secondary determinant of T and N staging	Same	Signifies a locally advanced lesion; dominant prognostic factor for grouping stages I, II, and III
Mitotic rate per square millimeter	Not used	Used for categorizing T1 melanoma	Mitosis $\geq 1/mm^2$ used as a primary criterion for defining T1b melanoma
Satellite metastases	In N category	Same	Merged with in-transit lesions
Immunochemical detection of nodal metastases	Not included	Included	Must include at least 1 melanoma-associated marker (eg, HMB-45, Melan-A, MART-1) unless diagnostic cellular morphology is present
0.2 mm threshold of defined N+	Implied	No lower threshold of staging N+ disease	Isolated tumor cells or tumor deposits <0.1 mm meeting the criteria for histologic or immunohistochemical detection of melanoma should be scored as N+
Number of nodal metastases	Primary determinant of N staging	Same	Thresholds of 1 v 2–3 v 4+ nodes
Metastatic volume	Included as a second determinant of N staging	Same	Clinically occult (microscopic) nodes are diagnosed at sentinel node biopsy v clinically apparent (macroscopic) nodes diagnosed by palpation or imaging studies or by the finding of gross (not microscopic) extracapsular extension in a clinically occult node
Lung metastases	Separate category as M1b	Same	Has a somewhat better prognosis than other visceral metastases
Elevated serum LDH	Included as a second determinant of M staging	Same	Recommend a second confirmatory LDH level if elevated
Clinical vs pathologic staging	Sentinel node results incorporated into definition of pathologic staging		Large variability in outcome between clinical and pathologic staging; sentinel node staging encouraged for standard patient care should be required before entry into clinical trials

Abbreviation: LDH, lactate dehydrogenase.
Adapted from Balch CM, Gershenwald JE, Soong SJ, et al. Melanoma of the skin. In: Edge SB, Byrd DR, Compton CC, et al, editors. AJCC staging manual. 7th edition. New York: Springer; 2010. p. 325–44; with permission.

Table 4
Multivariate Cox regression analysis of prognostic factors in 10,233 patients with localized cutaneous melanoma (stage I and II)

Variable	Chi-Square Value (1 df)	P	HR	95% CI
Tumor thickness	84.6	<.0001	1.25	1.19–1.31
Mitotic rate	79.1	<.0001	1.26	1.20–1.32
Ulceration	47.2	<.0001	1.56	1.38–1.78
Age	40.8	<.0001	1.16	1.11–1.22
Gender	32.4	<.0001	0.70	0.62–0.79
Site	29.1	<.0001	1.38	1.23–1.54
Clark level	8.2	.0041	1.15	1.04–1.26

Abbreviations: CI, confidence interval; HR, hazard ratio.
Adapted from Balch CM, Gershenwald JE, Soong SJ, et al. Melanoma of the skin. In: Edge SB, Byrd DR, Compton CC, et al, editors. AJCC staging manual. 7th edition. New York: Springer; 2010. p. 325–44; with permission.

spot. Using the hot spot as the focal point, the number of mitotic figures is then counted in the hot spot and then the count is extended to adjacent fields until an area of 1 mm^2 has been evaluated. If a hot spot cannot be identified, a representative mitosis is chosen as the focal point for the count.[6] The analysis of the 2008 AJCC melanoma staging database revealed a worsening prognosis with increasing mitotic rate. The 5-year survival ranged from 97% with less than 1 mitosis/mm^2 to 60% with greater than 20 mitoses/mm^2 for stage I and II disease (**Table 7**).[6,8] However, through the examination of multiple mitotic rate thresholds, a mitotic rate of greater than or equal to 1/mm^2 had the most significant correlation with survival.[4] The 10-year survival rate decreases to 87% in T1b patients whose Breslow thickness is 0.5 to 1.0 mm

Table 5
Clark levels of invasion

I	Tumor confined to the epidermis
II	Tumor invading into the upper papillary dermis
III	Tumor filling the papillary dermis with no extension into the reticular dermis
IV	Tumor invading into the reticular dermis
V	Tumor invading into the subcutaneous tissue

Data from Clark WH Jr, et al. The histogenesis and biologic behavior of primary human malignant melanomas of the skin. Cancer Res 1969;29:705–26.

compared with a 93% survival rate in T1a patients with the same depth. In addition, preliminary evidence suggests that there is an approximate 10% risk of finding occult metastasis on sentinel lymph node biopsy in T1 melanomas greater than 0.76 mm with a mitotic rate greater than or equal to 1/mm^2.[6] Although the data show a worsening prognosis with increasing mitotic rates and the AJCC staging manual (seventh edition) states, "Mitotic rate should be addressed on all primary melanomas,"[6] mitotic rate is not included in the current AJCC T2–4 classification.

The presence of ulceration was previously included as a prognostic criterion in the sixth edition of the AJCC melanoma staging classification and there were no changes to its use in the current edition. Ulceration is defined as being present if there is a full-thickness epidermal defect; reactive changes, such as fibrin deposition and neutrophils; and effacement of the surrounding epidermis or reactive hyperplasia in the absence of trauma or a recent surgical procedure. Ulceration predicts a clinically significant lower survival rate for tumors of the same T category, raising them to the next T category's risk level. For example, a T2a melanoma (stage IB) has a 5-year survival rate of 91%, whereas T2b and T3a melanomas (stage IIA) have similar 5-year survival rates of 82% and 79%, respectively.[6] Although the AJCC defines melanoma ulceration by the presence or absence of ulceration, a recent single-institution retrospective study of 235 patients suggests that the percentage of surface ulceration provides an increased prognostic significance.[9] In this study, the percentage of ulceration was determined by comparing the diameter of the ulceration and the surface diameter overlying the vertical growth phase of the tumor. In tumors with less than 5% ulceration, the overall survival was 80.7%, whereas tumors with greater than 5% had a survival of 66.7% using a univariate Cox regression analysis ($P = .0006$).

Combining the 3 components of the T classification, the 2009 AJCC melanoma staging 5- and 10-year survival rates range from 97% and 93% in patients with T1a melanoma to 53% and 39%, respectively, in patients with T4b melanoma (P<.0001). When comparing the survival rates published in the 2001 and 2009 AJCC staging manuals, similar 5-year survival rates were found in all categories, including the T1b category, despite the change in category criteria (**Table 8**).[6,10]

N Regional Lymph Node Involvement Classification

For more advanced disease, the determination of lymph node involvement is the first step in

Table 6
Multivariate Cox regression analysis of pathologic factors by T category for stage I and II melanoma

T Category	Tumor Thickness		Ulceration		Mitotic Rate		Clark Level	
	χ^2	P	χ^2	P	χ^2	P	χ^2	P
T1	12.8	.0003	3.8	.05	20.8	<.0001	1.9	.17
T2	4.9	.03	16.2	<.0001	15.9	<.0001	0.2	.65
T3	4.1	.04	15.4	<.0001	12.2	.0005	1.4	.24
T4	0.2	.69	14.2	.0002	9.1	.003	2.7	.10

Adapted from Balch CM, Gershenwald JE, Soong SJ, et al. Final version of 2009 AJCC melanoma staging and classification. J Clin Oncol 2009;27:6199–206; with permission.

evaluating for systemic involvement and predicting survivability.[4,11,12] The seventh edition of the AJCC melanoma staging manual defines nodal involvement by the number of nodes involved and whether the nodal involvement is microscopic (micrometastasis) versus clinically evident (macrometastasis). The number of nodes involved, along with ulceration and Breslow thickness, have been shown to be the most predictive independent factors for survival in patients with regional nodal or in-transit/satellite (stage III) metastatic disease in the Cox multivariate analysis of the melanoma staging database (P<.001, **Table 9**).[4] The current AJCC melanoma staging manual lists 5-year

Table 7
2008 AJCC melanoma staging database data on mitotic rate and survival

Number of Mitoses/mm²	n	Survival Rate ± SE	
		5 y	10 y
0–0.99	3312	0.973 ± 0.004	0.927 ± 0.007
1.00–1.99	2117	0.920 ± 0.007	0.842 ± 0.012
2.00–4.99	3254	0.869 ± 0.007	0.754 ± 0.012
5.00–10.99	2049	0.781 ± 0.011	0.680 ± 0.018
11.00–19.99	673	0.695 ± 0.022	0.576 ± 0.027
≥20.0	259	0.594 ± 0.039	0.476 ± 0.050
Total	11,664[a]		

[a] Includes patients with mitosis, tumor thickness, and follow-up information available.
Adapted from Balch CM, Gershenwald JE, Soong SJ, et al. Melanoma of the skin. In: Edge SB, Byrd DR, Compton CC, et al, editors. AJCC staging manual. 7th edition. New York: Springer; 2010. p. 325–44; with permission.

overall survival ranges from 78% in nonulcerated stage IIIA to 40% in stage IIIC.

In a recent study evaluating 2313 patients with stage III disease (81% with micrometastasis and 19% with macrometastasis) in the 2008 AJCC melanoma staging database, there was an overall 5-year survival of 67% in patients with nodal micrometastases and 43% with nodal macrometastases (P<.001).[13] When stratified by the number of tumor-positive nodes and tumor burden, the 5-year survival rates for patients with 1, 2, or 3 tumor-positive nodes (microscopic vs macroscopic) were 71% versus 50% (P<.001), 65% versus 43% (P<.001), and 61% versus 40% (P<.004), respectively. However, when there were 4 or more nodes involved, the 5-year survival was 36% regardless of microscopic or macroscopic disease.

New to the seventh edition of the AJCC melanoma staging manual, the N classification is the acceptance of immunohistochemical (IHC) stains alone in determining the presence of a tumor. Also, the lower threshold (previously 0.2 mm) of the melanoma tumor burden to define the presence of significant lymph node metastasis when evaluating microscopic disease has been eliminated. Hematoxylin and eosin stained sections have traditionally been the standard for evaluating lymph node pathologic specimens; but in the current AJCC melanoma staging manual, lymph node positivity can be determined solely by IHC stain if at least one melanoma-associated marker (human melanin black [HMB-45], Melan-A/MART-1) is positive.[14] These IHC stains are able to detect micrometastases less than 0.1 mm. However, although the 0.2-mm threshold has been removed, no lower tumor burden lacking significance has been defined. The seventh edition of the AJCC staging manual cites 2 opposing studies with clinically significant data on this issue[15,16] and concludes that the significance of a lower threshold of isolated tumor cells

Table 8
Comparison of the 2001 and 2009 AJCC melanoma staging database T classification survival rates in patients with localized melanoma (stage I and II)

Stage	T Classification	2002 AJCC 5-Year Survival	2009 AJCC 5-Year Survival
IA	T1a	95%, n = 4510	97%, n = 9452
IB	T1b[a]	91%, n = 1380	94%, n = 2389
	T2a	89%, n = 3285	92%, n = 6429
IIA	T2b	77%, n = 958	82%, n = 1517
	T3a	79%, n = 1717	79%, n = 3127
IIB	T3b	63%, n = 1523	68%, n = 2164
	T4a	67%, n = 563	71%, n = 1064
IIC	T4b	45%, n = 978	53%, n = 1397

[a] 2002 T1b criteria used Clark level of invasion, whereas the 2009 T1b criteria uses mitotic rate.

Data from Balch CM, Gershenwald JE, Soong SJ, et al. Melanoma of the skin. In: Edge SB, Byrd DR, Compton CC, et al, editors. AJCC Staging manual. 7th edition. New York: Springer; 2010. p. 325–44; and Balch CM, Atkins MB, JE, et al. Melanoma of the skin. In: Green FL, Page DL, Fleming ID, et al, editors. AJCC staging manual. 6th edition. New York: Springer; 2002. p. 209–20.

in the lymph nodes cannot be substantiated at this time.

To address this issue, a recent study evaluated the prognostic value of sentinel lymph node positivity using the Dewar and Rotterdam criteria.[17] This study was a retrospective study of 1009 patients that had a positive sentinel lymph node biopsy (SLNB) followed by completion lymph node dissection (CLND). The Dewar criteria define the tumor location in the lymph node (subcapsular, combined, parenchymal, multifocal, extensive, unknown) and the Rotterdam criteria evaluate the size of the tumor deposits (<0.1 mm, 0.1–1.0 mm, and >1.0 mm). Although this study confirmed the data that larger

tumor sizes portended a worsening prognosis,[18] the most significant finding resulted from a subgroup analysis that combined the Rotterdam and Dewar criteria. This subgroup, called the Rotterdam-Dewar combined (RDC) criteria, compared a less than 0.1-mm tumor load in the subcapsular versus nonsubcapsular areas. Comparing the melanoma-specific survival (MSS) of the subcapsular versus nonsubcapsular areas with a tumor load of less than 0.1 mm, the 5-year MSS rates were 95% versus 88%, respectively (P<.001%); whereas the 10-year MSS rates were 95% and 80%, respectively (P<.001). The nonsentinel node positivity rate on CLND was 2% versus 16%, respectively, for the

Table 9
Multivariate Cox regression analysis of prognostic factors in 1338 stage III patients in the 2008 melanoma staging database

	Chi-Square Values (1 df)		
Variable	All Patients with Stage III (n = 1338)	Patients with Micrometastasis (n = 1070)	Patients with Macrometastasis (n = 268)
Number of positive nodes	27.4	27.8	5.0
Ulceration	17.5	13.5	2.1
Tumor thickness	9.1	9.4	1.1
Tumor burden (micro vs macro)	4.7	—	—
Mitotic rate	4.4	12.7	0.2
Age	24.8	15.8	7.1
Site	4.3	4.7	0.4
Gender	0.5	0.4	0.2
Clark level	0.l	0.0	0.2

Adapted from Balch CM, Gershenwald JE, Soong SJ, et al. Melanoma of the skin. In: Edge SB, Byrd DR, Compton CC, et al, editors. AJCC staging manual. 7th edition. New York: Springer; 2010. p. 325–44; with permission.

2 groups (P<.001). This retrospective study recommends using the RDC criteria to evaluate micrometastasis less than 1 mm based on its location in the subcapsular versus nonsubcapsular areas; a micrometastasis tumor load of less than 1 mm in the subcapsular area may not benefit from CLND, whereas a tumor load less than 1 mm in a nonsubcapsular area is likely to benefit from CLND. It is anticipated that the prospective randomized controlled Multicenter Selective Lymphadenectomy trial II will further address this lower threshold issue.

Regarding intralymphatic metastasis, as with the previous AJCC staging manual, the presence of clinical or histologic satellites or in-transit metastases is included in the N classification as N2c when nodal metastases are absent or N3 if there is concurrent nodal disease. In-transit metastases and satellites (clinical or histologic) are grouped together because of similar prognostic outcomes. The presence of intralymphatic metastases increases the risk of regional recurrence and carries a 5-year survival rate of 69%. The prognosis of intralymphatic metastases is absent in the setting of concurrent nodal disease is defined by the presence of nodal involvement and is classified as stage IIIC.[6]

M Distant Metastases Classification

Melanoma is capable of spreading to any distant site; the most common locations are the skin, soft tissues, lung, liver, brain, bone, and gastrointestinal tract.[6,19] When analyzing prognosis by anatomic metastatic site, significant differences were found only when the sites are arranged into 3 categories: distant skin/subcutaneous tissue/distant lymph nodes (M1a), the lungs (M1b), or any other visceral site (M1c).[20–22] Based on the 2008 AJCC melanoma staging database of 7972 patients with stage IV melanoma, survival was clinically significant at the 1-year mark with reported rates of 62%, 53%, and 33% for the 3 categories, respectively (P<.0001).

Beyond 1 year, patients with an M1a classification had slightly better survival rates than patients with M1b and M1c classifications, but the difference is not significant.[6]

In addition to the classification based on the anatomic site of metastasis, the presence of an elevated serum lactase dehydrogenase (LDH) with metastasis in any site will upstage patients to the M1c classification. It is unclear how the LDH is involved in survival, but if the LDH is elevated more than a laboratory's reference standard, survival rates decrease regardless of the site of distant metastatic disease. The AJCC staging database found 1- and 2-year overall survival rates of 65% and 40%, respectively, with a normal LDH compared with 32% and 18% overall survival rates with an elevated LDH. Median survival has been found to be 16, 14, and 9 months for the M1a, M1b, and M1c categories, respectively, with a normal LDH, whereas an elevated LDH decreased survival to 9, 9, and 5 months, respectively, for the 3 categories (Table 10).[22]

The number of metastases has been found to be significant in several studies and confirmed using the 2008 AJCC melanoma staging database. A recent single institution's multivariate analysis found a hazard ratio (HR) of 1.27 (P = .04, 95% confidence interval [CI], 1.01–1.60) when more than one organ is involved and an HR of 2.27 (P<.001, 95% CI, 1.65–3.14) when more than one metastases is found.[22] However, because of the significant variability in the use of diagnostic tests to diagnosis distant disease, the AJCC did not include the number of metastatic sites into the staging classification.

Although there are survival differences between the M categories at 1 year, the differences are clinically insignificant for the TNM staging purposes. The overall staging prognostic value of the M classification is determined by the presence versus the absence of distant metastasis. One important consideration when determining metastatic disease is the occurrence of metastatic melanoma in the

Table 10
Impact of serum LDH on median survival by site of disease

Site of Disease	LDH <200 U/L			LDH >200 U/L			P Value
	Number of Patients	Number of Deaths	Median Survival	Number of Patients	Number of Deaths	Median Survival	
Skin/subcutaneous/ distant nodal	49	32	16 (13–21)	5	5	9 (2−n/r)	.10
Lung	83	71	14 (12–17)	15	12	9 (4–17)	.008
Other viscera	114	91	9 (7–10)	105	95	5 (4–7)	.003

Adapted from Neuman HB, Patel A, Ishill M. A single-institution validation of the AJCC staging system for stage IV melanoma. Ann Surg Oncol 2008;15:2034–41; with permission.

setting of an unknown primary site. According to the seventh edition of the AJCC melanoma staging manual, prognosis is based on the location of the initial metastatic disease. When metastatic disease is found in the skin, subcutaneous tissue, or a localized lymph node, the applied stage is stage III if no further disease is found. Metastatic disease to a visceral site is treated as stage IV disease. When placing melanoma of unknown primary into either stage III or stage IV disease, its prognosis has been found to be the same or slightly better than that found for patients in whom the primary tumor site is known.[23–25]

AN ELECTRONIC PREDICTION TOOL BASED ON THE 2008 AJCC MELANOMA DATABASE

The AJCC has created an online melanoma prediction tool (www.melanomaprognosis.org) to more accurately determine melanoma prognosis for localized and regional disease. The prediction tool expands on the AJCC melanoma staging system by generating a prognostic analysis based on the patient's individual characteristics. For localized disease, the Cox regression model was used to analyze the AJCC melanoma staging data set of 14,760 patients with localized melanoma. Tumor thickness (χ^2 = 232.9, $P<.000001$), ulceration (χ^2 = 126.2, $P<.000001$), age (χ^2 = 91.9, $P<.000001$), lesion site (χ^2 = 45.5, $P<.00001$), sex (χ^2 = 23.9, $P<.00001$), and level of invasion (χ^2 = 21.2, $P<.00001$) were the 6 factors identified that significantly affected survival.[26] For regional disease, the number of lymph nodes involved (χ^2 = 46.84, $P<.00001$) and lymph node tumor burden (micrometastasis vs macrometastasis; χ^2 = 28.03, $P<.0001$)[27] were added to the model to predict 1-year, 2-year, 5-year, and 10-year overall survival rates at the 95% CI. The mitotic rate was not included in this prognostic model. Validation of the 2008 AJCC melanoma staging data was conducted by comparing the data set with a similarly large database maintained by the Sydney Melanoma Unit in Australia.[26,27] The Sydney Melanoma Unit provided data from 10,974 patients with melanoma to evaluate the AJCC localized disease model, making this the first local and regional melanoma predictive model that is validated by an equally large independent data set.[26]

Exclusion of the Mitotic Rate in the AJCC Predictive Model

The primary reason that the mitotic rate was not included in the predictive model for localized and regional melanoma was that more than 60% of the patients in the database did not have their melanoma's mitotic rate recorded (Soong SJ, personal communication, November 1, 2011). Including missing data of mitotic rate in the multivariate statistical modeling would significantly reduce the sample size for the model development. However, the model developers concluded that even without the mitotic rate included in the 2010 melanoma predictive model, the model would still be valid. Because the mitotic rate is significantly correlated with other key prognostic factors, such as tumor thickness, ulceration, and age, some significant predictability of the mitotic rate was represented by the combination of the previously mentioned factors. Mitotic rate is planned to be included in future predictive models once adequate data are available.

Age as a Melanoma Prognostic Factor

According to the AJCC's recent multivariate Cox regression analysis of prognostic factors in 10,233 patients with localized cutaneous melanoma, age is fourth in the list of prognostic indications (χ^2 = 40.8, $P<.0001$, see **Table 4**).[6] A recent study of 4785 patients with cutaneous melanoma focusing on age and gender as independent prognostic factors found patients aged older than 65 years had a lower 10-year disease-specific survival (DSS) than younger patients (81.8% vs 88.4%, $P<.001$).[28] In particular, patients with melanoma aged 65 years or older carried a 1.45-fold increased risk of death in 5 years compared with younger patients. This study also demonstrated that patients aged more than than 65 years compared with younger patients presented more frequently with thicker (>1 mm) lesions (63.3% vs 46.9%, $P<.001$) and ulcerated tumors (9.9% vs 4.7%, $P<.001$). The rate of developing metastasis was also significantly higher in patients aged more than 65 years (21.1% vs 16.3%, $P<.05$). Regarding the patterns of metastasis, older patients present more frequently with in-transit disease (34.3% vs 20.0%, $P<.001$) and less frequently with metastasis in the regional lymph nodes (37.7% vs 50.9%, $P<.001$) compared with younger patients. The occurrence of distant metastasis as the first site of recurrence is not significantly different between older and younger patients. However, when it does occur, older patients more frequently present with liver metastasis (18.2% vs 7.5%, $P<.05$) and brain metastasis (24.7% vs 15.2%, $P<.05$). Recent Surveillance, Epidemiology, and End Results (SEER) program data confirm that older age portends a worse prognosis.[29]

Regarding the significance of age as it relates to patients younger than 21 years of age, conflicting data exist on the outcome of pediatric melanoma compared with older patients. Smaller case series report a better prognosis in patients aged less than 10 years despite a higher median thickness, but the validity of the results is limited because of the low case numbers.[30] A larger case series found that younger patients with melanoma were found to have a higher incidence of positive lymph nodes at initial presentation compared with adults (17.8% vs 9.6% respectively), but this finding was not clinically significant and the overall survival was the same.[31] If younger patients are stratified into 2 groups comprised of patients aged younger than 10 years and patients aged 10 to 18 years, a recent study showed that 57% of the patients in the younger group had tumors greater than or equal to 2.01 mm, whereas 56% of the patients in the older group had tumors less than or equal to 1.0 mm (P<.05). However, as seen in the larger studies, although the incidence of SLNB positivity was higher for the younger patients, it was not clinically significant and the overall survival was still the same.[32]

Gender's Role in Melanoma Prognosis

Gender follows age in the AJCC 2008 multivariate Cox regression analysis of localized melanoma prognostic factors ($\chi^2 = 32.4$, P<.0001, see **Table 4**).[6] Overall, men have a greater risk for having advanced disease with a poorer outcome. Using 68,495 invasive melanoma cases diagnosed from 1992 to 2005 in the SEER database, the risk of death for women was lower than for men (HR 0.76, 95% CI, 0.71–0.81).[29] In another study investigating gender's influence in cutaneous melanoma, 11,774 melanoma cases were analyzed for survival and disease progression by gender.[33] This study found that women compared with men had a higher MSS (HR 0.62, 95% CI, 0.56–0.70). They also had lower risks of progression (HR 0.68, 95% CI, 0.62–0.75), lymph node metastasis (HR 0.58, 95% CI, 0.51–0.65), and visceral metastasis (HR 0.56, 95% CI, 0.49–0.65). In addition, women continued to have a significant survival advantage after the first progression (HR 0.81, 95% CI, 0.71–0.92) and lymph node metastasis (HR 0.80, 95% CI, 0.66–0.96). However, the significance decreased with visceral metastasis (HR 0.88, 95% CI, 0.76–1.03).

Although a favorable outcome seems to be significant for women overall, whether there is a significant difference in women aged more than 65 years is unclear because age may be the more powerful prognostic factor in this age group. Overall, 10-year disease-free survival (DFS) has been shown to be significantly lower in men (75.8%, 95% CI, 73.4–78.2) compared with women (82.7%, 95% CI, 80.9–84.5, P<.0001),

and 10-year DSS was significantly lower in men (83.5%, 95% CI, 81.5–85.5) compared with women (88.5%, 95% CI, 88.5–91.3, P<.0001).[28] However, when age stratification was introduced, there was no significant difference in either DFS or DSS in patients aged more than 65 years. Independent of age, this study showed that when recurrence occurred, women presented more frequently with local disease (30.5% vs 15.9%, P<.001) and less frequently with regional lymph node (43.8% vs 50.3%, P<.001) or distant recurrence (25.6% vs 35.1%, P<.001). If distant relapse did occur in women, the survival was not significantly different between genders.

The Influence of Primary Tumor Location on Melanoma Survival

The location of the cutaneous melanoma ranks sixth in the AJCC 2008 multivariate Cox regression analysis of localized melanoma prognostic factors ($\chi^2 = 29.1$, P<.0001, see **Table 4**).[6] The electronic melanoma prediction tool divides anatomic location into 2 categories: axial versus extremity. An axial lesion site is defined by the presence of the melanoma on the trunk, head, or neck.[26] Studies have shown the presence of a melanoma on an axial site conferred a worse prognosis than an extremity site.[3,21] A recent study reported survival by anatomic site was similar for melanoma diagnosed on the face/ears, trunk, and extremities (5-year MSS 90.2%, 91.2%, 92.5%, respectively) but decreased for melanoma on the scalp and neck (5-year MSS 82.6%).[29] Using the SEER database during the years of 1992 to 2003 to further explain the aggressiveness of the scalp and neck location, patients with scalp and neck melanomas were older (mean age at diagnosis, 58.8 vs 55.1 years), had thicker tumors (median thickness, 0.80 mm vs 0.63 mm), and were more commonly men (74% vs 54%) compared with melanomas in the face/ears, trunk, and extremities (P<.001 for all comparisons).[34] These melanomas were also more likely to be ulcerated (7% vs 5%), to have positive lymph nodes (7% vs 4%), and to be classified as a nodular melanoma (10% vs 8%) or a lentigo maligna melanoma (12% vs 6%). This study also found 5- and 10-year Kaplan-Meier survival rates for patients with scalp/neck melanoma of 83.1% and 76.2%, respectively, compared with 92.1% and 88.7%, respectively, for melanomas at the other sites (P<.001). Patients with scalp/neck melanoma died of melanoma at an increased rate (HR 1.84, 95% CI, 1.62–2.10) compared with the rate of patients with extremity melanomas. Patients with melanomas located on the trunk versus the extremities also died of melanoma at an increased rate (HR 1.27, 95% CI, 1.16–1.40) but not those with melanomas of the face and ears compared with the extremities (HR 0.95, 95% CI, 0.83–1.09).

OTHER COMMON HISTOLOGIC AND CLINICAL PROGNOSTIC FACTORS

In addition to the AJCC melanoma staging criteria, numerous clinical and histologic prognostic factors have been found to influence outcome, but multivariate analysis has shown that most variables are not independent prognostic factors or the data are inconclusive. Regardless, these prognostic factors can still assist in clinical decision making. The following is a discussion on the most commonly discussed prognostic factors along with clinical scenarios with important survival implications.

Melanoma Prognostic Factors in the Dermatopathology Report

According to the American Academy of Dermatology's "Guidelines of Care for the Management of Primary Cutaneous Melanoma,"[35] the recommended essential histologic features of primary melanoma to be included in the pathology report are tumor thickness, ulceration, mitotic rate, margin status, Clark level of invasion, and microsatellitosis. The optional features include angiolymphatic invasion, histologic subtype, neurotropism, regression, T-stage classification, tumor infiltrating lymphocytes, and vertical growth phase. The prognostic values of the "essential" histologic features of melanoma listed in a pathology report have been discussed above, whereas the rest of the "optional" features were recently reviewed in *Clinics in Dermatology* in 2009.[8] **Table 11** summarizes the 2009 *Clinics in Dermatology* review article's prognostic findings on these optional histologic features.

Transplant Patients

Melanoma occurring with immunosuppression in transplant patients is a controversial topic. Particular concern arises when considering a transplant in patients with a previous history of melanoma (pretransplant melanoma) because of the potential for immunosuppression causing recurrence or progression of the melanoma. In addition, in patients without a history of melanoma undergoing a solid organ transplant, the risk for developing melanoma related to the immunosuppressed state (posttransplant melanoma) has recently become a prominent concern.[36–38] Statistically significant data have previously been limited for both

scenarios. Because there are large variances in the collection of prognostic factors in several small case series, it is difficult to control for different immunosuppressive protocols. In the case of pretransplant melanomas, there is a tendency for selection bias toward thinner melanomas. Recently, a review of melanoma in transplant patients compared SEER melanoma data with organ transplant consolidated case series data.[39] Sixty-one melanoma cases from 59 transplant patients before receiving a solid organ transplant and 724 melanoma cases from 638 transplant patients after receiving a solid organ were reviewed, representing the largest series of cases to date. Using matched controls from the SEER data, prognostic analyses of overall and MSS by Breslow thickness and Clark level of invasion were performed. A 1-sample log-rank test was used to determine whether the observed survival of the study cohort differed from the expected survival. This study showed that 3-year overall survival, regardless of Breslow thickness or the Clark level, was worse in all posttransplant patients with melanoma (**Table 12**). Three-year MSS for posttransplant patients with melanoma was found to be significant in melanomas 1.51 to 3.00 mm in thickness or Clark level III or IV (3-year study MSS = 73.2%; control MSS = 91.0%; *P* = .002). A subgroup analysis of posttransplant patients with melanoma with higher immunosuppression (ie, cardiac transplant patients) demonstrated a statistically significant difference in MSS only for Breslow thickness greater than 1.51 mm (3-year study MSS = 45.2%; control MSS = 78.9%; *P* = .009). As for pretransplant patients with melanoma, there was no significant difference in survival outcomes.

Patients with HIV

Patients who are HIV positive with melanoma follow a similar pattern as solid organ transplant patients.[40] In a study evaluating 17 patients who were HIV positive with melanoma matched with patients who were HIV negative, overall survival was evaluated controlling for melanoma subtype, tumor thickness, Clark level, sex and age of the patients, and anatomic location of the primary tumor.[41] This study found a significant reduction of overall survival compared with matched controls with a median overall survival of approximately 2.8 years for patients who were HIV positive versus 6.4 years for patients who were HIV negative (*P* = .002). Despite this survival difference, there was no association between CD4 cell counts and tumor thickness in patients with melanoma who were HIV positive at the time of melanoma diagnosis. However, there was an inverse

Table 11
Optional melanoma histologic features with prognostic value found in the dermatopathology report

Histologic Feature	Description	Impact on Prognosis
Angiolymphatic Invasion	Presence of tumor cells within a vessel lumen	Potential marker for hematologic/lymphatic spread of melanoma cells, but there is a high potential for misinterpretation in the presence of torturous vessels; Prognostic power overlaps with angiotropism
Histologic Subtype	SSM NM LMM ALM	LMM and SSM have been found to have a better prognosis than NM and ALM, but when controlling for tumor thickness, studies have not consistently found a significant difference between the subtypes There is also significant variance in categorization criteria among dermatopathologists
Neurotropism	Neoplastic infiltration of nerve fibers	Found to increase risk for local recurrence with an unclear role in metastatic disease, but there is limited data reported in the literature
Regression	Partial or complete absence of tumor cells in both the dermis and epidermis found within a melanoma; There is a residual variable combination of fibrosis, degenerative melanoma cells, melanophages, lymphocytes, and telangiectasia. Thought to be caused by interaction between the host immune response and the tumor cells	Unclear prognostic value because of inconsistencies in definition and measurement and lack of control of other histologic variables Several studies have shown that severe regression correlates with a worsening DFS, whereas other studies have found that regression in thin melanomas had a decreased metastatic risk
Angiotropism	Melanoma cells cuffing the external surface of vessels	Potential source for hematologic spread of melanoma cells, but there is limited data to evaluate whether angiotropism is an independent risk factor for metastasis or survival
Tumor Infiltrating Lymphocytes	Brisk: diffuse infiltrate of lymphocytes throughout the dermal tumor cells or the presence of lymphocytes along 90% of the circumference of the lesion base Non-Brisk: focal infiltrate of lymphocytes Absent: no lymphocytes are admixed with melanoma cells, but may be present perivascularly	Presence of a host inflammatory response is generally associated with a better prognosis, but prognostic power is limited because of the inconsistency in controlling for other prognostic features in previous studies There is lack of research on the functional status of lymphocytic infiltrates to determine whether they are operating as an active vs anergic immune response
Vertical Growth Phase	Presence of aggregates of tumor cells in the dermis with at least one nest in the dermis being larger than the largest intraepidermal nest, or the presence of mitoses	Indicates a worse prognosis, but its value as an independent risk factor has not been consistently validated; confounding factors are Breslow thickness and mitotic rate, with significant controversy in thin melanomas

Abbreviations: ALM, acral-lentiginous melanoma; LMM, lentigo maligna melanoma; NM, nodular melanoma; SSM, superficial spreading melanoma.
Data from Payette MJ, Katz M, Grant-Kels JM. Melanoma prognostic factors found in the dermatopathology report. J Clin Dermatol 2009;27:53–74.

Table 12
Three-year survival rates for patients with melanoma after solid organ transplantation compared with SEER data

Feature	3-Year Overall Survival (%)			3-Year MM Cause-Specific Survival (%)		
	Study Cohort (95% CI)	Expected Derived from SEER	P Value	Study Cohort (95% CI)	Expected Derived from SEER	P Value
Breslow thickness (mm)						
≤0.75[a]	88.2 (79.0–98.5)	96.7	<.001	97.8 (93.7–100)	98.8	.70
0.76–1.50	80.8 (65.4–99.7)	93.3	<.001	89.4 (76.5–100)	96.6	.08
1.51–3.00	51.2 (32.4–80.9)	87.4	<.001	73.2 (53.2–100)	91.0	.002
>3.00	55.3 (37.1–82.4)	76.2	.007	73.9 (56.4–96.6)	81.0	.31
Clark level[b]						
I	87.6 (75.3–100)	98.2	<.001	100	99.8	.002
II	87.9 (77.4–99.8)	96.7	.002	97.4 (92.4–100)	99.3	.19
III	59.1 (41.2–85.0)	94.9	<.001	82.8 (65.3–100)	97.4	<.001
IV	49.6 (36.3–67.8)	88.9	<.001	65.8 (51.8–83.7)	92.4	<.001

[a] Includes in situ in the sample of patients who received organ transplants. For comparison with the Breslow thickness–specific expected survival derived from SEER data for 1988 to 2006, 1 patient in the study sample who received a diagnosis in the early 1980s with a Breslow thickness of 0.75 mm or smaller was excluded.
[b] Results are not presented for Clark level V because of the small number of patients in the study cohort (n = 12).

Adapted from Brewer JD, Christenson LJ, Weaver AL, et al. Malignant melanoma in solid transplant recipients: collection of database cases and comparison with surveillance, epidemiology, and end results data for outcome analysis. Arch Dermatol 2011;147:790–6; with permission.

relationship between CD4 cell counts and time to first melanoma recurrence. These data demonstrate a more aggressive course with an increased risk of mortality among patients who are HIV positive with melanoma, necessitating antiretroviral therapy and close surveillance to detect the presence of metastatic disease.

Pregnancy

Several retrospective reviews with small case numbers from the 1970s and 1980s indicated that melanoma in pregnancy portended a worse prognosis than in nonpregnant women,[42–44] but when controlling for age, race, stage, and tumor thickness, no significant difference is found.[45,46] There is some debate on disease-free intervals (DFI) for melanoma that occurs during pregnancy, but the overall survival is not significantly different for melanoma diagnosed before, during, or after pregnancy compared with age-matched nonpregnant women.[47] The current recommendation of waiting 2 to 3 years to become pregnant after a diagnosis of melanoma is based on recurrence data for all patients. It is not based on data indicating a worse outcome with pregnancy, but the literature on the prognosis of melanoma occurring before pregnancy is limited.[48]

As for the effect of maternal melanoma on the fetus, the prognosis for the fetus is not significantly different unless the mother has widespread metastatic disease. When evaluating the rate of Cesarean delivery, length of stay, risk of low birth weight or very low birth weight, prematurity, hospital charges, or neonatal death, no significant difference has been found compared with controls.[45] Regarding the risk for metastasis to the fetus, this risk is difficult to ascertain because few cases of metastasis to the placenta and subsequently to the fetus have been reported in the literature. According to the available studies, when placental melanoma metastasis is found, metastasis to the fetus is reported to occur 25% of the time.[48] The pathologist should be alerted to examine the placenta carefully in women with metastatic melanoma.

Race and Ethnicity

Melanoma occurs most commonly among whites (95%), followed by Hispanics, American Indians/Alaskan Natives, Asians/Pacific Islanders, and blacks; with a higher percentage of advanced and thicker melanomas occurring among nonwhite individuals. In the most recent study on different ethnic groups with invasive melanoma in the United States, the 5-year MSS were calculated for the previously mentioned groups using 38 population-based cancer registries (National Program of Cancer Registries and SEER programs) containing 288,741 melanoma cases from 1999 to 2006.[49] The study population was comprised of 95% white, 0.5% black, 0.3% Asian/Pacific Islander, and 0.2%

American Indians/Alaskan Natives. Metastatic melanoma was found in 4% of cases among whites and 7% to 13% in nonwhite patients. Melanomas less than 1.0 mm occurred 63% of the time in white patients and only 38% to 48% in the other ethnic groups. Whites and Hispanics had lower rates of melanomas thicker than 4 mm (5% and 8%, respectively) compared with 11% in each of the other racial groups. Overall 5-year MSS was lowest for blacks (78.2%), followed by Asian/Pacific Islanders (80.7%), American Indian (84.9%), and highest for whites (90.0%). The 5-year MSS was similar for localized melanoma among all racial and ethnic groups except blacks, which was slightly lower, whereas there were no significant differences in the 5-year MSS for advanced melanomas.

Socioeconomic Status

A study taking a socioeconomic perspective on melanoma prognosis compared 17,702 melanoma cases in the SEER database from 1988 to 1993 with sociodemographic data from the 1990 US census. It revealed education level, ethnicity, and income to be significant prognostic indicators.[50] This study found that patients with melanoma who live in areas where greater than 79% of the population has more than a high school level of education (odds ratio [OR] 0.4, 95% CI, 0.3–0.5), more than 85% of the population are white residents (OR 0.7, 95% CI, 0.5–0.8), or the median income is greater than $28,750 (OR 0.4, 95% CI, 0.2–0.5) were less likely to have a poor prognosis. Education seems to be the strongest predictor of melanoma survival, demonstrating 3.3 times more variance than race and 1.9 times more than income.

MELANOMA GENETIC BIOMARKERS

Molecular biomarkers are defined as a biologic component that can be used as an indicator of a disease or physiologic state. They are typically genes, gene products, enzymes, or hormones.[51] Numerous melanoma biomarkers have been identified,[52–55] with most of the early research focused on protein biomarkers, such as LDH. LDH is the only molecular biomarker used in the AJCC 2009 melanoma staging system, and its presence in stage IV disease indicates a worsening prognosis, as described earlier. Aside from LDH, inconsistent results between studies caused by critical methodological differences have limited the usefulness of previously proposed biomarkers.[56] In more recent years, through applying stricter study methodology and an increased understanding of cancer's genetic pathways, more clinically significant data on melanoma biomarkers have been

produced and a shift has occurred toward identifying prognostic genetic biomarkers.[57]

Melanoma Genetic Biomarkers

In recent years, medical science's understanding of a cancer's potential to grow and evade the body's immune system has evolved from an anatomic and histologic level to a biomolecular approach. Revisiting Dr William Clark's early attempts to quantify melanoma's aggressive nature through differentiating radial and vertical growth phases, he hoped to capture genetic aberrations through a more comprehensive quantification of their histologic manifestations.[3] Through this early work, Dr Clark and several other notable melanoma researchers introduced the concept that that the mere presence of cancer on the anatomic or histologic level may not be as important as what its presence and descriptive features represent.[58] Essentially, this work proposed the view that the anatomic and histologic features of melanoma can serve as manifestations of a cancer's biologic aggressiveness and their presence or numerical measurement should not be the sole focus.[5] Although it is important that a melanoma *has* invaded to a certain depth, it may be more significant that a melanoma *can* invade to a certain depth.[3] Current prognostic factors, such as the Breslow thickness, predict a certain overall survival, whereas the identification of the tumor's genetic composition will potentially define the risk of being in the proportion that does not survive, thus creating a new model for prognosis in patients with melanoma.[58,59]

The Prognosis of Mutated-BRAF Melanomas

By identifying the major genetic pathways that contribute to the development of melanoma,[60] the genes involved in these pathways have become a prime target for therapy and prognosis indication.[61] The current most promising prognostic genetic biomarker is the *BRAF* oncogene.[62] The *BRAF* oncogene, which codes a serine-threonine protein kinase, is found in the Ras/mitogen-activated protein kinase (*MAPK*) pathway. Mutated *BRAF* has been reported to be present in 33% to 47% of primary melanomas and 41% to 55% of metastatic melanomas.[63] Particular emphasis has been placed on the mutated *BRAF* oncogene because its presence is successfully used by the new targeted molecular therapies.[64]

In a recent study, *BRAF* and *NRAS* oncogene mutation status was evaluated in 302 archived tissue samples of primary cutaneous melanoma.[65] The most common mutations in *BRAF* and *NRAS* were evaluated to identify clinical and morphologic features correlated with the presence of these gene mutations. This study found that melanomas with a *BRAF* mutation (codon 600) were more likely than wild-type BRAF to have increased upward scatter and nest formation of intraepidermal melanocytes; thickening of the involved epidermis; sharp demarcation from the surrounding skin; the presence of a larger, rounder, and more pigmented tumor cells; and age less than 55 years (age was the strongest predictor of BRAF mutational status). However, no overall *BRAF* prognostic value was found in this study. Stage 4 patients with an *NRAS* Q61 mutation have a worse survival than patients with wild-type *NRAS*.

In a similar recent study evaluating 197 patients with metastatic melanoma, a comparison of melanomas with the two most common *BRAF* mutations (V600E and V600K) with wild-type *BRAF* was conducted.[63] Of the 197 patients, 48% of the patients were found to have a *BRAF* mutation. The most significant ($P<.05$) associations found in mutated *BRAF* melanomas were histopathologic subtype (superficial spreading or nodular melanoma), presence of mitoses, single or occult primary melanoma, truncal location, and age less than 50 years at the time of diagnosis. A lack of chronic sun damage was also found to correlate with the presence of a *BRAF* mutation, but the sample size (n = 25) limits this factor's validity. Important features that were not correlated with a *BRAF* mutation were an associated nevus, Breslow thickness, ulceration, gender, family history of melanoma, type of distant metastases, LDH status, Eastern Cooperative Oncology Group performance status (adjusted for age), development of brain metastases, and response to first-line chemotherapy. Similar to previous studies regarding the prognostic value of *BRAF*, this study found that there was no significant difference in the DFI between mutated *BRAF* and wild-type *BRAF*. However, this study did show that there is a potential negative outcome when metastatic disease occurs in melanomas with the *BRAF* mutation. The median overall survival for the cohort of patients of melanoma with mutated *BRAF* not treated with a *BRAF* inhibitor compared with wild-type BRAF melanomas was 11.1 months versus 46.1 months ($P = .006$), respectively. When evaluating patients only with newly diagnosed metastatic melanoma during the study period, a more representative subgroup of the metastatic population, the median survival times were 5.7 months for patients with a *BRAF* mutation not treated with a BRAF inhibitor and 8.5 months for *BRAF* wild-type patients ($P = .147$). These data are limited because of the selection bias created from the subgroup of patients that were included in the *BRAF* inhibitor studies, but a trend is seen indicating a poorer prognosis in melanomas with a mutated *BRAF*. This trend necessitates further

research on outcomes before the use of *BRAF* inhibitors.

REFERENCES

1. Clark WH Jr, From L, Bernardino EA, et al. The histogenesis and biological behavior of primary human malignant melanomas of the skin. Cancer Res 1969;29:705–26.
2. Breslow A. Thickness, cross-sectional areas and depth of invasion in the prognosis of cutaneous melanoma. Ann Surg 1970;172:902–8.
3. Clark WH Jr, Elder DE, Guerry D 4th, et al. Model predicting survival in stage I melanoma based on tumor progression. J Natl Cancer Inst 1989;81:1893–904.
4. Balch CM, Gershenwald JE, Soong SJ, et al. Final version of 2009 AJCC melanoma staging and classification. J Clin Oncol 2009;27:6199–206.
5. Spatz A, Batist G, Eggermont AM. The biology behind prognostic factors of cutaneous melanoma. Curr Opin Oncol 2010;22:163–8.
6. Balch CM, Gershenwald JE, Soong SJ, et al. Melanoma of the skin. In: Edge SB, Byrd DR, Compton CC, et al, editors. AJCC staging manual. 7th edition. New York: Springer; 2010. p. 325–44.
7. Balch CM, Gershenwald JE, Soong SJ, et al. Update on the melanoma staging system: the importance of sentinel node staging and primary tumor mitotic rate. J Surg Oncol 2011;104:379–85.
8. Payette MJ, Katz M, Grant-Kels JM. Melanoma prognostic factors found in the dermatopathology report. J Clin Dermatol 2009;27:53–74.
9. Sarpa HG, Reinke K, Shaikh L, et al. Prognostic significance of extent of ulceration in primary cutaneous melanoma. Am J Surg Pathol 2006;30:1396–400.
10. Balch CM, Atkins MB, Buzaid AC, et al. Melanoma of the skin. In: Green FL, Page DL, Fleming ID, et al, editors. AJCC staging manual. 6th edition. New York: Springer; 2002. p. 209–20.
11. Morton DL, Thompson JF, Cochran AJ, et al. Sentinel-node biopsy or nodal observation in melanoma. N Engl J Med 2006;355:1307–17.
12. Gershenwald JE, Ross MI. Sentinel-lymph-node biopsy for cutaneous melanoma. N Engl J Med 2011;364:1738–45.
13. Balch CM, Gershenwald JE, Soong SJ, et al. Multivariate analysis of prognostic factors among 2,313 patients with stage III melanoma: comparison of nodal micrometastases versus macrometastases. J Clin Oncol 2010;28:2452–9.
14. Ohsie SJ, Sarantopoulos GP, Ochran AJ, et al. Immunohistochemical characteristics of melanoma. J Cutan Pathol 2008;35:433–44.
15. Van Akkooi AC, de Wilt JH, Verhoef C, et al. Clinical relevance of melanoma micrometastases (<0.1 mm) in sentinel nodes: are these nodes to be considered negative? Ann Oncol 2006;17:1578–85.

16. Scheri RP, Essner R, Turner RR, et al. Isolated tumor cells in the sentinel node affect long-term prognosis of patients with melanoma. Ann Surg Oncol 2007;14: 2861–6.

17. van der Pleog AP, van Akkooi AC, Rutkowski P, et al. Prognosis in patients with sentinel node-positive melanoma is accurately defined by the combined Rotterdam tumor load and Dewar topography criteria. J Clin Oncol 2011;29:2206–14.

18. Satzger I, Volker B, Al Ghazal M, et al. Prognostic significance of histopathological parameters in sentinel nodes of melanoma patients. Histopathology 2007;50:764–72.

19. Balch CM, Soong SJ, Murad TM, et al. A multifactorial analysis of melanoma. IV. Prognostic factors in 200 melanoma patients with distant metastases (stage III). J Clin Oncol 1983;1:126–34.

20. Buzzell RA, Zitelli JA. Favorable prognostic factors in recurrent and metastatic melanoma. J Am Acad Dermatol 1996;34:798–803.

21. Balch CM, Soong SJ, Gershenwald JE. Prognostic factors analysis of 17,600 melanoma patients: validation of the American Joint Committee on Cancer melanoma staging system. J Clin Oncol 2001;19: 3622–34.

22. Neuman HB, Patel A, Ishill M. A single-institution validation of the AJCC staging system for stage IV melanoma. Ann Surg Oncol 2008;15:2034–41.

23. Rutkowski P, Nowecki ZI, Dziewirski W, et al. Melanoma without a detectable primary site with metastases to lymph nodes. Dermatol Surg 2010;36: 828–76.

24. Katz KA, Jonash E, Hodi FS, et al. Melanoma of unknown primary: experience at Massachusetts General Hospital and Dana-Farber Cancer Institute. Melanoma Res 2005;14:77–82.

25. Lee CC, Fairies MB, Wanek LA, et al. Improved survival for stage IV melanoma from an unknown primary site. J Clin Oncol 2009;27:3489–95.

26. Soong SJ, Ding S, Coit D, et al. Predicting survival outcome of localized melanoma: an electronic prediction tool based on the AJCC melanoma database. Ann Surg Oncol 2010;17:2006–14.

27. Soong SJ, Ding S, Coit D, et al. Models of predicting melanoma outcome. In: Balch CM, Houghton AN, Sober AJ, et al, editors. Cutaneous melanoma. 5th edition. St Louis (MO): Quality Medical Publishing; 2009. p. 87–104.

28. Lasithiotakis K, Leiter U, Meier f, et al. Age and gender are significant independent predictors of survival in primary cutaneous melanoma. Cancer 2008;112:1795–804.

29. Pollack LA, Li J, Berkowitz Z, et al. Melanoma survival in the United States, 1992 to 2005. J Am Acad Dermatol 2011;65:S78–86.

30. Ferrari A, Bono A, Baldi M, et al. Does melanoma behave differently in younger children than in adults? A retrospective study of 33 cases of childhood melanoma from a single institution. Pediatrics 2005;115:640–54.

31. Livestro DP, Kaine EM, Michaelson JS, et al. Melanoma in the young: differences and similarities with adult melanoma: a case-matched controlled analysis. Cancer 2007;110:614–24.

32. Moore-Olufemi S, Herzog C, Warneke C, et al. Outcomes in pediatric melanoma: comparing prepubertal to adolescent pediatric patients. Ann Surg 2011;253:1211–5.

33. Joosse A, de Vries E, Eckel R, et al. Gender differences in melanoma survival: female patients have a decreased risk of metastasis. J Invest Dermatol 2011;131:719–26.

34. Lachiewicz AM, Berwick M, Wiggins CL, et al. Survival differences between patients with scalp or neck melanoma and those with melanoma of other sites in the surveillance, epidemiology, and end results (SEER) program. Arch Dermatol 2008; 144:515–21.

35. Bichakjian CK, Halpern AC, Johnson TM, et al. Guidelines of care for the management of primary cutaneous melanoma. J Am Acad Dermatol 2011;65:1032–47.

36. Colegio OR, Proby CM, Bordeaux, et al. Prognosis of pretransplant melanoma, letter to the editor. Am J Transplant 2009;9:862.

37. Dapprich DC, Weenig RH, Rohlinger AL, et al. Outcomes of melanoma in recipients of solid organ transplant. J Am Acad Dermatol 2008;59:405–17.

38. Zwald FO, Christenson LJ, Billingsley EM, et al. Melanoma in solid organ transplant recipients. Am J Transplant 2010;10:1297–304.

39. Brewer JD, Christenson LJ, Weaver AL, et al. Malignant melanoma in solid transplant recipients: collection of database cases and comparison with surveillance, epidemiology, and end results data for outcome analysis. Arch Dermatol 2011;147:790–6.

40. Burke MM, Kluger HM, Golden M, et al. Case report: response to ipilimumab in a patient with HIV with metastatic melanoma. J Clin Oncol 2011;29:e792–4.

41. Rodrigues LK, Klencke BJ, Vin-Christian K, et al. Altered clinical course of malignant melanoma in HIV-positive patients. Arch Dermatol 2002;138: 765–70.

42. Shiu MH, Schottenfeld D, Maclean B, et al. Adverse effect of pregnancy on melanoma: a reappraisal. Cancer 1976;37:181–7.

43. Reintgen DS, McCarty KS, Vollmer R, et al. Malignant melanoma and pregnancy. Cancer 1985;55: 1340–4.

44. Houghton AN, Flannery J, Viola MV. Malignant melanoma of the skin occurring during pregnancy. Cancer 1981;48:407–10.

45. O'Meara AT, Cress R, Xing G, et al. Malignant melanoma in pregnancy: a population-based evaluation. Cancer 2005;103:1217–26.

46. Pages C, Robert C, Thomas L. Management and outcome of metastatic melanoma during pregnancy. Br J Dermatol 2010;162:274–81.

47. Jhaveri MB, Driscoll MS, Grant-Kels JM. Melanoma in pregnancy. Clin Obstet Gynecol 2011;54:537–45.

48. Driscoll MS, Grant-Kels JM. Hormones, nevi, and melanoma: an approach to the patient. J Am Acad Dermatol 2007;57:919–31.

49. Wu XC, Eide MJ, King J, et al. Racial and ethnic variations in incidence and survival of cutaneous melanoma in the United States, 1999-2006. J Am Acad Dermatol 2011;65:S26–37.

50. Eide MJ, Weinstock MA, Clark MA. Demographic and socioeconomic predictors of melanoma prognosis in the United States. J Health Care Poor Underserved 2009;20:227–45.

51. Grimm EA, Hoon DS, Duncan LM. Biomarkers for melanoma. In: Balch CM, Houghton AN, Sober AJ, et al, editors. Cutaneous melanoma. 5th edition. St Louis (MO): Quality Medical Publishing; 2009. p. 883–97.

52. Utikal J, Schadendorf D, Ugurel S. Serologic and immunohistochemical prognostic biomarkers. Arch Dermatol Res 2007;298:469–77.

53. Haass NK, Smalley KS. Melanoma biomarkers: current status and utility in diagnosis, prognosis, and response to therapy. Mol Diagn Ther 2009;13:283–96.

54. Gould-Rothberg BE, Bracken MB, Rimm DL. Tissue biomarkers for prognosis in cutaneous melanoma: a systematic review and meta-analysis. J Natl Cancer Inst 2009;101:452–74.

55. Gould-Rothberg BE, Rimm DL. Biomarkers: the useful and the not so useful - an assessment of molecular prognostic markers for cutaneous melanoma. J Invest Dermatol 2010;130:1971–87.

56. Schramm SJ, Mann GJ. Melanoma prognosis: a REMARK-based systematic review and bioinformatic analysis of immunohistochemical and gene microarray studies. Mol Cancer Ther 2011;10: 1520–8.

57. Schramm SJ, Campain AE, Scolyer RA, et al. Review and cross-validation of gene expression signatures and melanoma prognosis. J Invest Dermatol 2012; 132:274–83.

58. Elder DE. Prognostic models for melanoma: invited review. J Cutan Pathol 2010;37(Suppl 1):68–75.

59. Gershenwald JE, Soong SJ, Balch CM, et al. 2010 TNM staging system for cutaneous melanoma...and beyond [editorial]. Ann Surg Oncol 2010;17:1475–7.

60. Hocker TL, Singh MK, Tsao H. Melanoma genetics and therapeutic approaches in the 21st century: moving from the bench side to the bedside. J Invest Dermatol 2008;128:2575–95.

61. Smalley KS. Understanding melanoma signaling networks as the basis for molecular targeted therapy. J Invest Dermatol 2010;130:28–37.

62. Flaherty KT. Is it good or bad to find a BRAF mutation? J Clin Oncol 2011;29:1229–30.

63. Long GV, Menzies AM, Nagrial AM, et al. Prognostic and clinicopathologic associations of oncogenic BRAF in metastatic melanoma. J Clin Oncol 2011; 29:1239–46.

64. Flaherty KT, Puzanov I, Kim KB, et al. Inhibition of mutated, activated BRAF in metastatic melanoma. N Engl J Med 2010;363:809–19.

65. Amaya V, Fridlyand J, Bauer J, et al. Improving melanoma classification by integrating genetic and morphologic features. PLoS Med 2008;5:941–51.

Surgical Treatment of Malignant Melanoma
Practical Guidelines

Steven M. Levine, MD[a], Richard L. Shapiro, MD[b],*

KEYWORDS

- Malignant melanoma • Cutaneous malignany • Skin cancer • Surgical treatment

KEY POINTS

- Melanoma is currently the fifth and sixth most common solid malignancy diagnosed in men and women, respectively.
- Melanoma accounts for more than 75% of all deaths from skin cancer.
- Treatment of this malignancy relies on appropriate staging.
- Biopsy technique and tissue diagnosis are crucial to developing the appropriate treatment plan for melanoma.

INTRODUCTION

The incidence of cutaneous malignant melanoma has been rising steadily over the past century. In the United States, the lifetime risk of developing an in situ or invasive melanoma is now estimated to be 1 in 30 in comparison with 1 in 1500 in 1935.[1–4] Melanoma is currently the fifth and sixth most common solid malignancy diagnosed in men and women, respectively.[5] Although accounting for only 4% of cases of all cutaneous malignancies, melanoma accounts for more than 75% of all deaths from skin cancer.[6] In 2012, it is estimated that 70,230 Americans will be diagnosed with invasive melanoma as well as an additional 53,360 with in situ lesions, and 8790 people, 1 person every hour, will die.[7] Efforts during the past decade to make the clinical characteristics of early cutaneous melanoma more widely known[8,9] have resulted in most patients (82%) being diagnosed in the early stages, when the primary tumor is confined to the skin.[10] Five-year survival rates exceeding 90% are achieved in patients

with invasive melanomas confined to the skin in comparison with rates of approximately 60% and 5% in those with regional lymph node and distant metastases, respectively.[11]

EPIDEMIOLOGY AND RISK FACTORS

Melanoma is diagnosed within a broad range of ages beginning in the third decade of life, although occurring slightly more commonly in women younger than 40 and in men older than 40. Although the peak incidence is in the late 40s, melanoma is the commonest cancer diagnosed in young adults 25 to 29 years of age and the second most frequently diagnosed malignant tumor in patients 15 to 29 years of age. Melanoma most frequently arises on the skin of the back in men and on the lower extremities in women. In darker-skinned ethnic groups (African American, Asian, and Hispanic), melanoma frequently arises in the volar and plantar skin (acral) or in the nail bed (subungual). Although 95% of melanomas originate in the skin, they develop in other anatomic locations, such as the eye and mucous

[a] Institute of Reconstructive Plastic Surgery, Department of Plastic Surgery, New York University Langone Medical Center, New York, NY 10016, USA; [b] Division of Surgical Oncology, Department of Surgery, NYU Clinical Cancer Center, New York University Langone Medical Center, 160 East 34th Street, 4th Floor, New York, NY 10016, USA
* Corresponding author.
E-mail address: Richard.Shapiro@nyumc.org

Dermatol Clin 30 (2012) 487–501
doi:10.1016/j.det.2012.04.009

derm.theclinics.com

membranes, including the vagina and anus.[12] Approximately 3% to 10% of patients present with metastatic disease in the absence of a clinically identified primary melanoma.[13,14] Patients with metastases from an unknown or occult primary melanoma have the same prognosis and should be managed in the same manner as patients with known primary lesions.[15,16]

The typical patient with melanoma has light-colored eyes, reddish or blonde hair, and a fair or ruddy complexion that tans poorly and burns easily during brief periods of intense sun exposure.[9] Blistering sunburns sustained as a child or teenager are a significant risk factor for the development of melanoma and more deleterious than prolonged sun exposure in the later years.[17] More recently, an association between the exposure of teenagers and young adults to UV radiation through the use of tanning beds and the development of cutaneous malignancies including melanoma has been reported and is currently under intense scrutiny.[18]

The development of atypical (dysplastic) nevi is a significant risk factor for melanoma. Although patients with more than 100 dysplastic nevi (atypical mole syndrome) have a 10% to 15% incidence of melanoma in their lifetime, the presence of even a single atypical mole also increases the risk.[19-21] The prophylactic excision of dysplastic nevi is not justified, however, because in most patients melanoma arises from normal skin, as opposed to from within a preexisting benign nevus.[22,23] Children with large congenital nevi are at increased risk for melanoma, although this occurs uncommonly (10%–15%), and almost exclusively in patients with truncal lesions and within the first 2 decades of life.[24-26]

A thorough physical examination includes an inspection of the entire cutaneous surface (including the volar and plantar skin, webspaces, and mucous membranes) of a completely undressed patient under appropriate lightning conditions. The ABCDE rule helps to identify those pigmented lesions most likely to be melanoma.[27-30] Lesions that are Asymmetric have irregular Borders, Color variation, and Diameters exceeding 6 mm (the size of a pencil eraser) are considered to be suspicious. In addition, any pigmented lesion that Evolves (or becomes darker or lighter in color, increases in size or becomes raised, or itches or bleeds) should immediately arouse suspicion. The use of dermoscopy,[31] as well as more recently developed advanced computer-aided digital imaging tools,[32] may be used to more selectively identify lesions for biopsy that are more likely to be malignant, obviating the need for excision of less suspicious moles. Complete excisional biopsy, however, of any preexisting mole that has changed in appearance, itches, or bleeds is recommended.

Patients diagnosed previously with a melanoma have a 3% to 6% risk of developing a second primary cutaneous melanoma in the course of their lifetime.[33,34] In addition, there is a 3% to 10% incidence of melanoma in first-degree family members.[35] Formal genetics consultation should be considered in patients with significant family history of melanoma, as well as families affected by cancers of the breasts and ovaries. These patients may harbor a deleterious BRCA mutation that confers a risk of developing melanoma in addition to other known solid tumors.[36] Lifelong total cutaneous surveillance of all patients with melanoma and their immediate families is also strongly recommended.

PROPER BIOPSY TECHNIQUE

Accurate sampling of any lesion suspicious for melanoma may be considered adequate only if sufficient tissue is obtained to definitively confirm or exclude a histologic diagnosis of malignancy. The biopsy must accurately assess the depth of tumor penetration of the skin, which strongly determines the scope of the initial diagnostic evaluation, the extent of surgical resection in terms of margin width, and appropriateness of sentinel lymphadenectomy in newly diagnosed clinically node-negative patients.[37,38]

Complete surgical excision has long been considered the biopsy method of choice for all cutaneous lesions suspected of being melanoma.[39] This technique can be performed rapidly in the office setting using local anesthesia and enables complete assessment of tumor thickness, should the lesion indeed prove to be melanoma. Although punch and shave biopsies may be suboptimal because insufficient sampling of atypical elements may occur and/or tumor thickness in malignant lesions is underestimated, recent studies have confirmed the adequacy of these techniques when performed properly.[40] If a biopsy is nondiagnostic or significant clinical concern persists, complete excisional biopsy should be performed. Incisional biopsy of unusually large or broad lesions is acceptable only if the diagnosis of melanoma is confirmed and tumor thickness is assessed accurately. For extremity lesions, surgical biopsy incisions should always be oriented vertically so as not to interfere with or complicate subsequent definitive excision and reconstruction.

ADVANCED HISTOLOGIC EVALUATION OF BIOPSY MATERIAL

Immunohistochemistry is used routinely to complement standard histopathologic techniques in confirming the diagnosis of melanoma. The monoclonal antibody HMB-45[41,42] and the polyvalent antibody recognizing the S-100 antigen[43,44] are used most extensively. Although a combination of the 2 may improve the histopathologic characterization of difficult lesions, neither has proved to be completely reliable. For example, the S-100 protein, although expressed in almost all melanomas, is also detected in other tissues of neural crest derivation. Although HMB-45 staining may be used to distinguish unusual melanomas from unusual benign nevi, it is sometimes not identified in amelanotic and desmoplastic melanomas[42] nor in the metastatic lesions.

Further microscopic evaluation of melanoma to identify histologic evidence of ulceration and to quantify mitosis (if present), is now required to determine melanoma staging and plan surgery appropriately.[45,46] The presence of histologic regression may also indicate a more aggressive phenotype than a melanoma of equivalent thickness, and may influence the diagnostic evaluation and possibly the extent of surgery. The identification of unusual melanoma subtypes, such as nevoid, spitzoid, and desmoplastic variants, refines the diagnosis, and in some instances may also influence the scope of surgery. In patients with purely desmoplastic melanomas, wide margins should be maintained, but sentinel lymphadenectomy may be unnecessary in patients with lesions thinner than 4 mm, which are associated with increased rates of local recurrence, yet rarely metastasize to the regional nodes.[47] Malignancy is sometimes difficult to confirm in lesions exhibiting nevoid or spitzoid features especially when arising in children and teenagers. Obtaining additional expert dermatopathologic review is essential in many such cases.

Molecular profiling and the identification of biomarkers, such as mutations in BRAF and KIT, in thicker or locally advanced primary, recurrent, or metastatic lesions, is also now routinely requested to guide newly available adjuvant targeted therapies.[48,49]

ASSESSMENT OF TUMOR THICKNESS AND STAGING

Tumor thickness is a measure of the vertical growth phase of the melanoma and is a significant prognostic indicator of the potential for local recurrence, metastases, and death.[11] An accurate assessment of tumor thickness is therefore critical in the planning of an appropriate metastatic survey, surgery, adjuvant treatment, and follow-up schedule. Melanoma thickness is assessed in millimeters by ocular microscopy as described by Breslow[50] or by increasing levels of dermal penetration in the manner described by Clark and colleagues.[51] The

micro staging techniques of both Clark and colleagues[51] and Breslow[50] have enabled a more accurate grouping of patients with primary melanomas based on reproducible measurements of tumor thickness and are predictors of survival. Melanoma is staged according to published American Joint Committee on Cancer (AJCC) guidelines using the TNM system.[52] The AJCC staging system for melanoma has been officially revised and expanded in recent years.[53,54] The current 2010 version further stratifies groups of patients by including important prognostic factors, such as ulceration and the presence of mitoses in the primary lesion. The new classification revises the importance of Clark level in the T classification of tumor thickness, and further delineates the extent of nodal involvement by recognizing the extent of microscopic nodal involvement of the sentinel node and number of nodes affected.[55–57] Other parameters, such as lactate dehydrogenase (LDH) level and anatomic site of distant metastatic disease, are also maintained in this more recent staging system.[52] Patients seeking an opinion after lesion excision at another institution should be encouraged to submit all outside reports and biopsy slides for an in-house review to confirm not only the diagnosis of melanoma but also to precisely measure tumor thickness before planning definitive surgery.

PREOPERATIVE METASTATIC EVALUATION

Preoperative metastatic survey is determined primarily by the thickness and histologic features of the primary melanoma and disease stage at presentation. No laboratory or radiologic metastatic evaluation is required for patients with malignant melanoma in situ or invasive lesions thinner than 0.5 mm. Patients with invasive melanomas thicker than 0.5 mm but thinner than 1.0 mm undergo chest radiograph and routine blood chemistries (including LDH) primarily as a baseline, although the risk of distant metastases is minimal (<3%). Patients with intermediate-thickness lesions (1–4 mm) are also evaluated initially with chest radiography and routine blood chemistries, although the yield of confirming metastatic disease is low. Patients presenting with thick lesions (>4 mm), less thick lesions (>2 mm) with ulceration or mitoses, or in the presence of satellite or in-transit metastases have a significant risk of metastases to the regional nodes (60%–75%) and distant sites (30%–50%). These patients should be evaluated with advanced imaging modalities with intravenous contrast, which may include computed tomography (CT) or fluorodeoxyglucose (FDG)-based positron emission tomography (PET) CT scans, and magnetic resonance imaging (MRI) of the brain. Although the actual benefit of performing such advanced and often expensive examinations is controversial,[58] they do allow for more precise staging and allow for stratification on entry into clinical trials. The degree of suspicion with which ambiguous radiologic findings are viewed is dependent on the risk of metastases as assessed by physical examination, melanoma thickness, and disease stage. Indeterminate findings suspicious for metastases on any scan are investigated further and confirmed cytologically or histologically using image-guided needle aspiration biopsy.

EXCISION MARGINS

The propensity of melanoma to disseminate and recur locally is well documented and has historically influenced the surgical approach to this tumor.[59,60] The surgical treatment of melanoma in terms of margin excision width has been studied extensively in prospectively randomized trials. Appropriately, the margins recommended for definitive melanoma excison have become increasingly more conservative and esthetically sensitive over the past several decades (Table 1).[61–69] Excision margin width is determined primarily by lesion thickness as measured in millimeters. The peripheral border or edge of a faintly pigmented or regressed melanoma may be difficult to ascertain in some patients, especially in those with extremely sun-damaged skin. Examination of the lesion using dermoscopy or a Wood lamp may help delineate the periphery of these melanomas to avoid excising the lesion too narrowly, resulting in inadequate surgical margins.

Malignant melanoma in situ is excised with 5-mm margins. Mohs micrographic surgery has been attempted in the treatment of these early noninvasive lesions but the results have been disappointing, possibly owing to the presence of clinically occult discontinuous microscopic foci of disease.[70] Thin (<1 mm) melanomas have an extremely low rate of local recurrence (<2%) and are excised with 1-cm margins.[67,71,72] For intermediate-thickness (1–4 mm) lesions, the safety of 2-cm excision margins has been confirmed in prospectively randomized studies.[69] Excision of narrower 1-cm margins have also more recently been shown to be adequate for lesions thinner than 2 mm in prospective randomized trials. Despite a slightly higher rate of local recurrence, there appears to be no significant impact on overall survival.[65,73] These data support the use of narrower excision margins for selected lesions and may greatly enhance the cosmetic result in anatomic areas such as the face. For thicker melanomas (>4 mm) the guidelines are less certain. Whereas 2-cm margins may be appropriate for these lesions based on currently available data, in selected circumstances (very thick lesions or in the presence of multiple satellite metastases) many surgeons advocate wider excision margins of 3 cm. It is unlikely, however, that margins exceeding 2 cm significantly impact on the higher rates of local recurrence (12%) and poor survival (55% at 5 years) with which these lesions are associated.[74] The failure of more radical procedures using wider (3–5 cm) excision margins, or in the past, limb amputation,[75] to diminish local recurrence rates and increase survival in patients with thick (>4 mm) melanomas, is further evidence that local recurrence reflects the biologic aggressiveness of the primary lesion, not the inadequacy of the primary excision.

Most excision site defects may be closed primarily, although split- or full-thickness skin grafting, or flap closure, may be required for the reconstruction of larger defects. In patients requiring a skin graft for closure of a wound located on the extremity, skin should not be harvested from an area in close proximity to the melanoma, as this could potentially reintroduce tumor cells into the reconstructed wound. Similarly, the changing of gloves and surgical instruments is prudent and should be performed routinely after melanoma excision to avoid wound contamination.

TREATMENT OF THE REGIONAL LYMPH NODES
Clinically Negative Regional Lymph Nodes

Most patients with newly diagnosed melanoma exhibit no evidence of regional lymph node metastases. The potential for regional lymph node metastases is assessed most accurately by tumor thickness. Malignant melanoma in situ by definition has no significant potential for lymph node metastases. For thin melanomas (<1 mm) the risk of nodal metastases is minimal (<5%) and therefore the complete elective dissection of the regional lymph

Table 1	
Guidelines for excision margins for primary cutaneous melanoma	
Melanoma Thickness	Excision Margin
In situ	5 mm
<1 mm	1 cm
≥1 to <4 mm	2 cm[a]
≥4 mm	2 cm[b]

[a] May be 1-cm margin for lesions thinner than 2 mm in aesthetically sensitive areas.
[b] Margin should be no less than 2 cm, although when available, a 3-cm margin is often used.

nodes is not required. Patients with intermediate-thickness lesions (1–4 mm) have a 20% to 25% incidence of microscopic regional disease and a 3% to 5% risk of distant metastases. For these reasons, this group is traditionally thought to most likely derive a therapeutic benefit from elective lymph node dissection. Prospectively randomized studies, however, have consistently failed to demonstrate a significant survival advantage with elective lymph node dissection in most patients.[61,72,76–79]

Sentinel Lymph Node Biopsy

Sentinel lymph node biopsy (SLNB) has effectively replaced elective lymph node dissection for the evaluation of clinically negative regional lymph nodes in patients with invasive primary cutaneous malignant melanoma. The technical details of intraoperative lymphatic mapping, with vital blue dye and filtered technetium radiolabeled sulfur colloid, and sentinel lymph node biopsy have been well described.[80–83] The safety, reproducibility, and validity of the procedure has been demonstrated through the results of the prospectively randomized Multicenter Selective Lymphadenectomy Trial I (MSLT I).[84,85] Precisely which specific patients will derive the greatest benefit from the sentinel lymph node biopsy procedure is less clear.

The *ideal* candidate for SLNB is the patient with a melanoma at least 1-mm thick in the absence of clinical or radiologic evidence of regional lymph node or distant metastases (**Table 2**). Lymphoscintigraphy performed before surgery must clearly demonstrate the lymphatic drainage

pathway and regional nodal drainage basin to precisely localize and excise the appropriate sentinel node. As the risk of metastasis to the regional lymph nodes is closely correlated with the thickness of the primary lesion, planning definitive surgery may be problematic for melanomas sampled incompletely by punch or shave biopsy, especially when they are thinner than 0.76 mm but extend to a biopsy margin. Repeat biopsy or complete excision of these lesions may ultimately be required to more precisely assess thickness.

Regional lymph node metastasis occurs rarely (<5%) in patients with melanomas thinner than 1.00 mm, and most often with melanomas thicker than 0.85 mm, and in lesions with extensive ulceration and mitoses.[86] In our own unpublished series of 100 SLNBs in patients with melanomas thinner than 1.00 mm, only 3 patients had positive nodes, and all 3 had primary lesions thicker than 0.85 mm. Although unproven by clinical trials, it would therefore seem reasonable to defer SLNB in patients with melanomas thinner than 0.86 mm in the absence of significant ulceration or mitoses. Melanomas with predominantly desmoplastic features similarly appear to be associated with a diminished propensity to metastasize to the regional nodes, making SLNB less compelling especially in those patients with thinner (<4 mm) desmoplastic lesions.[87] Patients with thick primary melanomas (>4 mm) and no evidence of regional lymph node metastases are still at high (50%–75%) risk to have microscopic nodal metastases and are also appropriate candidates for intraoperative lymphatic mapping and sentinel lymphadenectomy in the absence of documented distant metastatic disease or limited life expectancy from associated comorbidities.

Intraoperative lymphatic mapping and SLNB may be suboptimal for technical reasons in the following groups: patients who have already undergone definitive wide and deep excision of the melanoma (≥2 cm margins or flap closures), when lymphoscintigraphy demonstrates multiple (>2) potential regional nodal drainage basins, in patients with melanomas situated in close proximity or directly over the regional nodal drainage basin such that the weaker signal from the sentinel node is obscured by the stronger primary injection ("shine-through effect"), or when a head and neck melanoma maps to an intraparotid sentinel node (risk of facial nerve branch injury). SLNB should not be performed if lymphoscintigraphy does not clearly demonstrate a regional lymph node drainage basin and sentinel node, in patients with confirmed regional nodal or distant metastases, or in patients with limited life expectancy from melanoma or associated medical conditions.

Table 2 Sentinel lymph node biopsy for melanoma	
Melanoma Thickness[a] (mm)	SLN Biopsy
<0.76 mm	No
<0.76 mm, (+)ulceration, mitotic rate >1, tumor extends to deep biopsy margin	No
≥0.76 to <0.85 mm, no ulceration, regression, or mitoses	No
≥0.76 to <0.85 mm, (+) ulceration, regression, or mitoses	Yes
≥0.85 to <1.00 mm	Yes
≥1.00 mm	Yes

[a] Guidelines refer to thickness determined after final excision. When the melanoma extends to the deep margin of the biopsy, actual tumor thickness may be underestimated.

Intraoperatively, the sentinel node is sent immediately for microscopic examination, which may include touch preparation, frozen section analysis, or rapid immunostains. If no definitive evidence of metastatic melanoma is noted, wide and deep excision is performed as planned and the procedure is terminated. If micro metastases are confirmed in the sentinel lymph node, then formal (therapeutic) lymphadenectomy is performed at this time. Postoperatively, the sentinel lymph node is serially sectioned and examined in greater detail using standard hematoxylin and eosin staining and S-100 and HMB-45 immunostaining. The utility and clinical relevance of staging the sentinel node further on a molecular level using advanced techniques, such as reverse polymerase chain reaction, is currently being evaluated.[88–90]

Complications of SLNB are fortunately rare but should be discussed with the patient preoperatively and include, but are not limited to, dye reactions (<1%),[91] wound complications, seroma formation, the development of lymphedema (<5%), and a false-negative sentinel node (5%–15%).

Sentinel lymph node metastasis has proven to be a powerful independent predictor of subsequent disease progression and survival when confirmed histologically, immunologically, or on a molecular level.[80] Metastasis to the SLN also provides useful information, allowing for improved tumor staging that led to several major revisions of the AJCC staging system for melanoma beginning in 2002. Unfortunately, no histologic factors have been identified to date to consistently predict which patients have microscopically positive sentinel node involvement as an isolated event and which patients have additional nonsentinel node metastases.[92–94] Although the risk of additional nonsentinel lymph node metastasis appears to be low (<15%) in patients with positive sentinel nodes, it is currently recommended that patients with confirmed micrometastases in the sentinel node undergo complete regional lymph node dissection as a second procedure. The efficacy and precise role of a complete lymph node dissection in these patients is unclear and is currently being evaluated in the prospective randomized Multicenter Selective Lymphadenectomy Trial II (MSLT II).

Clinically Positive Lymph Node Metastases

Any palpable lymph node in a patient with melanoma should be considered indicative of metastasis until proved otherwise. Fine-needle aspiration biopsy is an accurate, reliable method of confirming metastatic melanoma.[95,96] If the fine-needle aspiration is biopsy is not available or results are indeterminate, excisional biopsy of the lymph node is performed. Patients presenting with or subsequently developing regional lymph node metastases are at high risk for distant metastases and should undergo advanced imaging including CT scanning (with intravenous contrast) of the chest, abdomen, and pelvis or FDG-PET scanning and MRI scanning of the brain. In patients with cytologically or histologically proven regional nodal metastases, formal complete lymph node dissection is performed. The development of palpable lymph node metastases is correlated significantly with substantially diminished survival (10%–50%), which is influenced strongly by the number of and the extent to which the lymph nodes are involved, as well as the primary melanoma thickness.[15,97]

Regional lymph node dissection should not be performed routinely in patients with documented distant metastases that are extensive or in those patients with large lymph node metastases fixed to adjacent structures. Significant palliation of inoperable bulky or bleeding regional nodal metastases may be achieved with radiation therapy in such situations, which are associated with an extremely poor prognosis.

TREATMENT OF LOCAL RECURRENCE

Local recurrence in a patient with malignant melanoma is an ominous clinical event and is almost always associated with the development of systemic metastases. The survival of these patients is extremely poor, averaging less than 5% at 10 years.

Primary melanoma thickness remains the most significant prognostic indicator of local recurrence and death, with other important predictive variables being the presence of ulceration and anatomic location of the primary lesion.[11] Large multi-institutional randomized trials confirm that local recurrence, and the incidence of in-transit, regional lymph node, and distant metastases, rises significantly with increasing primary melanoma thickness.

Local recurrence most often appears clinically as a blue-tinged subcutaneous nodule, arising in close proximity (within 2–5 cm) to an excision site of a primary melanoma (satellite metastasis), or en route to the regional lymph node basin (in-transit metastasis). Any subcutaneous nodule arising in the vicinity of a melanoma excision site should be considered to be disease recurrence or progression until proved otherwise. Diagnosis is accomplished rapidly and accurately by fine-needle aspiration biopsy. Excisional biopsy of the nodule under local anesthesia may sometimes be required for diagnostic confirmation. A complete metastatic survey, including CT or MRI and FDG-PET scans, should then be performed because most of these patients will now also have evidence of systemic metastases.

SURGICAL TREATMENT OF LOCALLY RECURRENT MALIGNANT MELANOMA

Although no standardized surgical approach to all patients with locally recurrent melanoma has been established, treatment guidelines have been developed based on clinical trials in patients selected by the extent and specific anatomic site of the disease recurrence. The realization that local recurrence is not simply the result of inadequate surgical excision but is an outward manifestation of the biologic aggressiveness of the primary melanoma has led to a more rational approach to the treatment of these patients.

Complete surgical resection with primary wound closure is the most straightforward means of treating single recurrent lesions. Patients with multiple subcutaneous metastases grouped within a single focus can similarly be treated with wide local excision with skin grafting or flap closures necessary for wound coverage. Although wide resection margins are not as well defined in the resection of locally recurrent disease as they are in the treatment of primary cutaneous melanoma, recurrent lesions should be resected with a margin of normal tissue if possible. Fracturing of the tumor mass is often followed by further rapid local recurrence. The changing of surgical instruments and gloves immediately after surgical resection or debulking of extensive metastases is recommended because rapid recurrence in the surgical wound and surrounding soft tissues is not uncommon.

Despite complete surgical resection of multiple cutaneous metastases, further local and regional recurrence may occur in up to 67% of patients and is strongly associated with subsequent disease progression,[98] with as many as 70% to 82% of such patients ultimately succumbing to distant metastases.[99]

SPECIAL CLINICAL SITUATIONS
Subungual Melanoma

Subungual melanoma is rare clinical entity representing up to 3% of cases of melanoma in whites, but a higher proportion of melanomas (15%–35%) in dark-skinned ethnic groups.[99,100] More than 75% of subungual melanomas involve either the great toe or the thumb. Early signs of this lesion include a darkening of the nail bed. Dark pigmentation of the proximal nail fold, Hutchinson sign, is a classic stigmata of

subungual melanoma. Many patients with subungual melanoma report a recent history of trauma to the digit and attribute the lesion to a poorly healing wound. The differential diagnosis of subungual melanoma includes benign pigmented lesions of the nail bed mechanism (melanonychia striata),[101] chronic bacterial fungal infection, and subungual hematoma.

The major pitfall in the diagnosis of subungual melanoma is an inadequate biopsy. Although nodular and amelanotic lesions do occur, most subungual hematomas appear as a sharply demarcated blue-black to brown discoloration of the nail, which does not involve the adjacent cuticle. A diagnosis of subungual hematoma may be confirmed by releasing the clotted blood through a large-bore puncture (trephination) or partial removal of the nail plate. Formal biopsy of the nail bed is performed under digital or regional anesthesia block in the office or as an outpatient procedure in the operating room. The nail plate is then elevated carefully from the nail bed and the lesion in question is clearly visualized. An elliptical incision in the nail bed down to the underlying periosteum is then performed allowing for complete excisional biopsy of the lesion and primary closure of the defect with fine absorbable sutures. Larger defects may be repaired with nail bed flaps or skin grafting. Generous incisional biopsy through the central portion of pigmentation is performed for larger lesions not amenable to simple excision.

Melanoma in situ of the nail bed is treated with complete wide local excision, including the entire nail bed and proximal matrix. Negative surgical margins of at least 5 mm are optimal. The surgical defect may be repaired with a local flap of skin or may require skin grafting.

Invasive subungual melanomas of the lower extremity are treated most easily with amputation of the toe. The appropriate surgical resection margin width of 1 or 2 cm for lesions with thickness less than 1 mm or greater than or equal to 1 mm, respectively, is achieved through complete amputation of the affected toe. Ray amputation may be required for lesions extending into the webspace. In most patients, the resulting surgical defect closes easily, heals well, and allows for ambulation without a specialized prosthesis or orthotic device, even when complete or partial amputation of the great toe is required. For upper extremity subungual invasive melanomas, surgical treatment is more individualized. Amputation is performed through the joint most proximal to the lesion, which represents a more conservative and functionally superior approach to the more radical amputations performed in the recent past.[102] Wound closure is achieved with a flap of volar tissue while ideally maintaining a margin of at least 1 cm of normal tissue. For subungual melanomas of the thumb, a reconstruction is performed by webspace deepening using a Z-plasty, reducing the length of digit loss by approximately 50%.[101]

Sentinel lymph node mapping and excision is performed according to guidelines established for the treatment of melanomas of equivalent thickness and histology arising in the skin in the absence of clinically palpable regional nodes. Patients presenting with palpable nodal metastases undergo concurrent complete regional lymphadenectomy.

Plantar Melanoma

Melanoma arising on the sole of the foot, characteristically in an acral lentiginous growth pattern, is a rare clinical entity in whites, accounting for only 2% to 8% of melanoma cases in that population.[103] In dark-skinned ethnic groups, such as patients of African American, Asian, or Hispanic descent, however, melanoma arises on the plantar surface of the foot in 35% to 90% of patients diagnosed with melanoma in those populations.[104]

Although the metastatic potential of these lesions is correlated significantly with the thickness of the primary melanoma, as it is for cutaneous melanomas arising elsewhere, these lesions are often diagnosed at later stages and therefore generally have a less favorable prognosis. The frequent delay in diagnosis of plantar lesions may be explained in part by their rarity and their unusual and infrequently examined anatomic location. In addition, the increased thickness of the epidermis of the plantar surface may obscure the characteristic clinical appearance of the melanoma. Even melanomas that appear flat may be revealed after adequate biopsy to be thick lesions. A major pitfall in the early diagnosis of this lesion, however, is the failure to obtain a satisfactory biopsy specimen for histologic confirmation of malignancy. The extreme thickness of the plantar epidermis limits the use of shave biopsy as a diagnostic modality. In addition, the haphazard pigment pattern of these lesions also makes accurate diagnosis and assessment of lesion thickness by other techniques, such as punch or even incisional biopsy, less likely to be successful.

The preferred method of biopsy for these difficult lesions is complete excisional biopsy. Definitive wound closure may be deferred until rapid histologic diagnosis and margin inspection are complete. Once the diagnosis of melanoma is confirmed, the lesion is excised and staged according to guidelines established for other cutaneous primary melanomas of comparable thickness. Sentinel lymph node mapping and excision are performed according to guidelines established for the treatment of melanomas of equivalent thickness and histology arising in other cutaneous sites in the absence of clinically palpable regional nodes. Patients presenting with palpable nodal metastases undergo concurrent complete regional lymphadenectomy.

Dissection of the deep inguinal nodes is performed in patients with involvement of Cloquet node or extensive disease in the upper aspect of the femoral triangle. Lesions confirmed to be melanomas on shave, punch, or incisional biopsy that approach or exceed 1 mm in thickness may be treated definitively as outlined previously and may not require a preliminary excisional biopsy procedure.

Wound closure of the plantar surface requires special consideration. The exact location of the melanoma on the plantar surface, stage of disease, age, associated medical conditions, and lifestyle of the patient must be considered in the determination of wound closure. Defects on non–weight-bearing aspects of the plantar surface or those in patients with sedentary lifestyles, significant medical comorbidities, or advanced metastatic disease may be closed most easily primarily or more commonly with split-thickness or full-thickness skin grafts. Closure of defects on the weight-bearing surface of the plantar region in ambulatory patients is accomplished with a variety of flap reconstructive procedures. These include relatively straightforward cutaneous rotational or advancement flaps and more complex reconstructive procedures, such as musculocutaneous free flaps with microvascular anastomosis. These latter procedures are usually performed with a plastic reconstructive surgeon who ideally has been involved in the care of the patient once the diagnosis of melanoma has been confirmed.

Locally advanced, recurrent, or metastatic acral lentigenous melanomas should also be evaluated for mutations in KIT, which are more frequently noted in acral lentigenous and mucosal melanomas than in lesions arising elsewhere in the skin. Demonstration of KIT mutations may make the patient a candidate for targeted therapy with imatinib (Gleevec), developed originally for the treatment of central nervous system and hematologic malignancies, that now shows promise in melanoma.[48]

Melanoma on the Face

Melanoma occurs rather commonly on the face often as a broad, somewhat ill-defined situ lesion, known traditionally as a Hutchinson melanotic freckle or lentigo maligna.[105] Despite their diminished biologic aggressiveness, however, the cosmetic and functional considerations of performing tumor surgery on the face makes treating these thin lesions especially challenging.

Biopsy should be performed to fully assess melanoma thickness to plan definitive surgical treatment appropriately and to determine the risk of regional lymph node metastases and the need for additional procedures, such as lymphatic mapping and sentinel lymphadenectomy. As in other anatomic locations, complete excisional biopsy or extensive and deep shave biopsy is required to confirm the diagnosis of melanoma and tumor thickness. Other techniques, such as punch and incisional biopsy, clearly have a role in certain circumstances but are less optimal because melanocytic neoplasms arising on the face, especially on significantly sun-damaged skin, are often far more extensive microscopically in terms of their radial extension than they appear clinically. If complete excisional biopsy of such a large lesion is required, and the defect created is not amenable to cosmetically acceptable primary closure, then a moist, sterile dressing should be placed until the pathologic examination of the surgical specimen is complete. Care should be taken, however, with any biopsy technique chosen, to avoid injury to the branches of the facial nerve. The marginal mandibular division, because of its superficial location and diminutive size, is particularly at risk. The possibility of facial nerve injury should be discussed with the patient and documented appropriately before any biopsy procedure.

On the face, achieving an appropriately wide resection margin may be particularly challenging for melanomas located in close proximity to structures, such as the eye, nose, and mouth. A good rule of practice is to obtain as close to the desired surgical margin as possible based on the thickness of the melanoma when excising invasive melanomas thinner than 2 mm arising in cosmetically important areas of the face. This practice is a reasonable approach in such circumstances because prospective randomized trials designed to define the width of melanoma excision have demonstrated that although narrower margins obtained for melanomas thicker than 1 mm but thinner than 2 mm are associated with slightly higher local recurrence rates, they have no significant impact in long-term survival.[72]

Traditional resection margin widths for the excision of in situ and thin invasive melanomas have been challenged by investigators advocating the technique of Mohs micrographic surgery as an alternative to wider local excision.[106] Although study is ongoing, the efficacy and overall safety of this technique in the treatment of melanoma of the face remains unproven and is not recommended.

A plastic reconstructive surgeon should be included in the planning and performance of any resection of a melanoma on the face that will result in a significant surgical defect. A range of reconstructive techniques is now widely available to make the final cosmetic and functional surgical result more acceptable. All patients should have the advantage of such a multidisciplinary approach, including the dermatologist, surgical oncologist, and plastic reconstructive surgeon.

As in other anatomic areas, patients with melanomas on the face approaching 1 mm in thickness are at risk for occult micrometastases in the regional lymph nodes. The advent and refinement of cutaneous lymphoscintigraphy has better delineated the often-complex lymphatic drainage patterns unique to this region. Accordingly, elective lymph node dissection of presumed sites of micrometastatic disease in the head and neck region has been replaced by cutaneous lymphoscintigraphy and sentinel lymphadenectomy using a radiolabeled tracer substance, such as technetium sulfur colloid alone. The additional use of vital blue dyes to perform sentinel lymphadenectomy is often superfluous in this region and carries with it a remote risk of permanent discoloration of the skin, necrosis, or anaphylaxis.[91,107–109] Regional lymphadenectomy is performed selectively in those patients with histologically confirmed micrometastases in the sentinel nodes. Superficial parotidectomy with dissection of all facial nerve branches is recommended for patients with micrometastases in periparotid nodes. Selective cervical lymph node dissection based on the precise location of a positive cervical sentinel node has replaced more traditional modified radical and formal radical neck dissections. Patients presenting with or developing palpable lymph node metastases in the absence of significant distant metastases should undergo formal regional lymphadenectomy.

In a small but not insignificant number of patients with melanoma of the face, preoperative cutaneous lymphoscintigraphy reveals a complex pattern of lymphatic drainage from the primary lesion to multiple sentinel nodes widely dispersed throughout the head and neck region. The diagnostic accuracy may decline and risk of facial or spinal accessory nerve injury rises, as the complexity and number of individual sentinel nodes to be identified and excised increases. It seems reasonable to forgo sentinel lymphadenectomy in individualized circumstances when multiple sentinel node sites are revealed by preoperative cutaneous lymphoscintigraphy. The reasons for this decision and the risks and benefits of not identifying potential microscopic regional nodal metastases should be discussed fully with the patient and carefully documented.

SURGICAL TREATMENT OF UNUSUAL ATYPICAL MELANOCYTIC CUTANEOUS LESIONS OF UNCERTAIN DIAGNOSIS

Occasionally, unusual melanocytic lesions pose serious diagnostic challenges even though the histopathologic criteria of melanoma have been well described. In these difficult clinical situations, a second (or third) dermatopathologic opinion is prudent. Whenever possible, additional material should be acquired and a new set of slides prepared from the original cell blocks and histologic and immunohistochemical staining repeated. If any of the original lesion of concern remains at the primary site, a complete excisional biopsy should be performed in an attempt to secure an accurate diagnosis.

The treatment of patients with lesions that have not been definitively confirmed to be melanoma or a benign lesion, as well as those lesions generating divergent dermatopathologic diagnoses, is difficult; however, some guidelines may be established. A detailed discussion should be initiated with the patient, family, and referring physicians, which addresses specifically the advantages and disadvantages of treating the lesion as a melanoma as opposed to a benign lesion. The management of lesions suspicious for melanoma in situ is usually handled easily with complete surgical reexcision, maintaining 5-mm margins if possible. Complete wide and deep excision, maintaining 1-cm margins, is also recommended for lesions that may possibly represent invasive melanomas less than 1 mm in Breslow thickness. In anatomic areas where 1-cm surgical margins cannot be obtained easily because of cosmetic or functional considerations, such as on the face or near the mouth, nose, or in proximity to the eye, complete excision is still advisable with as wide (although <1 cm) a margin as is reasonably possible.

Lesions thought to represent, but not definitively confirmed to be, invasive melanoma greater than or equal to 1 mm are more difficult to manage because of the more complex surgery required and potential metastatic capability of lesions of this thickness. Once again, a detailed discussion with the patient and all parties concerned carefully delineating the pros and cons of treating such a lesion is essential and should be well documented in the official patient care record. For those lesions arising in such anatomic areas as the chest wall, back, abdominal wall, or thigh, surgical excision with 2-cm margins seems reasonable because primary closure with an acceptable cosmetic and functional outcome can almost always be achieved. Although complete excision of the lesion with clear margins should be performed, in those anatomic areas where 2-cm excisional margins leave a defect not amenable to simple primary wound closure and necessitate more complex reconstructions or result in significant functional or cosmetic deformity, the actual excision margin width should be individualized and planned and discussed carefully with the patient preoperatively. Sentinel lymph node mapping and biopsy may also be offered to patients with lesions that may represent melanomas greater than or equal to 1 mm in thickness. The risks and benefits of undergoing or declining this procedure should also be discussed carefully with the patient and family.

Any patient who undergoes excision of a lesion of uncertain malignant potential should be followed carefully postoperatively, as if the lesion were definitively proved to be melanoma. This includes routine physical examination and periodic laboratory and radiologic assessment appropriate for a patient with a melanoma of that particular thickness.

MELANOMA IN PREGNANCY

Approximately one-third of the increasing numbers of women diagnosed with melanoma each year are of childbearing age, and melanoma accounts for about 8% of malignancies diagnosed during pregnancy.[110] The overall incidence of melanoma in pregnancy is estimated to be 0.14 to 0.28 cases per 1000 births.[111] Although occurring extremely rarely, melanoma is one of the most common tumors known to metastasize to the placenta and fetus.[112,113]

Although melanocytic nevi commonly become larger and darker under the hormonal influence of pregnancy, presumably because of increased levels of estrogen and melanocyte-stimulating hormone,[114,115] there exists no conclusive evidence that pregnancy significantly affects the biologic aggressiveness of a melanoma in terms of increasing the incidence of metastasis or lowering overall survival.[116–118] Moreover, pregnancy occurring either before or after the diagnosis and treatment of melanoma, similarly seems to have no significant effect on the clinical course of the disease.[118,119] Based on the data presently available, the termination of pregnancy of a patient recently diagnosed with melanoma, as a therapeutic measure, cannot be recommended. Because the overwhelming (>75%) majority of melanoma recurrences happen within 2 to 3 years after treatment of the primary lesion, many women are encouraged to avoid becoming pregnant during that period of time postoperatively.

The frequent observation that melanocytic lesions may become more pronounced during pregnancy makes the diagnosis of melanoma even more difficult. As in any other patient, however, any cutaneous lesion suspicious for melanoma in a pregnant patient should undergo biopsy without delay. This is accomplished with shave, punch, incisional, or, preferably, complete excisional biopsy, which may be performed safely in the pregnant patient under local lidocaine anesthesia, without the addition of epinephrine. Although most of these biopsy procedures may be performed safely and rapidly in the office setting, the excision of larger lesions may be performed more prudently in the ambulatory surgery unit with an anesthesiologist who is knowledgeable in the care of the pregnant patient, as well as with intraoperative fetal monitoring in patients with viable pregnancies.

Once the diagnosis of the melanoma is confirmed histologically, an abbreviated metastatic survey may be ordered, but surgical treatment is planned commensurate with the thickness of the primary lesion and clinical lesion and clinical stage if disease. Routine laboratory tests, including determination of LDH level should be ordered. Radiologic workup should be reviewed with the patient's obstetrician and may include radiographs of the chest, which may be performed safely during pregnancy with the appropriate shielding. In patients with thicker melanomas or those presenting with palpable regional nodal metastases, a search for metastases is more individualized and may include abdominal ultrasound or MRI.

Wide local excision with 5-mm margins is performed under local anesthesia in patients with melanoma in situ. Invasive melanomas thinner than 1 mm are similarly treated under local anesthesia in the ambulatory surgery suite, with appropriate maternal fetal monitoring, with wide and deep excision maintaining 1-cm margins.

Patients with melanomas greater than or equal to 1 mm thick undergo wide and deep excision, maintaining 2-cm margins. These larger excisions may require additional anesthesia given by an anesthesiologist with experience in the care of the obstetric patient. Formal therapeutic regional lymph node dissection is performed concurrently in the presence of palpable nodal metastases. Lymphatic mapping and sentinel lymph node biopsy in clinically node-negative pregnant patients with a variety of malignancies, such as breast cancer, appears to be safe and technically accurate and are performed with technetium radiolabeled sulfa colloid alone. Vital blue dyes including isosulfan blue

(Lymphazurin) are not recommended for use in pregnant patients.[120–122] It would seem prudent that the surgical approach to evaluating the regional lymph nodes in pregnant patients be individualized and commensurate with the risk of concurrent subclinical regional nodal disease, however, with all possible outcomes discussed in detail with the patient and her family and the obstetrician of record. In concerned patients or in those in the more tenuous early stages of pregnancy, a reasonable approach is to perform an appropriate wide and deep excision of the primary melanoma and defer lymphatic mapping and sentinel node biopsy to be performed as a second procedure after completion of the pregnancy. Complete regional node dissection should be performed during pregnancy in those patients presenting with or developing confirmed regional nodal metastases.

REFERENCES

1. Landis SH, Murray T, Bolden S, et al. Cancer statistics, 1999. CA Cancer J Clin 1999;49:8–31, 31.
2. Forty-five years of cancer incidence in Connecticut: 1935-79. Natl Cancer Inst Monogr 1986;70: 1–706.
3. Glass AG, Hoover RN. The emerging epidemic of melanoma and squamous cell skin cancer. JAMA 1989;262:2097–100.
4. Rigel DS. Trends in dermatology: melanoma incidence. Arch Dermatol 2010;146:318.
5. Rigel DS. Epidemiology of melanoma. Semin Cutan Med Surg 2010;29:204–9.
6. Cummins DL, Cummins JM, Pantle H, et al. Cutaneous malignant melanoma. Mayo Clin Proc 2006; 81:500–7.
7. American Academy of Dermatology. Melanoma fact sheet. Schaumburg (IL): American Academy of Dermatology; 2010.
8. Friedman RJ, Rigel DS, Kopf AW. Early detection of malignant melanoma: the role of physician examination and self-examination of the skin. CA Cancer J Clin 1985;35:130–51.
9. Rhodes AR, Weinstock MA, Fitzpatrick TB, et al. Risk factors for cutaneous melanoma. A practical method of recognizing predisposed individuals. JAMA 1987;258:3146–54.
10. Weir HK, Thun MJ, Hankey BF, et al. Annual report to the nation on the status of cancer, 1975-2000, featuring the uses of surveillance data for cancer prevention and control. J Natl Cancer Inst 2003; 95:1276–99.
11. Balch CM, Soong SJ, Shaw H, et al. An analysis of prognostic factors in 8500 patients with cutaneous melanoma. In: Balch CM, Houghton A, Milton G, et al, editors. Cutaneous melanoma. 2nd edition. Philadelphia: JB Lippincott; 1992. p. 165–87.

12. Ross MI, Stern SJ, Wanebo HJ. Mucosal melanomas. In: Balch CM, Houghton A, Milton G, et al, editors. Cutaneous melanoma. 2nd edition. Philadelphia: JB Lippincott; 1992. p. 325–35.

13. Reintgen DS, McCarty KS, Woodard B, et al. Metastatic malignant melanoma with an unknown primary. Surg Gynecol Obstet 1983;156:335–40.

14. Giuliano AE, Moseley HS, Morton DL. Clinical aspects of unknown primary melanoma. Ann Surg 1980;191:98–104.

15. Balch CM, Soong SJ, Murad TM, et al. A multifactorial analysis of melanoma: III. Prognostic factors in melanoma patients with lymph node metastases (stage II). Ann Surg 1981;193: 377–88.

16. Milton GW, Shaw HM, McCarthy WH. Occult primary malignant melanoma: factors influencing survival. Br J Surg 1977;64:805–8.

17. Gilchrest BA, Eller MS, Geller AC, et al. The pathogenesis of melanoma induced by ultraviolet radiation. N Engl J Med 1999;340:1341–8.

18. Mogensen M, Jemec GB. The potential carcinogenic risk of tanning beds: clinical guidelines and patient safety advice. Cancer Manag Res 2010;2: 277–82.

19. Rigel DS, Rivers JK, Kopf AW, et al. Dysplastic nevi. Markers for increased risk for melanoma. Cancer 1989;63:386–9.

20. MacKie RM, Freudenberger T, Aitchison TC. Personal risk-factor chart for cutaneous melanoma. Lancet 1989;2:487–90.

21. Ackerman AB. What naevus is dysplastic, a syndrome and the commonest precursor of malignant melanoma? A riddle and an answer. Histopathology 1988;13:241–56.

22. Rigel DS, Friedman RJ, Kopf AW, et al. Precursors of malignant melanoma. Problems in computing the risk of malignant melanoma arising in dysplastic and congenital nevocytic nevi. Dermatol Clin 1985; 3:361–5.

23. Gruber SB, Barnhill RL, Stenn KS, et al. Nevomelanocytic proliferations in association with cutaneous malignant melanoma: a multivariate analysis. J Am Acad Dermatol 1989;21:773–80.

24. Hendrickson MR, Ross JC. Neoplasms arising in congenital giant nevi: morphologic study of seven cases and a review of the literature. Am J Surg Pathol 1981;5:109–35.

25. Illig L, Weidner F, Hundeiker M, et al. Congenital nevi less than or equal to 10 cm as precursors to melanoma: 52 cases, a review, and a new conception. Arch Dermatol 1985;121:1274–81.

26. Rhodes AR, Melski JW. Small congenital nevocellular nevi and the risk of cutaneous melanoma. J Pediatr 1982;100:219–24.

27. Koh HK. Cutaneous melanoma. N Engl J Med 1991;325:171–82.

28. Mihm MC, Fitzpatrick TB, Brown MM, et al. Early detection of primary cutaneous malignant melanoma. A color atlas. N Engl J Med 1973;289: 989–96.

29. Wick MM, Sober AJ, Fitzpatrick TB, et al. Clinical characteristics of early cutaneous melanoma. Cancer 1980;45:2684–6.

30. Rigel DS, Russak J, Friedman R. The evolution of melanoma diagnosis: 25 years beyond the ABCDs. CA Cancer J Clin 2010;60:301–16.

31. Oh TS, Bae EJ, Ro KW, et al. Acral lentiginous melanoma developing during long-standing atypical melanosis: usefulness of dermoscopy for detection of early acral melanoma. Ann Dermatol 2011;23:400–4.

32. Monheit G, Cognetta AB, Ferris L, et al. The performance of MelaFind: a prospective multicenter study. Arch Dermatol 2011;147:188–94.

33. Scheibner A, Milton GW, McCarthy WH, et al. Multiple primary melanoma—a review of 90 cases. Australas J Dermatol 1982;23:1–8.

34. Veronesi U, Cascinelli N, Bufalino R. Evaluation of the risk of multiple primaries in malignant cutaneous melanoma. Tumori 1976;62:127–30.

35. Reimer RR, Clark WH Jr, Greene MH, et al. Precursor lesions in familial melanoma. A new genetic preneoplastic syndrome. JAMA 1978;239:744–6.

36. Mai PL, Chatterjee N, Hartge P, et al. Potential excess mortality in BRCA1/2 mutation carriers beyond breast, ovarian, prostate, and pancreatic cancers, and melanoma. PLoS One 2009;4: e4812.

37. Warycha MA, Zakrzewski J, Ni Q, et al. Meta-analysis of sentinel lymph node positivity in thin melanoma (<or=1 mm). Cancer 2009;115:869–79.

38. Porter GA, Ross MI, Berman RS, et al. How many lymph nodes are enough during sentinel lymphadenectomy for primary melanoma? Surgery 2000; 128:306–11.

39. Harris MN, Gumport SL. Biopsy technique for malignant melanoma. J Dermatol Surg 1975;1:24–7.

40. Zager JS, Hochwald SN, Marzban SS, et al. Shave biopsy is a safe and accurate method for the initial evaluation of melanoma. J Am Coll Surg 2011;212: 454–60 [discussion: 460–2].

41. Gown AM, Vogel AM, Hoak D, et al. Monoclonal antibodies specific for melanocytic tumors distinguish subpopulations of melanocytes. Am J Pathol 1986;123:195–203.

42. Wick MR, Swanson PE, Rocamora A. Recognition of malignant melanoma by monoclonal antibody HMB-45. An immunohistochemical study of 200 paraffin-embedded cutaneous tumors. J Cutan Pathol 1988;15:201–7.

43. Cochran AJ, Wen DR. S-100 protein as a marker for melanocytic and other tumours. Pathology 1985; 17:340–5.

44. Nakajima T, Watanabe S, Sato Y, et al. Immunohistochemical demonstration of S100 protein in malignant melanoma and pigmented nevus, and its diagnostic application. Cancer 1982;50:912–8.

45. Thompson JF, Soong SJ, Balch CM, et al. Prognostic significance of mitotic rate in localized primary cutaneous melanoma: an analysis of patients in the multi-institutional American Joint Committee on Cancer melanoma staging database. J Clin Oncol 2011;29:2199–205.

46. Callender GG, McMasters KM. What does ulceration of a melanoma mean for prognosis? Adv Surg 2011;45:225–36.

47. Maurichi A, Miceli R, Camerini T, et al. Pure desmoplastic melanoma: a melanoma with distinctive clinical behavior. Ann Surg 2010;252:1052–7.

48. Carvajal RD, Antonescu CR, Wolchok JD, et al. KIT as a therapeutic target in metastatic melanoma. JAMA 2011;305:2327–34.

49. Scheier B, Amaria R, Lewis K, et al. Novel therapies in melanoma. Immunotherapy 2011;3:1461–9.

50. Breslow A. Thickness, cross-sectional areas and depth of invasion in the prognosis of cutaneous melanoma. Ann Surg 1970;172:902–8.

51. Clark WH, From L, Bernardino EA, et al. The histogenesis and biologic behavior of primary human malignant melanomas of the skin. Cancer Res 1969;29:705–27.

52. Edge SB, American Joint Committee on Cancer. AJCC cancer staging manual. 7th edition. New York, London: Springer. p. xiv, 648.

53. Balch CM, Gershenwald JE, Soong SJ, et al. Final version of 2009 AJCC melanoma staging and classification. J Clin Oncol 2009;27:6199–206.

54. Gershenwald JE, Soong SJ, Balch CM. 2010 TNM staging system for cutaneous melanoma and beyond. Ann Surg Oncol 2010;17:1475–7.

55. Gershenwald JE, Thompson W, Mansfield PF, et al. Multi-institutional melanoma lymphatic mapping experience: the prognostic value of sentinel lymph node status in 612 stage I or II melanoma patients. J Clin Oncol 1999;17:976–83.

56. Buzaid AC, Colome M, Bedikian A, et al. Phase II study of neoadjuvant concurrent biochemotherapy in melanoma patients with local-regional metastases. Melanoma Res 1998;8:549–56.

57. Ye X, Yang Q, Wang Y, et al. Electrochemical behaviour of gold, silver, platinum and palladium on the glassy carbon electrode modified by chitosan and its application. Talanta 1998;47:1099–106.

58. Yancovitz M, Finelt N, Warycha MA, et al. Role of radiologic imaging at the time of initial diagnosis of stage T1b-T3b melanoma. Cancer 2007;110:1107–14.

59. Handley W. The bunterian lectures on the pathology of melanocytic growths in relation to their operative treatment. Lancet 1907;169:927–33.

60. Pemberton O. Observations on the history, pathology, and treatment of cancerous diseases. Part I: melanosis. London: Churchill; 1858.

61. Cascinelli N, Morabito A, Santinami M, et al. Immediate or delayed dissection of regional nodes in patients with melanoma of the trunk: a randomised trial. WHO Melanoma Programme. Lancet 1998;351:793–6.

62. Cohn-Cedermark G, Rutqvist LE, Andersson R, et al. Long-term results of a randomized study by the Swedish Melanoma Study Group on 2-cm versus 5-cm resection margins for patients with cutaneous melanoma with a tumor thickness of 0.8-2.0 mm. Cancer 2000;89:1495–501.

63. Khayat D, Rixe O, Martin G, et al. Surgical margins in cutaneous melanoma (2 cm versus 5 cm for lesions measuring less than 2.1-mm thick). Cancer 2003;97:1941–6.

64. Karakousis CP, Balch CM, Urist MM, et al. Local recurrence in malignant melanoma: long-term results of the multiinstitutional randomized surgical trial. Ann Surg Oncol 1996;3:446–52.

65. Thomas JM, Newton-Bishop J, A'Hern R, et al. Excision margins in high-risk malignant melanoma. N Engl J Med 2004;350:757–66.

66. Breslow A, Macht SD. Optimal size of resection margin for thin cutaneous melanoma. Surg Gynecol Obstet 1977;145:691–2.

67. Veronesi U, Cascinelli N. Narrow excision (1-cm margin). A safe procedure for thin cutaneous melanoma. Arch Surg 1991;126:438–41.

68. Harris MN, Shapiro RL, Roses DF. Malignant melanoma. Primary surgical management (excision and node dissection) based on pathology and staging. Cancer 1995;75:715–25.

69. Balch CM, Urist MM, Karakousis CP, et al. Efficacy of 2-cm surgical margins for intermediate-thickness melanomas (1 to 4 mm). Results of a multi-institutional randomized surgical trial. Ann Surg 1993;218:262–7 [discussion: 267–9].

70. Lang PG. Current concepts in the management of patients with melanoma. Am J Clin Dermatol 2002;3:401–26.

71. Roses DF, Harris MN, Rigel D, et al. Local and in-transit metastases following definitive excision for primary cutaneous malignant melanoma. Ann Surg 1983;198:65–9.

72. Veronesi U, Cascinelli N, Adamus J, et al. Thin stage I primary cutaneous malignant melanoma. Comparison of excision with margins of 1 or 3 cm. N Engl J Med 1988;318:1159–62.

73. Sladden MJ, Balch C, Barzilai DA, et al. Surgical excision margins for primary cutaneous melanoma. Cochrane Database Syst Rev 2009;4:CD004835.

74. Heaton KM, Sussman JJ, Gershenwald JE, et al. Surgical margins and prognostic factors in patients with thick (>4mm) primary melanoma. Ann Surg Oncol 1998;5:322–8.

75. Jaques DP, Coit DG, Brennan MF. Major amputation for advanced malignant melanoma. Surg Gynecol Obstet 1989;169:1–6.

76. Balch CM, Soong SJ, Bartolucci AA, et al. Efficacy of an elective regional lymph node dissection of 1 to 4 mm thick melanomas for patients 60 years of age and younger. Ann Surg 1996;224:255–63.

77. McCarthy WH, Shaw HM, Milton GW. Efficacy of elective lymph node dissection in 2,347 patients with clinical stage I malignant melanoma. Surg Gynecol Obstet 1985;161:575–80.

78. Milton GW, Shaw HM, McCarthy WH, et al. Prophylactic lymph node dissection in clinical stage I cutaneous malignant melanoma: results of surgical treatment in 1319 patients. Br J Surg 1982;69:108–11.

79. Sim FH, Taylor WF, Ivins JC, et al. A prospective randomized study of the efficacy of routine elective lymphadenectomy in management of malignant melanoma. Preliminary results. Cancer 1978;41:948–56.

80. Murali R, Haydu LE, Quinn MJ, et al. Sentinel lymph node biopsy in patients with thin primary cutaneous melanoma. Ann Surg 2012;255(1):128–33.

81. Lourari S, Paul C, Gouraud PA, et al. Sentinel lymph node biopsy for melanoma is becoming a consensus: a national survey of French centres involved in melanoma care in 2008. J Eur Acad Dermatol Venereol 2011. [Epub ahead of print].

82. Bichakjian CK, Halpern AC, Johnson TM, et al. Guidelines of care for the management of primary cutaneous melanoma. J Am Acad Dermatol 2011;65:1032–47.

83. Wen DR, Cochran AJ, Huang RR, et al. Clinically relevant information from sentinel lymph node biopsies of melanoma patients. J Surg Oncol 2011;104:369–78.

84. Callender GG, McMasters KM. Early versus delayed complete lymphadenectomy in melanoma: insight from MSLT I. Ann Surg Oncol 2011;18:306–8.

85. Twomey P. Sentinel node biopsy for early-stage melanoma: accuracy and morbidity in MSLT-1, an international multicenter trial. Ann Surg 2007;245:156–7.

86. Wong SL, Brady MS, Busam KJ, et al. Results of sentinel lymph node biopsy in patients with thin melanoma. Ann Surg Oncol 2006;13:302–9.

87. Schmidt CR, Panageas KS, Coit DG, et al. An increased number of sentinel lymph nodes is associated with advanced Breslow depth and lymphovascular invasion in patients with primary melanoma. Ann Surg Oncol 2009;16:948–52.

88. Wang X, Heller R, VanVoorhis N, et al. Detection of submicroscopic lymph node metastases with polymerase chain reaction in patients with malignant melanoma. Ann Surg 1994;220:768–74.

89. Blaheta HJ, Schittek B, Breuninger H, et al. Lymph node micrometastases of cutaneous melanoma: increased sensitivity of molecular diagnosis in comparison to immunohistochemistry. Int J Cancer 1998;79:318–23.

90. Li W, Stall A, Shivers SC, et al. Clinical relevance of molecular staging for melanoma: comparison of RT-PCR and immunohistochemistry staining in sentinel lymph nodes of patients with melanoma. Ann Surg 2000;231:795–803.

91. Bezu C, Coutant C, Salengro A, et al. Anaphylactic response to blue dye during sentinel lymph node biopsy. Surg Oncol 2011;20:e55–9.

92. Cascinelli N, Bombardieri E, Bufalino R, et al. Sentinel and nonsentinel node status in stage IB and II melanoma patients: two-step prognostic indicators of survival. J Clin Oncol 2006;24:4464–71.

93. Satzger I, Meier A, Hoy L, et al. Sentinel node dissection delays recurrence and prolongs melanoma-related survival: an analysis of 673 patients from a single center with long-term follow-up. Ann Surg Oncol 2011;18:514–20.

94. McMasters KM, Wong SL, Edwards MJ, et al. Frequency of nonsentinel lymph node metastasis in melanoma. Ann Surg Oncol 2002;9:137–41.

95. Basler GC, Fader DJ, Yahanda A, et al. The utility of fine needle aspiration in the diagnosis of melanoma metastatic to lymph nodes. J Am Acad Dermatol 1997;36:403–8.

96. Doubrovsky A, Scolyer RA, Murali R, et al. Diagnostic accuracy of fine needle biopsy for metastatic melanoma and its implications for patient management. Ann Surg Oncol 2008;15:323–32.

97. Callery C, Cochran AJ, Roe DJ, et al. Factors prognostic for survival in patients with malignant melanoma spread to the regional lymph nodes. Ann Surg 1982;196:69–75.

98. Hafstrom L, Rudenstam CM, Blomquist E, et al. Regional hyperthermic perfusion with melphalan after surgery for recurrent malignant melanoma of the extremities. Swedish Melanoma Study Group. J Clin Oncol 1991;9:2091–4.

99. Wong JH, Cagle LA, Kopald KH, et al. Natural history and selective management of in transit melanoma. J Surg Oncol 1990;44:146–50.

100. Briggs JC. Subungual malignant melanoma: a review article. Br J Plast Surg 1985;38:174–6.

101. Glat PM, Spector JA, Roses DF, et al. The management of pigmented lesions of the nail bed. Ann Plast Surg 1996;37:125–34.

102. Ebskov LB. Major amputation for malignant melanoma: an epidemiological study. J Surg Oncol 1993;52:89–91.

103. Reintgen DS, McCarty KM Jr, Cox E, et al. Malignant melanoma in black American and white

American populations. A comparative review. JAMA 1982;248:1856–9.

104. Krementz ET, Feed RJ, Coleman WP 3rd, et al. Acral lentiginous melanoma. A clinicopathologic entity. Ann Surg 1982;195:632–45.

105. Clark WH Jr, Mihm MC Jr. Lentigo maligna and lentigo-maligna melanoma. Am J Pathol 1969;55: 39–67.

106. Zitelli JA, Brown C, Hanusa BH. Mohs micrographic surgery for the treatment of primary cutaneous melanoma. J Am Acad Dermatol 1997;37:236–45.

107. Jangjoo A, Forghani MN, Mehrabibahar M, et al. Anaphylaxis reaction of a breast cancer patient to methylene blue during breast surgery with sentinel node mapping. Acta Oncol 2010;49:877–8.

108. Kaufman G, Guth AA, Pachter HL, et al. A cautionary tale: anaphylaxis to isosulfan blue dye after 12 years and 3339 cases of lymphatic mapping. Am Surg 2008;74:152–5.

109. Neves RI, Reynolds BQ, Hazard SW, et al. Increased post-operative complications with methylene blue versus lymphazurin in sentinel lymph node biopsies for skin cancers. J Surg Oncol 2011;103:421–5.

110. Kjems E, Krag C. Melanoma and pregnancy. A review. Acta Oncol 1993;32:371–8.

111. Wong DJ, Strassner HT. Melanoma in pregnancy. Clin Obstet Gynecol 1990;33:782–91.

112. Baergen RN, Johnson D, Moore T, et al. Maternal melanoma metastatic to the placenta: a case report and review of the literature. Arch Pathol Lab Med 1997;121:508–11.

113. Dildy GA 3rd, Moise KJ Jr, Carpenter RJ Jr, et al. Maternal malignancy metastatic to the products of conception: a review. Obstet Gynecol Surv 1989;44:535–40.

114. Ances IG, Pomerantz SH. Serum concentrations of beta-melanocyte-stimulating hormone in human pregnancy. Am J Obstet Gynecol 1974;119: 1062–8.

115. Sanchez JL, Figueroa LD, Rodriguez E. Behavior of melanocytic nevi during pregnancy. Am J Dermatopathol 1984;6(Suppl):89–91.

116. Wong JH, Sterns EE, Kopald KH, et al. Prognostic significance of pregnancy in stage I melanoma. Arch Surg 1989;124:1227–30 [discussion: 1230–1].

117. Houghton AN, Flannery J, Viola MV. Malignant melanoma of the skin occurring during pregnancy. Cancer 1981;48:407–10.

118. Reintgen DS, McCarty KS Jr, Vollmer R, et al. Malignant melanoma and pregnancy. Cancer 1985;55:1340–4.

119. Lederman JS, Sober AJ. Effect of prior pregnancy on melanoma survival. Arch Dermatol 1985;121: 716.

120. Krag DN, Weaver DL, Alex JC, et al. Surgical resection and radiolocalization of the sentinel lymph node in breast cancer using a gamma probe. Surg Oncol 1993;2:335–9 [discussion: 340].

121. Arcan P, Ibis E, Aras G, et al. Identification of sentinel lymph node in stage I-II breast cancer with lymphoscintigraphy and surgical gamma probe: comparison of Tc-99m MIBI and Tc-99m sulfur colloid. Clin Nucl Med 2005;30:317–21.

122. Lin KM, Patel TH, Ray A, et al. Intradermal radioisotope is superior to peritumoral blue dye or radioisotope in identifying breast cancer sentinel nodes. J Am Coll Surg 2004;199:561–6.

Mohs Micrographic Surgery for the Treatment of Melanoma

Andrea M. Hui, MD[a],*, Michael Jacobson, MD[a],
Orit Markowitz, MD[a,b], Norman A. Brooks, MD[c],
Daniel M. Siegel, MD[a]

KEYWORDS

- Mohs • Surgery • Melanoma • Immunostaining • Zinc chloride paste • Fresh tissue • Fixed tissue

KEY POINTS

- MMS for melanoma offers complete histological margin examination of excised tissue, providing tissue conservation with similar or superior cure rates when compared with standard wide local excision.
- Several immunohistochemical stains are available for MMS for melanoma. These improve melanoma detection and may be concurrently performed with routine histopathology.
- Challenges to MMS for melanoma include: difficulty with interpretation of frozen section and surgical margins, the potentially noncontiguous quality of melanoma, and the need for further clinical trials.

INTRODUCTION

Mohs micrographic surgery (MMS), originally developed by Dr Frederic Mohs in the 1930s, is a technique designed to examine histologically 100% of the margins, peripheral and deep, of excised tissue. MMS has been extensively used and studied for the treatment of nonmelanoma skin cancer (NMSC), particularly at sites where tissue conservation is vital. The use of MMS for the treatment of melanoma has yet to become widely accepted owing to difficulties in histologic interpretation, among other factors. However, continued advances in MMS technique and immunohistochemical staining have allowed MMS for melanoma to gain further support.

Mohs first used this technique for treatment of melanoma in 1937, when it achieved fewer local recurrences and improved survival when compared with historical controls for standard excision.[1] One contrasting feature between MMS and standard wide local excision is the minimization of sacrificed healthy tissue with similar or superior cure rates.[2]

MMS can be performed on either fixed or fresh tissue. Working on fixed tissue was the first area explored by Mohs. In these cases, the tissue to be excised was fixed in place using a vehicle (zinc chloride paste), with each fixed plane being removed for histologic analysis. Issues with the paste (eg, pain, local inflammation, and lymphadenopathy) and the need to wait for the paste to penetrate and fix tissue in situ during successive excisions, requiring multiple-day visits, led to the development of fresh-tissue methods. These methods, lacking the fixative paste and usually requiring only a single session for the procedure, have become the predominantly employed form of MMS.[3]

RATIONALE FOR USE

Since MMS was first described and its use firmly established for treatment of NMSC, MMS has become an area of active interest for the treatment of melanoma. Lentigo maligna (LM) is a common subtype of melanoma in situ (MIS), comprising

[a] Department of Dermatology, State University of New York Downstate Medical Center, Box 46, 450 Clarkson Avenue, Brooklyn, NY 11203, USA; [b] Department of Dermatology, Mount Sinai School of Medicine, 5 East 98th Street, 5th Floor, New York, NY 10021, USA; [c] Skin Cancer Medical Center, 16311 Ventura Boulevard, Suite 690, Encino, CA 91436, USA
* Corresponding author.
E-mail address: hui.andrea@gmail.com

Dermatol Clin 30 (2012) 503–515
doi:10.1016/j.det.2012.04.010
0733-8635/12/$ – see front matter Published by Elsevier Inc.

79% to 83% of MIS, and it is especially prevalent in the white men aged 65 years and older.[4] LM melanoma (LMM) is the invasive counterpart to LM and comprises 4% to 15% of cutaneous melanoma.[4] Both LM and LMM present as irregular asymmetric pigmented patches on chronically sun-damaged skin. In these cases, margins can be difficult to ascertain, and in LMM, there may be extensive subclinical disease.[5] Additionally, melanoma may occur on cosmetically sensitive areas of the head and neck and notably functional areas such as the eyelids, ears, nose, and perioral areas, where tissue conservation is of utmost importance.

Current excisional margin guidelines from the National Comprehensive Cancer Network are based on Breslow depth (**Table 1**). Standard wide local excision for melanoma in situ is followed by histopathologic examination. Conventional transverse (bread-loaf) vertical sections require stepwise evaluation of the excision specimen, allowing histologic examination of only 0.1% of the total margin.[6] This may result in false-negative margins and recurrence of melanoma. According to Kimyai-Asadi and colleagues,[7] step sections at 1 mm, 2 mm, 4 mm, and 10 mm intervals would have a 58%, 37%, 19%, and 7% chance, respectively, of detecting positive margins. By their calculations, step sections would need to be performed every 0.1 mm to detect 100% of positive margins.

Several studies have shown that as melanoma approaches more closely to the margin on standard excision specimens, the local recurrence rate increases.[8,9] The recurrence rate for melanoma in situ after wide local excision with standard 5 mm margins ranges from 8% to 20%.[10] This may be due to presence of melanoma at the unexamined interval margins between step sections in wide excision specimens. When melanoma recurs due to residual disease, it may present with a more invasive component. Debloom and colleagues[11]

performed a prospective analysis on 108 marginally recurrent melanomas treated with standard excision or fresh-tissue MMS and permanent section of debulked specimens; 23% of patients with melanoma in situ left at the margin progressed to invasive disease, with a mean Breslow depth of 0.94 mm. Additionally, 33% of patients with minimally invasive melanoma left at the margin progressed to a greater depth of invasion with changes in mean Breslow depth from 1.5 mm at the time of primary treatment to 2.8 mm at the time of recurrence.

LM demonstrates a high rate of local recurrence of 9% to 20% after standard excision, which may occur more than 5 years after initial excision of the lesion.[12] Osborne and colleagues[13] showed that even with clear margins on standard histopathologic examination, local recurrence rate was 20%, and LMM developed in 1.5% of patients. Other case series showed local recurrence rates of about 9%.[14,15]

Studies of MMS for LM have demonstrated significantly lower recurrence rates of 0.5% to 3%.[16–18] Zitelli and colleagues[19] studied 184 cases of melanoma in situ treated with fresh-tissue MMS, showing a local recurrence rate of 0.5%. Additionally, they treated 369 cases of invasive melanoma with fresh-tissue MMS, demonstrating a local recurrence rate of 0.5%. This was in contrast to local recurrence rates of 6% and 3% for in situ and invasive disease respectively after standard excisional surgery. They concluded that MMS is an effective treatment, especially in areas where tissue conservation is important. Bricca and colleagues[20] studied 625 patients treated with frozen section MMS for primary cutaneous melanoma of the head and neck, demonstrating a local recurrence rate of 0.2% versus 9% or higher for standard surgery, with a mean follow-up of 58 months.

However, controversy remains regarding MMS in treating melanoma. The success of the procedure depends on both the ability of the surgeon to accurately detect melanoma at the excised margin with frozen sections and whether the margins narrow enough to excise the primary melanoma alone are adequate to prevent recurrence.[19] Additionally, just as for MMS used for other neoplasms, the tumor growth pattern must be contiguous without skip areas.[2]

FIXED TISSUE SURGICAL TECHNIQUE

Permanent section surgical technique combined with zinc chloride fixative paste (for ingredients, please see **Table 2**) is an excellent method for removal of invasive cutaneous melanoma.[21] The procedure begins with a fresh-tissue biopsy of a suspected melanoma. A saucerized excisional biopsy is a preferred method, because this

Table 1
Current melanoma excisional margin guidelines

Tumor Thickness	Recommended Clinical Margins
In situ	0.5 cm
≤1.0 mm	1.0 cm
1.01–2 mm	1–2 cm
2.01–4 mm	2.0 cm
>4 mm	2.0 cm

Data from Network NCC. NCCN Clinical Practice Guidelines in Oncology (NCCN Guidelines) Melanoma Version 2.20122011:51.

Table 2
Mohs zinc chloride paste formula for compounding

Ingredient	Amount	Origin	Use
Stibnite	40 g	Sulfide mineral with the formula Sb_2S_3, ground to pass through an 80-mesh sieve. Molecular weight, 339.70 g	Inert vehicle
Sanguinaria canadensis	10 g	Powdered root of the plant Sanguinaria canadensis, containing the alkaloid sanguinarine	Apoptosis and other plant alkaloid effects to be elucidated
Zinc chloride saturated solution	34.5 mL	Molecular weight 136.32 g/mol	Destructively penetrates skin

Zinc chloride fixative paste can be prepared by a compounding pharmacy. Delasco, a medical supply company in Council Bluffs, Iowa, can compound the paste reliably.
Data from Mohs FE. Chemosurgery: microscopically controlled surgery for skin cancer. Springfield (IL): Charles C. Thomas; 1978.

technique not only facilitates the removal of the suspected lesion, but also provides an ideal surface for the direct application of zinc chloride fixative paste once invasive melanoma has been histologically confirmed.

Permanent section biopsy results may be available as early as 1 day, but a delay of several days or more is not a problem. Zinc chloride fixative paste is very powerful. Its penetration can be deep, depending on contact time and thickness of application.[22] It must not be applied until the diagnosis of invasive melanoma has been histologically confirmed. Bleeding may be stopped using direct pressure or aluminum chloride on a cotton-tipped applicator. Bleeding may also be controlled with the direct application of zinc chloride fixative paste and absorbable suture ligation, if necessary. The procedure is performed under local anesthesia. Analgesics are prescribed, but often are not necessary.

A dose of a pea size or less of zinc chloride paste is adequate for most melanomas.[21] The paste is applied directly to the biopsy wound site extending to the epidermal edge with a cotton-tipped applicator to a total thickness of up to approximately 1 mm. If the lesion overlies an important anatomic structure, less may be applied; for thicker melanomas, more may be applied. The thicker the layer of paste applied, the more rapidly and deeper it penetrates.

The paste is held in place over the wound for a duration varying from 3 minutes to 24 hours after application. Much of the zinc chloride penetration occurs in the first few minutes, but zinc chloride continues to penetrate slowly over 18 to 24 hours, at which time it reaches its maximum depth of penetration. A complete and deep fixation of

a biopsy site may occur in as little as 3 minutes with the paste held manually in place with a Telfa nonstick pad. For longer applications, a cotton ball covered with a commercially available transparent adhesive film can be used to hold the paste in place. In some cases, it may be convenient for the patient to return the following day before removing the dressing. When the dressing is removed, any remaining paste may be washed off with hydrogen peroxide or saline. If not done in the office, simple bathing at home with soap and water will have the same benefit. If the patient cannot return within a few days, he or she should be instructed to take any and all debris that comes off the site, place it in a plastic bag, and bring it to the office. Prolonged delays between paste application and excision of more than a week can result in spontaneous separation of the pasted tissue, and inadvertent specimen loss becomes a risk.

A wide local excision may be performed the same day as the paste application or may be delayed up to 1 week longer. Because zinc chloride fixative paste both kills and histologically fixes tissue, a conservative margin may be safely removed with no need to extend to the deep fascia. A saucerized excision using beveled Mohs margins, with mapping of the excised tissue specimens for permanent vertical or en-face sections, facilitates the wide local excision. If residual invasive melanoma is found, a delayed repeat excision may be performed.

The use of zinc chloride fixative paste (fixed-tissue micrographic surgery) has been shown by retrospective analysis to significantly improve overall 5-year survival compared with conventional surgery. Mohs reported a 30-year consecutive series of mostly advanced melanomas in which more than 1 out of every 5 patients treated with zinc chloride fixative paste had microscopically proven palpable regional lymph node metastases, and compared his results to simple primary melanomas treated by conventional surgery. Despite an expected far worse prognosis, 5-year survival was improved 53% in the melanomas treated with zinc chloride fixative paste.[23–26] This result suggests that zinc chloride fixative paste may have an antimelanoma vaccine-like systemic effect.

To determine if zinc chloride fixative paste could act as an immune adjuvant, Kalish and colleagues[27] performed a murine melanoma implantation study. Simple excision of implanted melanomas was compared with combined zinc chloride fixative paste and excision. Upon reimplantation of melanomas at a distant challenge site, 1 week after excision, there was a significant reduction of over 50% (69% vs 32%) in the development of new melanomas in the mice receiving the combined treatment. Most importantly, when poorly immunogenic melanomas were substituted in the experiment, this phenomenon did not occur, indicating that immune mechanisms were involved.

Additionally, there is 1 epidemiologic report suggesting that conventional surgery may spread melanoma. A data set of 1224 patients comparing the risk of metastases in thin melanomas within 1 year after surgery to the risk of metastases in thick melanomas before surgery indicated that surgical removal of primary melanoma may trigger metastatic dissemination or enhance growth of subclinical micrometastatic deposits, resulting in the development of clinically evident metastases.[28] Warr and colleagues[29] used a reverse transcriptase polymerase chain reaction (RT-PCR)-based assay to detect tyrosinase transcripts, a marker of occult melanoma cells, in peripheral blood during melanoma excisions. The study demonstrated that surgical intervention increased the presence of circulating tumor cells. The presence of tyrosinase transcripts in peripheral blood has been shown to be a useful marker of melanoma progression and poor prognosis.[30] Several animal models have shown that surgical manipulation can trigger metastases of various cancers.[31,32] However, the role of surgery as a contributing factor in the spread of melanoma metastases remains unknown. By killing tissue and stimulating immunity, zinc chloride fixative paste may help prevent the development of melanoma metastases.

FRESH-TISSUE SURGICAL TECHNIQUES

MMS for melanoma may be performed on fresh tissue under local anesthesia. According to 1 recent protocol, the first step is to mark the tumor's clinical extent. The margin used is between 1 and 6 mm,

depending on the location.[33] For example, a smaller margin might be required when functionally important structures, such as tear ducts, are present, and tissue preservation is important.[34]

Next, reference marks are placed at 12 o'clock, 3 o'clock, 6 o'clock, and 9 o'clock by making small nicks that overlap the visible tumor and perilesional skin. The clinically visible tumor is then excised/debulked, and a small (1 mm) central strip is removed from it. The central strip is then processed by frozen section to confirm the Breslow depth and to serve as a positive control against successive slides. The remainder of the surgical specimen is then submitted for processing of permanent sections and additional assessment of Breslow depth.[34]

The first Mohs layer is then harvested using an incision along the previously marked margin. This incision is carried down to the desired depth of removal, but the horizontal incision of the deep margin is not performed yet. The epidermal and dermal portions of the Mohs layer are then removed together first, so as to be processed separately from the fat. This separation is important, because it allows for delicate 4 μm tissue sections needed for successful immunostaining. The strip itself is usually divided into 2 substrips, but more may be necessary if the tumor is large. Following the removal of the epidermal/dermal strip, the deep component of the specimen, consisting of the subcutaneous fat, is then excised parallel to the plane of the tissue surface.[34]

All the excised tissue is then mapped relative to the reference marks, and the nonepidermal tissue is inked in 2 colors to facilitate mapping of the tumor. The specimen is oriented on a cold glass slide; embedding medium is applied, and then the specimen is adhered to a cryostat specimen object disc. Following this, the slide is warmed to separate it from the specimen, and the block is then cut at 4 μm step sections at intervals of 50 μm until all of the epidermis is visible. The slide is then stained with hematoxylin and eosin, and immunostains may be performed at this time as well. The surgeon analyzes the slides and marks any areas positive for tumor on the map. If any tumor is found, additional excision and processing stages are performed until the tumor is completely removed.[34]

CHALLENGES OF MMS IN THE MANAGEMENT OF MELANOMA

The superior cure rates of MMS for melanoma depend on unequivocal evaluation of 100% of the surgical margins. This is only possible if the melanoma can be clearly discriminated from surrounding nonmalignant tissue. There are several concerns regarding the use of MMS for melanoma.

Challenges with Interpretation of Frozen Sections

There is significant challenge in identification of the pathologic changes of melanoma on frozen sections compared with atypical melanocytic hyperplasia in sun-damaged skin. Zitelli and colleagues noted sensitivity and specificity of 100% and 90%, respectively, of frozen sections for melanoma in a study comparing interpretations of 221 frozen and permanent sections. In this study, melanoma was defined as nests of atypical cells within the dermis or epidermis, or as atypical melanocytic hyperplasia. At the margin, single isolated atypical melanocytes were not identified as melanoma, because they are routinely found bordering benign lesions as well as actinically damaged skin.[35] When scattered atypical melanocytes were scored as benign, 3 or more serial sections or deeper cuts required further examination. If the diagnosis of melanoma could not be unequivocally reached, the section was marked as positive to ensure re-excision. Areas of suspected regression of melanoma, defined as dermal melanophages, fibrosis, and lymphohistiocytic infiltrate, were also considered positive, although no melanoma was seen. Additionally, no attempt was made to distinguish between benign and malignant melanocytic lesions, resulting in excision of benign nevi at the margins.[36]

In a study by Zitelli and colleagues, 535 primary cutaneous melanomas treated with MMS using frozen section stained with routine hematoxylin and eosin demonstrated excellent prognosis and a local recurrence rate of 0.5%. The study showed that 83% of melanomas were excised with a 6 mm margin, 95% with a 9 mm margin, and 97% with a 1.2 cm margin. Margin recommendations for complete excision for melanoma on the head and neck, comparing data by Zitelli and colleagues and the World Health Organization (WHO), are summarized in **Table 3**.[20] Greater margins were required for melanomas on the head/neck and acral areas, than on the trunk. Margin size was directly related to the clinical diameter of the melanoma. There was no significant relationship between required surgical margins and Breslow depth. Importantly, LM, with its typically large clinical diameter, was found to require greater than the recommended 5 mm margins to ensure complete removal. Additionally, because conventional excision relies on surgical margin width rather than clear histologic margins, a 9 mm margin is necessary for complete excision rate of 96.5%. Five-year survival and metastatic rates were comparable or favorable compared with wide local excision.[37]

In contrast, a study by Cohen and colleagues[38] comparing 107 frozen and permanent sections from 45 LM or LMM demonstrated 73% sensitivity and 68% specificity of frozen sections for melanoma. In this study, LM was defined as contiguous pleomorphic melanocytes in the basal layer of an atrophic dermis, infiltration of atypical melanocytes, and dermal solar elastosis with variable chronic inflammation. LMM was diagnosed if any melanoma was present in the dermis. Nests were not part of the criteria for diagnosis of LM or LMM. The false-positive rate of 17% was related to atypical melanocytic hyperplasia in sun-damaged skin without melanoma. This discordance may be explained by comparison of permanent sections that were peripheral to the frozen sections instead of mirror images to them. Both Zitelli and Cohen noted particular difficulty in differentiating melanoma in situ from severely sun-damaged skin.[37,38]

MMS using frozen sections alone may be inadequate for detecting single atypical melanocytes at margins of melanoma in situ. Barlow and colleagues[39] examined 154 frozen sections of melanoma in situ; from this total, 50 specimens considered difficult to interpret were subsequently thawed and sent for routine processing. These specimens were then examined by a dermatopathologist. The sensitivity and specificity of frozen sections were poor, at 59% and 81%, respectively. Another study comprising 330 evaluations (22 cases, 15 dermatopathologists) revealed a diagnostic discrepancy of 40% when comparing frozen sections and perpendicular paraffin-embedded sections in the same lesion.[40]

Challenges with Interpretation and Review of Surgical Margins

The potentially noncontiguous quality of melanoma and its predilection for early metastasis are additional concerns when considering MMS for melanoma. Initially, it was thought that wide surgical margins would augment excision of contiguous microsatellites, but several large studies have failed

---

Table 3
Comparison of MMS margin recommendations to completely excise head and neck melanomas

Tumor Thickness	Zitelli[37]	WHO
In situ	9 mm	5 mm
≤1.0 mm	9 mm	10 mm
1.01–2 mm	12 mm	10 mm
2.01–4 mm	12 mm	20 mm
>4 mm	>12 mm	20 mm

Data from Bricca GM, Brodland DG, Ren D, et al. Cutaneous head and neck melanoma treated with Mohs micrographic surgery. J Am Acad Dermatol 2005;52(1):92–100.

to demonstrate improved cure rates.[41–44] Microsatellites within primary melanoma excisions were more highly associated with risk for regional nodal metastases than primary melanoma thickness.[45] If the only goal of treatment were complete removal of melanoma to clear histologic margins, then MMS would be the preferred treatment. However, if microsatellites are found within MMS sections, the dilemma then arises regarding the futility of MMS for the treatment of melanoma. Studies are needed addressing the presence of microsatellites and their effect on local recurrences and melanoma-related death.

As reviewed by Trotter and colleagues and others, LM presents difficulty with interpretation at the lesion periphery, as it is often poorly defined both clinically and histologically. Positive margins frequently overlap with normal sun-exposed skin, especially if sun-induced melanocytic hyperplasia is present. Focal contiguous melanocytes, melanocytic atypia, and follicular melanocytes may be found in these areas adjacent to melanomas and NMSCs.[20,46] No single feature is specific for LM.

There are additional problems with review of surgical margins. Each hematoxylin and eosin-stained frozen section must be painstakingly reviewed, especially when challenged with sun-damaged skin and melanoma in situ, freeze artifact, tissue folding, and other findings. Keratinocytes can develop vacuolization, which causes them to resemble melanocytes and can result in false-positive margins.[47] Margin review can be considerably more challenging and time-consuming compared with review of NMSCs. In response, several authors have instead used permanent sections as an alternative or adjunct to frozen sections when performing MMS for melanoma.[17,38,48,49]

Permanent sections have been considered the gold standard for diagnosis of melanoma. However, for MMS, use of permanent sections for margin evaluation results in an interruption between melanoma excision and ensuing repair. Even rush permanent sections still require overnight processing and delay of subsequent sectioning and repair. This delay to repair has not been shown to have adverse effects on morbidity on the patient and can indeed minimize the risk of having to undo a complex tissue rearrangement in critical anatomic areas.[50–53]

IMMUNOHISTOCHEMICAL STAINS AND RATIONALE FOR USE

The use of immunohistochemical stains significantly improves melanoma detection and differentiation between malignant cells and melanocytes,

and they can be used on both permanent sections and frozen sections.[54] Using immunohistochemical stains for frozen section abrogates the delay encountered between preparation of permanent section and subsequent repair during MMS for melanoma. The benefit of sparing of normal tissue through MMS is thus retained.

Immunohistochemical staining is performed side by side with routine histopathology, and slide preparation is identical. An additional hour is necessary for immunostaining, but new protocols have shortened this time to 20 minutes or less.[55] There are a variety of immunostains available for use for MMS for melanoma, and it is important to review the background and rationale for use for each immunostain.

IMMUNOHISTOCHEMICAL STAINS AND THEIR INTERPRETATION
S-100

Many studies have shown S-100 to be the most sensitive immunohistochemical stain for diagnosis of primary and metastatic melanoma, and it is especially useful for staining spindle cell and desmoplastic melanoma.[54,56,57] S-100 stains dermal components of melanoma strongly positive, but epidermal components are variably positive, which is an issue when staining for melanoma in situ.[58,59]

S-100 lacks specificity. S-100 stains almost all melanocytic lesions, benign and malignant, as well as dendritic cells, Schwann cells, histiocytes, glands, chondrocytes, lipocytes, muscle, and many others.[54,56,60] This creates significant background noise that interferes with accurate interpretation of melanomas, especially when considering S-100's variable epidermal melanocytic staining pattern. Still, S-100 offers strong positive staining for deep melanoma components, which may not be as strongly positive by other immunostains.

Human Melanoma, Black-45

Human melanoma, black-45 (HMB-45) is a useful marker for melanocytic differentiation, and it is used routinely in melanoma diagnosis. HMB-45 is a mouse monoclonal antibody that recognizes a 30 to 35 kDa melanosome-associated sialated glycoprotein gp100 localized to premelanosomes. Specifically, it is localized to stage 1 and 2 melanosomes in neoplastic melanocytes.[61,62] HMB-45 staining is independent of tyrosinase activity, and it is cytoplasmic and granular.[62] HMB-45 is positively staining in active early melanosome formation of immature or proliferating melanocytes, such as those in fetal and neonatal skin, inflamed skin, and primary melanomas.[56] HMB-45 has also been found to exhibit positive staining for melanoma, junctional nevi, atypical nevi, Spitz nevi, and blue nevi.[28,63–65] Unstimulated adult melanocytes, keratinocytes, and most dermal melanocytes do not stain with HMB-45.[60–62] Because HMB-45 does not stain keratinocytes, this implies that positivity is related to uptake by melanocytes. A rare group of tumors containing premelanosomes stains positively with HMB-45, including clear cell tumors of the lung, angiomyolipomas, and lymphangiomyomatosis.[66]

HMB-45 exhibits great specificity in identifying malignant melanomas from other nonmelanocytic malignancies.[61] HMB-45 is more specific than S-100 protein but less sensitive.[28,63,65,67] Several studies have shown the sensitivity of HMB-45 on paraffin-embedded melanoma sections to be 85% to 97%.[60,66,68,69]

There are several issues with the use of HMB-45. It may demonstrate variable, patchy staining within typical melanosomes.[56] Moreover, HMB-45 staining for spindle cell melanomas such as desmoplastic and neurotrophic melanomas, shows inconsistent focal staining to the dermal component, or no staining at all.[60,70] Newer antigen retrieval techniques have increased sensitivity to 75% in spindle cell melanomas.[71]

The most problematic issue concerning HMB-45 is its inconsistency in identifying pseudonevoid nests at the base of a malignant melanoma. This may result in mistakenly labeling these nests as benign mature nests and subsequent errors in Breslow depth, surgical margins, and prognosis.

Mel-5

Mel-5 is a mouse monoclonal antibody against pigmentation-associated glycoprotein g75 of melanocytes and human melanoma.[72] Mel-5 is a member of the tyrosine-related family of proteins (TRP-1), and it is present in abundant quantities on the membrane of stage 3 and 4 melanosomes.[58,72,73] Mel-5 stains all melanocyte-containing cells, including normal epidermal melanocytes, epidermal components of benign nevi, and 95% of melanomas.[74]

In contrast to HMB-45, Mel-5 stains both proliferating and mature melanocytes. Mel-5 also offers an advantage over S-100 in that it more reliably and consistently stains epidermal melanocytes, and does not stain melanophages or Langerhans cells.[58] However, Mel-5 stains epithelial cells in the basal layer of the epidermis because of melanosome transfer.[75]

Mel-5 inconsistently stains dermal components for both benign and malignant melanocytic neoplasms. Additionally, it does not stain all amelanotic or desmoplastic melanoma,[58] or cultured melanoma cells with epithelioid morphology and no detectable pigment or tyrosinase activity.[72]

Compared with S-100, Mel-5 exhibited superior intensity and specificity with less background staining. However, HMB-45 was more specific.[69] Mel-5 stained nonmelanocytic lesions such as pigmented Bowen disease, pigmented actinic keratosis, and lichen planus-like keratosis.[58] Another confounding factor is that darker skin types stain more deeply than lighter skin types due to their greater number of melanosomes. Solar lentigines also stain more prominently.

Melanoma Antigen Recognized by T cells

The MART-1 antigen, also known as Melan-A antigen, is a 22-kDa cytoplasmic melanosome-associated glycoprotein recognized by mouse monoclonal antibodies A-103 and M2-7C10.[74] It is an antigen to melanocyte differentiation similar to gp100 and gp75 (recognized by HMB-45 and Mel-5, respectively). MART-1 is present in 80% to 100% of melanomas, nonproliferating adult melanocytes, and nevus cells in both epidermal and dermal components.[59,76–78] For primary melanomas, Blessing and colleagues noted 97% positivity for MART-1 and 90% positivity for HMB-45.[56] For metastatic melanomas, MART-1 stains with 81% to 89% positivity, compared with HMB-45, which stains 75% to 76% of tumors.[78,79]

MART-1 has demonstrated more consistent and intense staining than HMB-45 in several studies.[56,59,78] Jungbluth and colleagues[78] demonstrated homogenous staining, indicating greater than 75% reactive tumor cells, in 75% of melanomas stained with MART-1 compared with 51% of melanomas stained with HMB-45. Staining intensity was not affected by level of pigmentation in these melanomas.

Compared with all other melanocytic immunostains, MART-1 is considered the most accurate and reliable.[56,80] Zalla and colleagues[69] compared the effectiveness of MART-1 with 4 other in melanoma excisions of 68 patients (46 melanoma in situ and 22 invasive melanomas). A 64-minute staining protocol was used, comparing MART-1 with HMB-35, Mel-5, MART-1, and S-100. MART-1 was most reliable in epidermal staining and easiest to interpret compared with the other immunostains. Patients were followed for an average of 16 months (range 1–32 months), with no recurrences reported.

However, MART-1 may not be adequate for distinguishing melanoma in situ on sun-damaged skin from pigmented actinic keratosis. Pigmented actinic keratosis is considered a simulator of early melanoma in situ on sun-damaged skin due to difficulty in differentiating between pigmented keratinocytes and melanocytes. In a study by El Shabrawi-Calen and colleagues, 10 unequivocal cases of pigmented actinic keratosis were stained by MART-1 and compared with staining patterns by S-100, HMB-45, and tyrosinase. Areas of normal skin adjacent to the pigmented actinic keratosis showed prominent staining by MART-1, which could potentially result in false-positive margins. The other immunostains were only variably positive for intraepidermal melanocytes.[81] Therefore, MART-1 immunostains should be interpreted cautiously and in context of other immunostains.

Micropthalmia Transcription Factor

Micropthalmia transcription factor (MiTF) is a transcription factor that plays a role in the development and survival of melanocytes.[82] In mice, homozygous mutations cause accelerated age-dependent death of all melanocytes in the first months of life the in skin, choroid of the eye, and stria vascularis of the inner ear.[82] Heterozygous mutations of MiTF result in the autosomal dominant disorder Waardenburg syndrome type 2A, characterized by a white forelock and hearing loss.[83] Recently, MiTF was demonstrated as a transcriptional target of B-catenin/Wnt signaling in the zebra fish homolog, which is abnormally activated in many human melanomas.[84–86]

MiTF expression is conserved in both primary and metastatic melanomas, as well as benign nevi. King and colleagues[82] used MiTF antibody to immunostain 58 primary cutaneous melanomas of several types, including superficial spreading, LM, and nodular, and demonstrated 100% positive staining. Epithelioid and spindle cell-type melanomas in the dermal component were also MiTF positive. However, MiTF is of limited utility for staining desmoplastic melanomas; similar to other melanocyte-associated antigens, nearly all desmoplastic melanomas did not stain with MiTF antibody.

MiTF staining in melanocytes is nuclear, compared with cytoplasmic staining in the majority of other melanoma immunostains.[82] This characteristic is helpful for interpreting melanomas in which there is profuse pigment in the cytoplasm of the cells. Another benefit of MiTF nuclear staining is that the outline of the cell is clearly delineated, without cytoplasmic staining obscuring the tissue. Individual cells may therefore be identified. In cases of weak staining, comparison with bordering nuclei of other cells and structures such as keratinocytes and adnexal structures provides an adequate control.

MiTF is an excellent marker for quantification of melanocytes. For use in the often-challenging identification of solar lentigines and LM, Kim and colleagues[87] compared MiTF to Melan-A, HMB-45, and Mel-5 in a study of 43 lesions (20 melanomas in situ and 23 solar lentigos). The study demonstrated that Melan-A significantly overestimated the density of melanocytes within sun-damaged skin. MiTF provided superior contrast of melanocytes to keratinocytes with abundant cytoplasmic pigment.

Choosing Immunohistochemical Stains for Melanoma

Currently, there are many studies supporting MART-1 as the most accurate and reliable immunohistochemical stain for melanoma.[56,80] There may be some value in using combinations of stains for further confirmation of margins. For example, although S-100 produces the most background staining, it remains useful in the detection of desmoplastic melanomas, whereas the other stains are either inconsistent or do not stain desmoplastic melanomas at all. MiTF provides excellent contrast of melanocytes to keratinocytes in cases in which there is excessive cytoplasmic pigment. Each stain provides a unique quality that may compensate for other stains' deficiencies. More studies are necessary to determine the most appropriate stains for MMS for melanoma.

Improvements in Immunohistochemical Staining

Chang and colleagues[55] introduced a novel immunohistochemical staining technique that automates the performing of immunostains within 16 minutes. The group used a rapid automated instrument and performed immunostains with MART-1 on frozen sections, then compared the results with MART-1 stains of permanent sections, and hematoxylin and eosin (H&E) stains of frozen and permanent sections from positive or negative control specimens of the Mohs layers for melanoma. The rapid-stained frozen sections were significantly easier to interpret than the other sections, including the gold standard of permanent section stained with H&E. This automation has the potential to reduce variability between staining laboratories, technicians, and iterations during the Mohs process, thereby improving the quality of stains and accuracy of the analysis.

Challenges with Immunohistochemical Staining

Immunohistochemical staining is not currently considered cost-effective as costs per slide can be prohibitive, and quality control may also be an issue if not done frequently. Additionally, there may be additional Mohs technician training. After calculating the sum of supply costs and technician wages, the actual cost of preparing the immunohistochemical stained sections may be close to or below reimbursement levels.[88] With the development of newer, faster automated systems, immunohistochemical staining may soon become more cost-effective.

POSSIBLE ADJUNCTIVE MODALITIES TO MMS FOR MELANOMA
Topical Treatments

Several other treatments for melanoma in situ are available, but they should only be considered for cases in which surgery is impossible or may cause unacceptable morbidity to the area. Erickson and colleagues[89] performed a review of literature regarding treatments for melanoma in situ other than surgery, including topical imiquimod 5% cream and radiation therapy. For topical imiquimod therapy, several small case series with follow-up periods of 12 months or less showed relatively low cure rates of about 75% to 91%.

Radiation therapy with Grenz rays or soft radiographs provided cure rates of 86% to 95% in several small studies with follow-up times from 2 to 5 years. In general, these topical treatments provided viable noninvasive alternatives to therapy for patients who may be poor surgical candidates. There has been concern that imiquimod can mask invasive disease.[90–92]

Modified MMS Technique

Chang and colleagues[55] proposed a 6-step modification of the Mohs process that may help improve margin interpretation. This process uses a Woods lamp to improve delineation of the margin, and negative and positive control biopsies with the Mohs layer. The margin is then compared with the positive and negative control; if atypical melanocytic hyperplasia in the Mohs margin comparable to the negative control, then no additional layers are taken. If the margin is equivocal, then it is compared with the positive control. Finally, the block from the first stage of MMS and the positive control are submitted for permanent sectioning to further evaluate the Breslow depth and verify that the lesion is completely in situ.

Sentinel Lymph Node Biopsy

Sentinel lymph node (SLN) biopsy is the determination, through the use of radionuclides and dyes, of which lymph nodes are closest (sentinel) to the primary tumor. The identification and histopathologic examination of these nodes can aid in staging the cancer, as well as directing further treatment. With respect to malignant melanoma, there is currently controversy whether SLN is effective in increasing overall survival rates.

In 2006, Johnson and colleagues[93] performed a comprehensive review of 1198 articles evaluating the evidence base behind SLN biopsies for melanoma. They concluded that the available evidence overwhelmingly supported SLN status as the most significant independent factor predicting survival, with the highest sensitivity and specificity of any nodal staging test, and that results also improved regional disease control.

In 2006, Morton and colleagues[94] enrolled 1269 patients with intermediate thickness (1.2–3.5 mm) primary cutaneous melanomas as part of the Multicenter Selective Lymphadenectomy Trial-1 (MSLT-1). The authors determined that an immediate lymphadenectomy following a positive SLN result increased the 5-year survival rate (72% vs 52%) in those with primary melanoma. However, multiple commentaries on this report questioned the interpretation of the data in terms of increased morbidity with lymphadenectomy and no increase in survival rate based on the data presented.[95]

Confocal Microscopy

LM and LMM are particularly difficult to diagnose clinically and dermatoscopically. Among other reasons, this is because LMM occurs most commonly in highly photodamaged skin. In 2009, Ahlgrimm and colleagues[96] demonstrated the usage of in vivo reflectance confocal microscopy in the identification of LMM. With the goal of more accurately identifying, at a cellular level, atypical melanocytes and other known features of melanoma, these techniques have potential for adjunctive use with MMS as well.

SUMMARY

For the treatment of melanoma, the primary goal is complete removal with histologically negative margins. MMS, either with fixed tissue or frozen section technique aided by immunohistochemistry, allows for evaluation of 100% of the surgical margin and among many currently practiced techniques for melanoma surgery. MMS may offer lower recurrence rates and improved survival when compared with historical controls for standard excision. Additionally, fixed tissue technique may confer an immunologic advantage. MMS has been demonstrated as an acceptable option for treatment of melanoma, especially for lesions in functionally or cosmetically sensitive areas where tissue conservation is crucial. Further advances in MMS surgical techniques and immunohistochemical staining may promote MMS as a standard treatment for melanoma in the future; however, application of the techniques is currently limited to those with expertise in this evolving arena. Additionally, further clinical trials comparing long-term recurrence with MMS versus standard excision would be helpful.

REFERENCES

1. Chang KH, Dufresne R Jr, Cruz A, et al. The operative management of melanoma: where does Mohs surgery fit in? Dermatol Surg 2011;37(8):1069–79.

2. Whalen J, Leone D. Mohs micrographic surgery for the treatment of malignant melanoma. Clin Dermatol 2009;27(6):597–602.

3. Trost LB, Bailin PL. History of Mohs surgery. Dermatol Clin 2011;29(2):135–9.

4. Swetter SM, Boldrick JC, Jung SY, et al. Increasing incidence of lentigo maligna melanoma subtypes: northern california and national trends 1990-2000. J Invest Dermatol 2005;125(4):685–91.

5. Kwon SY, Miller SJ. Mohs surgery for melanoma in situ. Dermatol Clin 2011;29(2):175–83.

6. Abide JM, Nahai F, Bennett RG. The meaning of surgical margins. Plast Reconstr Surg 1984;73(3):492–7.

7. Kimyai-Asadi A, Katz T, Goldberg LH, et al. Margin involvement after the excision of melanoma in situ: the need for complete en face examination of the surgical margins. Dermatol Surg 2007;33(12):1434–9 [discussion: 1439–41].

8. McKinnon JG, Starritt EC, Scolyer RA, et al. Histopathologic excision margin affects local recurrence rate: analysis of 2681 patients with melanomas < or = 2 mm thick. Ann Surg 2005;241(2):326–33.

9. Ng AK, Jones WO, Shaw JH. Analysis of local recurrence and optimizing excision margins for cutaneous melanoma. Br J Surg 2001;88(1):137–42.

10. McKenna JK, Florell SR, Goldman GD, et al. Lentigo maligna/lentigo maligna melanoma: current state of diagnosis and treatment. Dermatol Surg 2006;32(4):493–504.

11. Debloom IJR, Zitelli JA, Brodland DG. The invasive growth potential of residual melanoma and melanoma in situ. Dermatol Surg 2010;36(8):1251–7.

12. Wildemore JK, Schuchter L, Mick R, et al. Locally recurrent malignant melanoma characteristics and outcomes: a single-institution study. Ann Plast Surg 2001;46(5):488–94.

13. Osborne JE, Hutchinson PE. A follow-up study to investigate the efficacy of initial treatment of lentigo maligna with surgical excision. Br J Plast Surg 2002;55(8):611–5.

14. Coleman WP 3rd, Davis RS, Reed RJ, et al. Treatment of lentigo maligna and lentigo maligna melanoma. J Dermatol Surg Oncol 1980;6(6):476–9.

15. Pitman GH, Kopf AW, Bart RS, et al. Treatment of lentigo maligna and lentigo maligna melanoma. J Dermatol Surg Oncol 1979;5(9):727–37.

16. Bhardwaj SS, Tope WD, Lee PK. Mohs micrographic surgery for lentigo maligna and lentigo maligna melanoma using mel-5 immunostaining: University of Minnesota experience. Dermatol Surg 2006;32(5):690–7.

17. Cohen LM, McCall MW, Zax RH. Mohs micrographic surgery for lentigo maligna and lentigo maligna melanoma. A follow-up study. Dermatol Surg 1998;24(6):673–7.

18. Walling HW, Scupham RK, Bean AK, et al. Staged excision versus Mohs micrographic surgery for lentigo maligna and lentigo maligna melanoma. J Am Acad Dermatol 2007;57(4):659–64.

19. Zitelli JA, Brown C, Hanusa BH. Mohs micrographic surgery for the treatment of primary cutaneous melanoma. J Am Acad Dermatol 1997;37(2 Part 1):236–45.

20. Bricca GM, Brodland DG, Ren D, et al. Cutaneous head and neck melanoma treated with Mohs micrographic surgery. J Am Acad Dermatol 2005;52(1):92–100.

21. Brooks NA. Chemosurgery for invasive melanoma. Dermatol Surg 2010;36(2):237–40.

22. McDaniel S, Goldman GD. Consequences of using escharotic agents as primary treatment for nonmelanoma skin cancer. Arch Dermatol 2002;138(12):1593–6.

23. Brooks NA. Fixed-tissue micrographic surgery in the treatment of cutaneous melanoma. An overlooked cancer treatment strategy. J Dermatol Surg Oncol 1992;18(11):999–1000.

24. Clark WH, From L, Bernardino EA, et al. The histogenesis and biologic behavior of primary human malignant melanomas of the skin. Cancer Res 1969;29(3):705–27.

25. Mohs FE. Chemosurgical treatment of melanoma; a microscopically controlled method of excision. Arch Derm Syphilol 1950;62(2):269–79.

26. Mohs FE. Chemosurgery: microscopically controlled surgery for skin cancer. Springfield (IL): Charles C. Thomas; 1978.

27. Kalish RS, Wood JA, Siegel DM, et al. Experimental rationale for treatment of high-risk human melanoma with zinc chloride fixative paste. Increased resistance to tumor challenge in murine melanoma model. Dermatol Surg 1998;24(9):1021–5.

28. Smolle J, Soyer HP, Smolle-Juttner FM, et al. Does surgical removal of primary melanoma trigger growth of occult metastases? An analytical epidemiological approach. Dermatol Surg 1997;23(11):1043–6.

29. Warr RP, Zebedee Z, Kenealy J, et al. Detection of melanoma seeding during surgical procedures—an RT-PCR based model. Eur J Surg Oncol 2002;28(8):832–7.

30. Kunter U, Buer J, Probst M, et al. Peripheral blood tyrosinase messenger RNA detection and survival in malignant melanoma. J Natl Cancer Inst 1996; 88(9):590–4.

31. Qadri SSA, Wang J-H, Coffey JC, et al. Can surgery for cancer accelerate the progression of secondary tumors within residual minimal disease at both local and systemic levels? Ann Thorac Surg 2005;80(3): 1046–51.

32. Nishizaki T, Matsumata T, Kanematsu T, et al. Surgical manipulation of VX2 carcinoma in the rabbit liver evokes enhancement of metastasis. J Surg Res 1990;49(1):92–7.

33. Etzkorn JR, Cherpelis BS, Glass LF. Mohs surgery for melanoma: rationale, advances and possibilities. Expert Rev Anticancer Ther 2011;11(7):1043–54.

34. Cherpelis BS, Fenske NA, Glass LF, et al. Mohs surgery for melanoma in situ: how we do it. J Drugs Dermatol 2010;9(7):786–8.

35. Montagna W, Kirchner S, Carlisle K. Histology of sun-damaged human skin. J Am Acad Dermatol 1989;21(5 Pt 1):907–18.

36. Zitelli JA, Moy RL, Abell E. The reliability of frozen sections in the evaluation of surgical margins for melanoma. J Am Acad Dermatol 1991;24(1):102–6.

37. Zitelli JA, Brown CD, Hanusa BH. Surgical margins for excision of primary cutaneous melanoma. J Am Acad Dermatol 1997;37(3):422–9.

38. Cohen LM, McCall MW, Hodge SJ, et al. Successful treatment of lentigo maligna and lentigo maligna melanoma with mohs' micrographic surgery aided by rush permanent sections. Cancer 1994;73(12): 2964–70.

39. Barlow RJ, White CR, Swanson NA. Mohs' micrographic surgery using frozen sections alone may be unsuitable for detecting single atypical melanocytes at the margins of melanoma in situ. Br J Dermatol 2002;146(2):290–4.

40. Prieto VG, Argenyi ZB, Barnhill RL, et al. Are en face frozen sections accurate for diagnosing margin status in melanocytic lesions? Am J Clin Pathol 2003;120(2):203–8.

41. Balch CM, Urist MM, Karakousis CP, et al. Efficacy of 2-cm surgical margins for intermediate-thickness melanomas (1 to 4 mm). Results of a multi-institutional randomized surgical trial. Ann Surg 1993;218(3):262–7 [discussion: 267–9].

42. Veronesi U, Cascinelli N. Narrow excision (1-cm margin) a safe procedure for thin cutaneous melanoma. Arch Surg 1991;126(4):438–41.

43. Elder DE, Guerry DT, Heiberger RM, et al. Optimal resection margin for cutaneous malignant melanoma. Plast Reconstr Surg 1983;71(1):66–72.

44. O'Brien CJ, Coates AS, Petersen-Schaefer K, et al. Experience with 998 cutaneous melanomas of the head and neck over 30 years. Am J Surg 1991; 162(4):310–4.

45. Harrist TJ, Rigel DS, Day CL Jr, et al. "Microscopic satellites" are more highly associated with regional lymph node metastases than is primary melanoma thickness. Cancer 1984;53(10):2183–7.

46. Trotter MJ. Melanoma margin assessment. Clin Lab Med 2011;31(2):289–300.

47. Cook J. Surgical margins for resection of primary cutaneous melanoma. Clin Dermatol 2004;22(3):228–33.

48. Dhawan SS, Wolf DJ, Rabinovitz HS, et al. Lentigo maligna: the use of rush permanent sections in therapy. Arch Dermatol 1990;126(7):928–30.

49. Johnson TM, Headington JT, Baker SR, et al. Usefulness of the staged excision for lentigo maligna and lentigo maligna melanoma: the "square" procedure. J Am Acad Dermatol 1997;37(5):758–64.

50. Escobar V, Zide MF. Delayed repair of skin cancer defects. J Oral Maxillofac Surg 1999;57(3):271–9.

51. David DB, Gimblett ML, Potts MJ, et al. Small margin (2 mm) excision of peri-ocular basal cell carcinoma with delayed repair. Orbit (Amsterdam, Netherlands) 1999;18(1):11–5.

52. Thomas JR, Frost TW. Immediate versus delayed repair of skin defects following resection of carcinoma. Otolaryngol Clin North Am 1993;26(2): 203–13.

53. Morris DS, Elzaridi E, Clarke L, et al. Periocular basal cell carcinoma: 5-year outcome following slow Mohs surgery with formalin-fixed paraffin-embedded sections and delayed closure. Br J Ophthalmol 2009; 93(4):474–6.

54. Ruiter DJ, Brocker EB. Immunohistochemistry in the evaluation of melanocytic tumors. Semin Diagn Pathol 1993;10(1):76–91.

55. Chang KH, Finn DT, Lee D, et al. Novel 16-minute technique for evaluating melanoma resection margins during Mohs surgery. J Am Acad Dermatol 2011;64(1):107–12.

56. Blessing K, Sanders DS, Grant JJ. Comparison of immunohistochemical staining of the novel antibody melan-A with S100 protein and HMB-45 in malignant melanoma and melanoma variants. Histopathology 1998;32(2):139–46.

57. Fernando SS, Johnson S, Bate J. Immunohistochemical analysis of cutaneous malignant melanoma: comparison of S-100 protein, HMB-45 monoclonal antibody and NKI/C3 monoclonal antibody. Pathology 1994;26(1):16–9.

58. Bhawan J. Mel-5: a novel antibody for differential diagnosis of epidermal pigmented lesions of the skin in paraffin-embedded sections. Melanoma Res 1997;7(1):43–8.

59. Busam KJ, Chen YT, Old LJ, et al. Expression of melan-A (MART1) in benign melanocytic nevi and primary cutaneous malignant melanoma. Am J Surg Pathol 1998;22(8):976–82.

60. Wick MR, Swanson PE, Rocamora A. Recognition of malignant melanoma by monoclonal antibody

HMB-45. An immunohistochemical study of 200 paraffin-embedded cutaneous tumors. J Cutan Pathol 1988;15(4):201–7.

61. Chiamenti AM, Vella F, Bonetti F, et al. Anti-melanoma monoclonal antibody HMB-45 on enhanced chemiluminescence-Western blotting recognizes a 30-35 kDa melanosome-associated sialated glycoprotein. Melanoma Res 1996;6(4):291–8.

62. Kikuchi A, Shimizu H, Nishikawa T. Expression and ultrastructural localization of HMB-45 antigen. Br J Dermatol 1996;135(3):400–5.

63. Palazzo J, Duray PH. Typical, dysplastic, congenital, and Spitz nevi: a comparative immunohistochemical study. Hum Pathol 1989;20(4):341–6.

64. Skelton HG 3rd, Smith KJ, Barrett TL, et al. HMB-45 staining in benign and malignant melanocytic lesions. A reflection of cellular activation. Am J Dermatopathol 1991;13(6):543–50.

65. Sun J, Morton TH Jr, Gown AM. Antibody HMB-45 identifies the cells of blue nevi. An immunohistochemical study on paraffin sections. Am J Surg Pathol 1990;14(8):748–51.

66. Bacchi CE, Gown AM. Specificity of antibody HMB-45. Arch Pathol Lab Med 1992;116(9):899–900.

67. Gown AM, Vogel AM, Hoak D, et al. Monoclonal antibodies specific for melanocytic tumors distinguish subpopulations of melanocytes. Am J Pathol 1986; 123(2):195–203.

68. Ordonez NG, Ji XL, Hickey RC. Comparison of HMB-45 monoclonal antibody and S-100 protein in the immunohistochemical diagnosis of melanoma. Am J Clin Pathol 1988;90(4):385–90.

69. Zalla MJ, Lim KK, DiCaudo DJ, et al. Mohs micrographic excision of melanoma using immunostains. Dermatol Surg 2000;26(8):771–84.

70. Longacre TA, Egbert BM, Rouse RV. Desmoplastic and spindle-cell malignant melanoma: an immunohistochemical study. Am J Surg Pathol 1996; 20(12):1489–500.

71. Miettinen M, Fernandez M, Franssila K, et al. Microphthalmia transcription factor in the immunohistochemical diagnosis of metastatic melanoma: comparison with four other melanoma markers. Am J Surg Pathol 2001;25(2):205–11.

72. Thomson TM, Mattes MJ, Roux L, et al. Pigmentation-associated glycoprotein of human melanomas and melanocytes: definition with a mouse monoclonal antibody. J Invest Dermatol 1985;85(2):169–74.

73. Vijayasaradhi S, Houghton AN. Purification of an autoantigenic 75-kDa human melanosomal glycoprotein. Int J Cancer 1991;47(2):298–303.

74. El Tal AK, Abrou AE, Stiff MA, et al. Immunostaining in Mohs micrographic surgery: a review. Dermatol Surg 2010;36(3):275–90.

75. Thomson TM, Real FX, Murakami S, et al. Differentiation antigens of melanocytes and melanoma: analysis of melanosome and cell surface markers of human pigmented cells with monoclonal antibodies. J Invest Dermatol 1988;90(4):459–66.

76. Chen YT, Stockert E, Jungbluth A, et al. Serological analysis of Melan-A(MART-1), a melanocyte-specific protein homogeneously expressed in human melanomas. Proc Natl Acad Sci 1996;93(12):5915–9.

77. Fetsch PA, Cormier J, Hijazi YM. Immunocytochemical detection of MART-1 in fresh and paraffin-embedded malignant melanomas. J Immunother 1997;20(1):60–4.

78. Jungbluth AA, Busam KJ, Gerald WL, et al. A103: an anti-Melan-A monoclonal antibody for the detection of malignant melanoma in paraffin-embedded tissues. Am J Surg Pathol 1998;22(5):595–602.

79. Cormier JN, Hijazi YM, Abati A, et al. Heterogeneous expression of melanoma-associated antigens and HLA-A2 in metastatic melanoma in vivo. Int J Cancer 1998;75(4):517–24.

80. Albertini JG, Elston DM, Libow LF, et al. Mohs micrographic surgery for melanoma: a case series, a comparative study of immunostains, an informative case report, and a unique mapping technique. Dermatol Surg 2002;28(8):656–65.

81. Shabrawi-Caelen LE, Kerl H, Cerroni L. Melan-A: not a helpful marker in distinction between melanoma in situ on sun-damaged skin and pigmented actinic keratosis. Am J Dermatopathol 2004;26(5):364–6.

82. King R, Googe PB, Weilbaecher KN, et al. Microphthalmia transcription factor expression in cutaneous benign, malignant melanocytic, and nonmelanocytic tumors. Am J Surg Pathol 2001;25(1):51–7.

83. Hughes AE, Newton VE, Liu XZ, et al. A gene for waardenburg syndrome type 2 maps close to the human homologue of the microphthalmia gene at chromosome 3p12-p14.1. Nat Genet 1994;7(4): 509–12.

84. Rimm DL, Caca K, Hu G, et al. Frequent nuclear/cytoplasmic localization of β-catenin without exon 3 mutations in malignant melanoma. Am J Pathol 1999;154(2):325–9.

85. Rubinfeld B, Robbins P, El-Gamil M, et al. Stabilization of β-catenin by genetic defects in melanoma cell lines. Science 1997;275(5307):1790–2.

86. Dorsky RI, Raible DW, Moon RT. Direct regulation of nacre, a zebrafish MITF homolog required for pigment cell formation, by the Wnt pathway. Genes Dev 2000;14(2):158–62.

87. Kim J, Taube JM, McCalmont TH, et al. Quantitative comparison of MiTF, Melan-A, HMB-45 and Mel-5 in solar lentigines and melanoma in situ. J Cutan Pathol 2011;38(10):775–9.

88. Bricca GM, Brodland DG, Zitelli JA. Immunostaining melanoma frozen sections: the 1-hour protocol. Dermatol Surg 2004;30(3):403–8.

89. Erickson C, Miller SJ. Treatment options in melanoma in situ: topical and radiation therapy, excision and Mohs surgery. Int J Dermatol 2010;49(5):482–91.

90. Turza K, Dengel LT, Harris RC, et al. Effectiveness of imiquimod limited to dermal melanoma metastases, with simultaneous resistance of subcutaneous metastasis. J Cutan Pathol 2010;37(1): 94–8.

91. Ugurel S, Wagner A, Pföhler C, et al. Topical imiquimod eradicates skin metastases of malignant melanoma but fails to prevent rapid lymphogenous metastatic spread. Br J Dermatol 2002;147(3): 621–3.

92. Kowalzick L, Eickenscheidt L. Progress of multiple cutaneous and subcutaneous melanoma metastases of the face during imiquimod treatment. J Dtsch Dermatol Ges 2009;7(6):538–40.

93. Johnson TM, Sondak VK, Bichakjian CK, et al. The role of sentinel lymph node biopsy for melanoma: evidence assessment. J Am Acad Dermatol 2006; 54(1):19–27.

94. Morton DL, Thompson JF, Cochran AJ, et al. Sentinel-node biopsy or nodal observation in melanoma. N Engl J Med 2006;355(13):1307–17.

95. Thomas JM, et al. Sentinel-node biopsy in melanoma. N Engl J Med 2007;356(4):418 [author reply: 419–21].

96. Ahlgrimm-Siess V, Massone C, Scope A, et al. Reflectance confocal microscopy of facial lentigo maligna and lentigo maligna melanoma: a preliminary study. Br J Dermatol 2009;161(6):1307–16.

Targeted Therapies for Metastatic Melanoma

Sunandana Chandra, MD[a], Anna C. Pavlick, BSN, MS, DO[b],*

KEYWORDS

- Metastatic melanoma • Targeted therapies • Immunotherapy • Signaling pathways

KEY POINTS

- Identifying genetic mutations in melanoma has permitted targeted therapies to impact treatment and survival of melanoma patients.
- Harnessing the activity of the immune system has been an effective means of impacting on the treatment and survival of melanoma patients.
- Combining targeted therapies and immunotherapeutic agents is the future of melanoma research.
- Despite the successful impact of vemurafenib and ipilimumab on the treatment and survival of melanoma patients, clinical trials must remain the "gold standard" in order to further improve patient outcomes.

INTRODUCTION

Disseminated malignant melanoma has been unresponsive to standard treatment and was associated with a dismal prognosis, with 5-year survivals at 10% to 25%[1] before the Food and Drug Administration (FDA) approval of 2 novel therapies in 2011. According to Surveillance, Epidemiology, and End Results (SEER) data, approximately 4% of melanomas are metastatic at the time of diagnosis. Systemic chemotherapy for disseminated melanomas has response rates of 6% to 15%, with median progression-free survival (PFS) of 2 to 3 months.[2] Until March of 2011, only 2 drugs were approved by the FDA in the United States for metastatic melanoma: interleukin 2 (IL-2) and dacarbazine, which is an alkylating agent. Temozolomide, an orally available congener of dacarbazine, was shown to be noninferior in efficacy in comparison with dacarbazine in a randomized phase III trial.[3] Until now, biochemotherapy and combination chemotherapy based on IL-2 and dacarbazine or temozolomide have not shown statistically significant improvement in overall survival (OS) and cannot be considered standard therapeutic options for metastatic melanoma. In 2011, 2 unique agents were FDA approved for the treatment of metastatic melanoma: ipilimumab and vemurafenib. Ipilimumab, an immunotherapy, and vemurafenib, a BRAF inhibitor, are further discussed in this article (Figs. 1 and 2).

TARGETED THERAPIES

As the molecular pathways involved in cell signaling are understood in greater detail, novel agents have been discovered. Some have been FDA approved, whereas others are in clinical trials alone or in combination therapy with chemotherapeutic or other biologic agents. Several oncogenic signaling pathways, such as mitogen-activated protein kinase (MAPK) and phosphoinositide 3-kinase (PI3K), are being targeted in melanoma to provide disease-specific killing of tumor cells. The binding of extracellular ligands to growth factor receptors, such as epidermal growth factor receptor (EGFR), c-kit, platelet-derived growth factor receptor (PDGFR), vascular endothelial growth factor receptor (VEGFR), fibroblast growth

a NYU School of Medicine, New York, NY 10016, USA; b NYU Melanoma Program, NYU Cancer Institute, 160 East 34th Street, 9th Floor, New York, NY 10016, USA
* Corresponding author. NYU Cancer Institute, 160 East 34th Street, 9th Floor, New York, NY 10016.
E-mail address: Anna.pavlick@nyumc.org

Dermatol Clin 30 (2012) 517–524
doi:10.1016/j.det.2012.05.001
0733-8635/12/$ – see front matter © 2012 Elsevier Inc. All rights reserved.

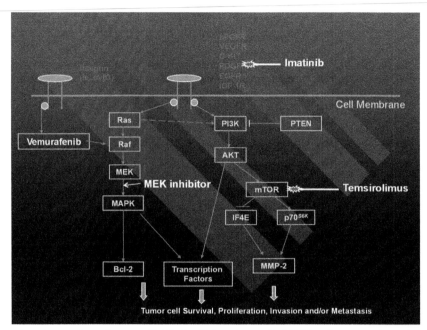

Fig. 1. Targeted pathways in melanoma. Bcl-2, B-cell lymphoma 2; MAPK, mitogen-activated protein kinase; MMP-2, matrix metalloproteinase-2; mTOR, mammalian target of rapamycin; PI3K, phosphoinositide 3-kinase.

factor receptor (FGFR), and FLIT-3, induces the receptor dimerization and activation of tyrosine kinases, which leads to intracellular phosphorylation cascades that lead to transcription factors that regulate cell proliferation, survival, and motility. Several tumor suppressor genes and oncogenes are known to be involved in melanoma pathogenesis, which likely leads to a functional redundancy of different signaling pathways.

The MAPK pathway is an essential regulator of cell growth, survival, and migration and is constitutively active in many human malignancies. This pathway has been of interest in melanoma since Davies and colleagues[4] reported in 2002 that more than 60% of melanomas harbor a specific missense mutation (V600E) in the BRAF gene. This mutation results in the MAPK pathway being constitutively active and drives melanoma growth.[5,6] Studies have revealed that some melanomas carry alterations in the PI3K pathway, such as a PTEN deletion, which is an inhibitor of upstream PI3K/AKT or AKT amplification, in addition to the BRAF^{V600E} mutation. These findings provide a rationale for combination therapy with targeted agents or the use of multi-target inhibitors in the treatment of melanoma.

AGENTS TARGETING THE MAPK PATHWAY

One of the earliest therapeutic drugs identified was sorafenib, a small-molecule, multi-targeted

tyrosine kinase inhibitor that blocks EGFR, c-kit, PDGF, VEGF, and BRAF. It is has no significant activity as a single agent in melanoma[7] and did not improve response rates or survival when used in combination therapy. A National Cancer Institute (NCI)–sponsored phase III randomized trial (E2603) comparing carboplatin, paclitaxel, and sorafenib with carboplatin, paclitaxel, and placebo in chemotherapy naïve patients demonstrated no benefit in the 3-drug versus the 2-drug combination, and the trial was terminated early.[8] In the paclitaxel and carboplatin with versus without sorafenib (second line) for advanced melanoma (PRISM) study, the addition of sorafenib to paclitaxel and carboplatin as a second-line treatment after chemotherapy with dacarbazine or temozolomide failed to improve PFS, tumor response rate, or the time to disease progression in metastatic melanoma.[9]

Since then, second-generation selective RAF inhibitors have been developed and are actively tested in various clinical trials. Vemurafenib is a highly selective oral inhibitor of the oncogenic V600E-mutant BRAF kinase, which showed promising results in early clinical studies. In a dose-finding phase I trial, 11 of 16 (68%) patients with mutant BRAF metastatic melanoma achieved a partial response (PR) and 4 patients had minor responses leading to a PFS of 8 to 9 months.[10] A dose-extension phase I trial with 32 patients demonstrated an objective response rate of 81%

(2 complete responses [CRs], 24 PRs).[8] The median PFS among these patients was more than 7 months. Vemurafenib was generally well tolerated; the most common side effects were rash, photosensitivity, arthralgia, and nausea. Of note, 31% of the patients developed grade 3 squamous cell carcinoma (SCC), keratoacanthoma (KA) type. The median time to the appearance of a cutaneous SCC was 8 weeks, with no reported involvement of other organs. The treatment with vemurafenib was not interrupted by the appearance of these skin lesions and most of them were resected.[8] The phase II trial of vemurafenib in previously treated patients with melanoma (BRAF inhibitor in melanoma [BRIM 2]) demonstrated an OS of 16.9 months, which is unprecedented in melanoma trials.[11] The phase III trial (BRIM 3) comparing vemurafenib with dacarbazine in untreated patients with BRAF V600E–mutant metastatic melanoma demonstrated improvement in PFS and OS for patients receiving vemurafenib. The trial was closed early because of the significant benefit of vemurafenib, and patients randomized to dacarbazine were then crossed over to the vemurafenib arm so that they could obtain the benefit of that therapy.[12] The robust data generated in this phase III trial were the basis for FDA approval of vemurafenib in patients with V600E-mutated metastatic melanoma.

GlaxoSmithKline 2118436 is another oral, highly potent, and selective inhibitor of the V600E/K/D-mutant BRAF. In a phase I/II study, the treatment with GSK 2118436 led to a decrease in fluorodeoxyglucose positron emission tomography (FDG-PET) metabolic uptake, with 11 of 14 (79%) patients with melanoma showing a decrease from baseline (range 5%–100%) and 18 of 30 (60%) patients demonstrated a greater than 20% tumor decrease by Response Evaluation Criteria In Solid Tumors (RECIST) at the first restaging (8–9 weeks). GSK 2118436 showed good tolerability and low-grade nausea, vomiting, fatigue, headaches, and skin changes (including low-grade SCC) were the main adverse effects.[13] A phase II study of GSK2118436 as the salvage therapy (NCT01153763) and a phase III study of GSK2118436 versus dacarbazine (NCT01227889) as the front-line therapy for patients with mutant-BRAF metastatic melanoma have been completed and results are pending publication.

MEK INHIBITORS

The serine/threonine tyrosine kinase MEK acts downstream from RAF in the RAF/MEK/ERK pathway; its inhibition is an attractive anticancer strategy because it has the potential to block upregulated signal transduction through this pathway regardless of the upstream position of the oncogenic aberration. AZD6244 (ARRY-142886) is a selective MEK1/2 inhibitor that has shown preclinical activity[14] and demonstrated clinical activity in a phase I study with a benign toxicity profile.[15–17] These results led to a randomized phase II trial comparing AZD6244 with temozolomide in chemotherapy naïve patients with advanced melanoma.[18] A total of 200 patients were enrolled, with 104 and 96 patients randomized to AZD6244 and temozolomide respectively; those who progressed on temozolomide could crossover to AZD6244. Results showed a trend toward OS in patients with BRAF mutations in the AZD6244 arm.[18] At the 2010 American Society of Clinical Oncology (ASCO) annual meeting, the early results of a phase I study with AZD6244 in combination with docetaxel, dacarbazine, or temsirolimus suggest that the presence of a BRAF mutation was significantly associated with clinical responses and an increased time to progression.[19] Several phase II studies of AZD6244 are underway for patients with advanced melanoma with BRAF mutations as the front-line therapy: for treatment-naïve patients versus temozolomide (NCT00338130), in combination with dacarbazine versus dacarbazine alone (NCT00936221), and as salvage therapy (NCT00866177). GSK1120212 is another potent and selective inhibitor of the MEK1/2 enzymes with promising antitumor activity in a phase I clinical trial, resulting in a response rate greater than 70% in patients with advanced melanoma with known BRAF mutations, including 1 patient who was previously treated with PLX4032.[20] This drug is currently being investigated in phase II and III clinical trials for patients with advanced BRAF-mutant melanomas who were either previously treated with a BRAF inhibitor or not (NCT01245062, NCT01037127).

Although targeting the MAPK pathway is a promising new therapeutic approach for the treatment of melanoma and treatment with selective BRAF and MEK inhibitors can induce high response rates, the limited duration of these responses in most patients, most likely because of the emerging resistance to these inhibitors, represents a significant clinical challenge. Molecular redundancy, partly caused by the existence of RAF isoforms and signaling through alternative oncogenic pathways, such as the PI3K/AKT/mammalian target of rapamycin (mTOR) pathway,[21,22] receptor tyrosine kinase (PDGFRβ)–dependent pathway,[23] and COT (MAP3K8),[24] may provide the melanoma cells escape mechanisms to specific pathway inhibitors and underscore their ability to adapt to pharmacologic challenges.[21,22] In preclinical models, it has been reported that the acquired resistance of melanoma cells to the BRAF inhibitors was associated with the rebound activation of the RAF/MEK/ERK pathway.[22] In line with this finding, activating signals to downstream MEK/ERK has been shown to switch to ARAF[25] or CRAF[25,26] via N-RAS upregulation[23] to overcome the effect of BRAF inhibition. Moreover, most melanoma cells harboring the BRAF V600E mutation retained the wild-type BRAF allele, which could be rescued from the effects of BRAF knockdown by extracellular growth factors, such as the basic fibroblast growth factor, hepatocyte growth factor, or endothelin-1.[27,28]

C-KIT INHIBITORS

Imatinib is a selective tyrosine kinase inhibitor with multiple targets, including c-kit and PDGFR receptors, and has been shown to be highly efficacious in chronic myelogenous leukemia and gastrointestinal stromal tumors.[29] The initial phase II trials with this agent in melanoma were disappointing with no objective responses.[30,31] However, gain-of-function mutations, gene amplifications, and overexpression of c-kit were subsequently reported in 30% to 40% of mucosal, acral, and cutaneous melanomas with chronic sun damage.[32] Impressive tumor regression was documented in a patient with mucosal melanoma who carried a mutation in the juxtamembranous domain of c-kit (exon 11) in response to single-agent imatinib.[33] Moreover, preclinical studies showed sensitivity of c-kit–mutant mucosal melanoma, providing a rationale for the use of imatinib in this melanoma type. Results of a phase II trial evaluating the effect of imatinib in patients with metastatic melanoma with c-kit aberrations were presented at the 2009 ASCO meeting. More than 30% of the patients achieved a response (CR and PR), whereas 50% had disease stability.[34] Another phase I/II study to define the safety and efficacy of imatinib in combination with temozolomide in patients with unresectable stage III/IV melanoma is currently underway. After the data on c-kit alterations became available when the trial was already in progress, patients with mucosal, acral, and chronic sun damage melanomas were preferentially enrolled in the phase II part of the study. Early results of the trial were presented at the 2008 ASCO meeting.[35] Of the 23 patients treated, 16 had been enrolled in phase I and 7 in phase II. The combination was well tolerated and demonstrated antitumor activity in melanoma. Of the 7 patients treated in the phase II trial, 1 patient had a CR and 6 had PRs.[36] Phase II studies with a second-generation c-kit inhibitor (nilotinib) in first- or second-line therapies for advanced melanomas with c-kit mutations or amplification are ongoing (NCT01168050, NCT01099514).

mTOR INHIBITORS

Resistance of mutant BRAF melanoma cells to RAF/MEK inhibition may also be caused by the activation of other survival signaling pathways, such as the PI3K/AKT/mTOR pathway (see **Fig. 1**) resulting in melanoma development and progression.[25,37,38] Recent reports suggested a significant correlation of increased PI3K-AKT activity with resistance to RAF/MEK inhibitors in melanoma[25,39,40] and that the inhibition of the PI3K/AKT/mTOR pathway could suppress MEK inhibitor–induced activation of AKT and resulted in synergistic cell killing with an MEK inhibitor (AZD6244).[39] This finding provides a rationale for combinatorial therapy leading to dual inhibition of both the RAF/MEK/ERK and PI3K/AKT/mTOR pathways. A phase II trial of the mTOR inhibitor temsirolimus (CCI-779) combined with the MEK inhibitor AZD6244 is currently recruiting treatment-naïve patients with BRAF-mutant advanced melanoma (NCT01166126). In addition, the inhibition of the PI3K/AKT/mTOR signaling pathway was found to sensitize melanoma cells to chemotherapeutic agents, such as cisplatin and temozolomide, in vitro as evidenced by enhanced apoptosis and suppressed invasive tumor growth.[41] A phase II study of mTOR inhibitor everolimus in combination with paclitaxel and carboplatin in patients with metastatic melanoma is in progress (NCT01014351).

IMMUNOTHERAPY
Anti–Cytotoxic T-Lymphocyte Antigen-4 Monoclonal Antibodies

Increasing knowledge of T-cell regulation has uncovered potential immunologic targets for the treatment of melanoma. The interaction between antigen-presenting cells (APC) and T lymphocytes is crucial for inducing melanoma-specific T-cell responses. In addition to the antigen-specific interaction between the human leukocyte antigens (HLA) peptide complex on the APC and the T-cell receptor (TCR), several different co-stimulatory and co-inhibitory molecules modulate the T-cell response. For instance, the T-cell surface molecule CD28 interacts with the B7 receptor on the APC to mediate a co-stimulatory signal (which is necessary in addition to the HLA-peptide-TCR interaction for efficient priming of the T cell), whereas the T-cell cytotoxic T-lymphocyte antigen-4 (CTLA-4) interacts with B7 to downregulate T-cell activation, acting as a natural checkpoint on the T-cell–mediated immunologic response. Blocking the interaction between CTLA-4 and B7 can overcome this checkpoint

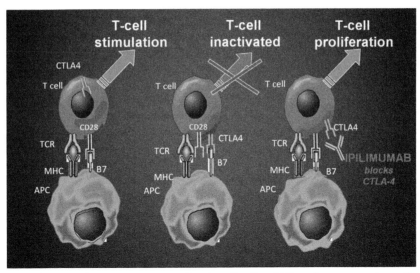

Fig. 2. Mechanism of action of anti–CTLA-4 monoclonal antibodies. APC, antigen-presenting cells; CTLA-4, cytotoxic T-lymphocyte antigen-4; MHC, major histocompatibility complex; TCR, T-cell receptor.

and enhance T-cell–mediated antitumor activity. This action can be achieved by an anti–CTLA-4 monoclonal antibody (moAb). To date, 2 fully human anti–CTLA-4 moAbs have been developed for metastatic melanoma: tremelimumab (CP-675, 206) and ipilimumab (MDX-010).

In the initial phase I study, tremelimumab was well tolerated and demonstrated encouraging clinical activity, including several CRs. However, in a randomized phase III study comparing single-agent tremelimumab with either dacarbazine or temozolomide in patients with advanced melanoma, tremelimumab failed to demonstrate a significant improvement in OS in comparison with standard chemotherapy.[42]

Another anti–CTLA-4 agent, ipilimumab, in a randomized phase III clinical trial comparing ipilimumab alone with gp100 vaccine alone to the combination of ipilimumab and gp100 vaccine, resulted in improved OS of nearly 4 months (median survival duration of 10.1 and 10.0 months in the ipilimumab arm and the combined arm, respectively) in comparison with 6.4 months in the vaccination alone arm (hazard ratio [HR] 0.66; 95% confidence interval [CI] 0.51–0.87; $P = .033$ and HR 0.68; 95% CI 0.55–0.85; $P<.001$, respectively). Included in this study were 676 patients who were HLA-A*0201 positive (necessary only because of the vaccine randomization) with unresectable stage III or IV melanoma whose disease had progressed after they had received a previous therapeutic regimen containing one or more of the following: dacarbazine, temozolomide, fotemustine, carboplatin, or IL-2. This trial was the first randomized clinical trial that showed a statistically significant improvement in OS for metastatic melanoma.[43]

This agent has now received FDA approval for use in metastatic melanoma.

The activity and side-effect profile of anti–CTLA-4 antibodies have several characteristics that reflect their immune-mediated mechanism of action. Objective responses observed in patients with metastatic melanomas with either tremelimumab or ipilimumab were seen in approximately 7% to 10% of patients. Remarkably, as much as 70% of the responses were durable.[42,43] The unique pattern of response to CTLA-4 moAbs, such as the initial apparent progression of disease, even with the emergence of new lesions, followed by regression and responses over the course of several months to years, has been seen with these agents.[44] The recognition of this unusual kinetics of response has led to a proposal of immune-related response criteria (irRC) when evaluating treatment responses to anti–CTLA-4 moAbs.[45,46] The irRC should replace currently accepted RECIST for the evaluation of patients with melanoma treated with immunotherapy.

The growing clinical experience with anti–CTLA-4 moAbs also identifies a constellation of autoimmune side effects, which have been designated immune-related adverse events (irAEs).[47] The irAEs are thought to be a result of nonspecific or cross-reactive tissue damage caused by activated T cells. These irAEs, including rash, autoimmune colitis, hepatitis, and, less frequently, hypophysitis and uveitis, tend not to be harmful provided the clinician is aware of these unusual side effects, monitors the symptoms adequately, and knows when to intervene. The treatment of any moderate to severe toxicity is with corticosteroids.

Anti–Programmed Death 1 Monoclonal Antibodies

The programmed death 1 (PD-1) receptor is a negative regulator of antigen-activated T cells.[48] It bears homology to CTLA-4 but provides distinct co-inhibitory signals. The cytoplasmic domain of PD-1 contains 2 tyrosine-signaling motifs that can attenuate the TCR/CD28 signal.[49] There are 2 known ligands for PD1: B7-H1/PD-L1 (hereafter PD-L1), the predominant mediator of PD-1–dependent immunosuppression, and B7-DC/PD-L2. PD-L1 is expressed by many tumors, including melanoma, and its interaction with PD-1 resulted in tumor escape in experimental models.[50]

MDX-1106 (BMS-936558/ONO-4538) is a fully human immunoglobulin G4 (IgG4) moAb specific for PD-1. The drug binds PD-1 with high affinity and blocks its interaction with both PD-L1 and PD-L2. A phase I study of single-agent MDX-1106 in refractory solid tumors was conducted in 39 patients with advanced metastatic non–small cell lung carcinoma (NSCLC), melanoma, castrate-resistant prostate cancer, renal cell carcinoma (RCC), or colorectal carcinoma (CRC). Although efficacy was not the primary end point of this phase I study, of the 39 treated patients, 1 durable CR (CRC) and 2 PRs (melanoma, RCC) were seen. Two additional patients (melanoma, NSCLC) had significant lesional tumor regressions, which did not meet criteria for PR. This study suggested a more benign immune-related toxicity profile for anti–PD-1 moAb than one seen associated with anti–CTLA-4 moAb. Only 1 patient with metastatic ocular melanoma developed grade 3 inflammatory colitis following 5 doses (1 mg/kg) administered over 8 months, which responded to steroids and infliximab, whereas grade 2 irAEs occurred in 3 patients presenting with polyarticular arthropathies requiring oral steroids and hypothyroidism requiring hormone replacement.[51] Another phase I trial was conducted on 16 patients with metastatic disease, including melanoma. Objective responses were documented in 37.5% of the patients lasting 3 to 13+ months; half of the patients had melanoma and there were few irAEs.[52]

SUMMARY

The next few years may show that when the novel therapeutics reviewed in this article are used in thoughtful combinations, a new standard of care for the treatment of advanced melanoma will emerge. As more understanding is gained on the different signaling pathways for tumor cell growth and mechanisms of action of the different classes of drugs, the ability to identify different subsets of patients with differentially dysregulated oncogenic signaling pathways may allow for more individualized treatments of advanced melanoma in the near future, which will ultimately translate into improved survival.

REFERENCES

1. Balch CM, Gershenwald JE, Soong SJ, et al. Final version of 2009 AJCC melanoma staging and classification. J Clin Oncol 2009;27(36):6199–206.
2. Mays S, Nelson B. Current therapy of cutaneous melanoma. Cutis 1999;63:293–8.
3. Middleton MR, Grob JJ, Aaronson N, et al. Randomized phase III study of temozolomide versus dacarbazine in the treatment of patients with advanced metastatic malignant melanoma. J Clin Oncol 2000;18(1):158–66.
4. Davies H, Bignell GR, Cox C, et al. Mutations of the BRAF gene in human cancer. Nature 2002; 417(6892):949–54.
5. Brose MS, Volpe P, Feldman M, et al. BRAF and RAS mutations in human lung cancer and melanoma. Cancer Res 2002;62:6997–7000.
6. Carvajal RD, Antonescu CR, Wolchok JD, et al. KIT as a therapeutic target in metastatic melanoma. JAMA 2011;305(22):2327–34.
7. Ott PA, Hamilton A, Min C, et al. A phase II trial of sorafenib in metastatic melanoma with tissue correlates. PLoS One 2010;5(12):e15588.
8. Flaherty KT, Puzanov I, Kim KB, et al. Inhibition of mutated, activated BRAF in metastatic melanoma. N Engl J Med 2010;363(9):809–19.
9. Agarwala S, Keilholz U, Hogg C, et al. Randomized phase III study of paclitaxel plus carboplatin with or without sorafenib as second-line treatment in patients with advanced melanoma. J Clin Oncol 2007;25:abstract 8510.
10. Flaherty K, Puzanov I, Sosman J, et al. Phase I study of PLX4032: proof of concept for V600E BRAF mutation as a therapeutic target in human cancer. J Clin Oncol 2009;27(15s):ASCO Annual Meeting Abstract(suppl; abstr 9000).
11. Sosman JA, Kim KB, Schuchter L, et al. Survival in BRAF V600-mutant advanced melanoma treated with vemurafenib. N Engl J Med 2012;366(8):707–14.
12. Chapman PB, Hauschild A, Robert C, et al. BRIM-3 study group. Improved survival with vemurafenib in melanoma patients with BRAF V600E mutations. N Engl J Med 2011;364(26):2507–16.
13. Kefford R, Arkenau H, Brown MP, et al. Phase I/II study of GSK2118436, a selective inhibitor of oncogenic mutant BRAF kinase, in patients with metastatic melanoma and other solid tumors. J Clin Oncol 2010;28(15s). ASCO Annual Meeting, abstract 8503.

14. Yeh TC, Marsh V, Bernat BA, et al. Biological characterization of ARRY-142886 (AZD6244), a potent, highly selective mitogen-activated protein kinase kinase 1/2 inhibitor. Clin Cancer Res 2007;13(5):1576–83.

15. Adjei AA, Cohen RB, Franklin W, et al. Phase I pharmacokinetic and pharmacodynamic study of the oral, small-molecule mitogen-activated protein kinase kinase 1/2 inhibitor AZD6244 (ARRY-142886) in patients with advanced cancers. J Clin Oncol 2008;26(13):2139–46.

16. Agarwala SS, Kirkwood JM, Gore M, et al. Temozolomide for the treatment of brain metastases associated with metastatic melanoma: a phase II study. J Clin Oncol 2004;22(11):2101–7.

17. Amaravadi RK, Schuchter LM, McDermott DF, et al. Phase II trial of temozolomide and sorafenib in advanced melanoma patients with or without brain metastases. Clin Cancer Res 2009;15(24):7711–8.

18. Dummer R, Robert C, Chapman PB, et al. AZD6244 (ARRY-142886) vs temozolomide (TMZ) in patients (pts) with advanced melanoma: an open-label, randomized, multicenter, phase II study. J Clin Oncol 2008;26(May 20 Suppl):ASCO Annual Meeting, abstract 9033.

19. Patel SP, Lazar AJ, Mahoney S, et al. Clinical responses to AZD6244 (ARRY-142886_-based combination therapy stratified by gene mutations in patients with metastatic melanoma. J Clin Oncol 2010;28:15s.

20. Infante JR, Fecher LA, Nallapareddy S, et al. Safety and efficacy results from the first-in-human study of the oral MEK 1/2 inhibitor GSK1120212. J Clin Oncol 2010;28(15s):ASCO Annual Meeting, abstract 2503.

21. Jiang CC, Lai F, Thorne RF, et al. MEK-independent survival of B-RAFV600E melanoma cells selected for resistance to apoptosis induced by the RAF inhibitor PLX4720. Clin Cancer Res 2011;17(4):721–30.

22. Paraiso KH, Fedorenko IV, Cantini LP, et al. Recovery of phospho-ERK activity allows melanoma cells to escape from BRAF inhibitor therapy. Br J Cancer 2010;102(12):1724–30.

23. Nazarian R, Shi H, Wang Q, et al. Melanomas acquire resistance to B-RAF(V600E) inhibition by RTK or N-RAS upregulation. Nature 2010; 468(7326):973–7.

24. Johannessen CM, Boehm JS, Kim SY, et al. COT drives resistance to RAF inhibition through MAP kinase pathway reactivation. Nature 2010;468(7326):968–72.

25. Villanueva J, Vultur A, Lee JT, et al. Acquired resistance to BRAF inhibitors mediated by a RAF kinase switch in melanoma can be overcome by cotargeting MEK and IGF-1R/PI3K. Cancer Cell 2010;18(6): 683–95.

26. Montagut C, Sharma SV, Shioda T, et al. Elevated CRAF as a potential mechanism of acquired resistance to BRAF inhibition in melanoma. Cancer Res 2008;68(12):4853–61.

27. Christensen C, Guldberg P. Growth factors rescue cutaneous melanoma cells from apoptosis induced by knockdown of mutated (V 600 E) B-RAF. Oncogene 2005;24(41):6292–302.

28. Csete B, Lengyel Z, Kadar Z, et al. Poly(adenosine diphosphate-ribose) polymerase-1 expression in cutaneous malignant melanomas as a new molecular marker of aggressive tumor. Pathol Oncol Res 2009;15(1):47–53.

29. Heinrich MC, Griffith DJ, Drucker BJ, et al. Inhibition of c-kit receptor tyrosine kinase activity by STI-571, a selective tyrosine kinase inhibitor. Blood 2000; 96(3):925–32.

30. Ugurel S, Hildenbrand R, Zimpfer A, et al. Lack of clinical efficacy of imatinib in metastatic melanoma. Br J Cancer 2005;92(8):1398–405.

31. Wyman K, Atkins MB, Prieto V, et al. Multicenter phase II trial of high-dose imatinib mesylate in metastatic melanoma: significant toxicity with no clinical efficacy. Cancer 2006;106(9):2005–11.

32. Curtin JA, Busam K, Pinkel D, et al. Somatic activation of KIT in distinct subtypes of melanoma. J Clin Oncol 2006;24(26):4340–6.

33. Hodi FS, Friedlander P, Corless CL, et al. Major response to imatinib mesylate in KIT-mutated melanoma. J Clin Oncol 2008;26(12):2046–51.

34. Carvajal RD, Cahpman PB, Wolchok JD, et al. A phase II study of imatinib mesylate (IM) for patients with advanced melanoma harboring somatic alterations of KIT. J Clin Oncol 2009;27:ASCO Annual Meeting, abstract 9001.

35. Fecher LA, Amaravadi RK, Flaherty KT. The MAPK pathway in melanoma. Curr Opin Oncol 2008; 20(2):183–9.

36. Fecher LA, Nathanson K, Flaherty KT, et al. Phase I/II trial of imatinib and temozolomide in advanced unresectable melanoma. J Clin Oncol 2008;26:ASCO 2008 Meeting, abstract 9059.

37. Shao Y, Aplin AE. Akt3-mediated resistance to apoptosis in B-RAF-targeted melanoma cells. Cancer Res 2010;70(16):6670–81.

38. Stahl JM, Sharma A, Cheung M, et al. Deregulated Akt3 activity promotes development of malignant melanoma. Cancer Res 2004;64(19):7002–10.

39. Gopal YN, Deng W, Woodman SE, et al. Basal and treatment-induced activation of AKT mediates resistance to cell death by AZD6244 (ARRY-142886) in Braf-mutant human cutaneous melanoma cells. Cancer Res 2010;70(21):8736–47.

40. Hauschild A, Agarwala SS, Trefzer U, et al. Results of a phase III, randomized, placebo-controlled study of sorafenib in combination with carboplatin and paclitaxel as second-line treatment in patients with unresectable stage III or stage IV melanoma. J Clin Oncol 2009;27(17):2823–30.

41. Sinnberg T, Lasithiotakis K, Niessner H, et al. Inhibition of PI3K-AKT-mTOR signaling sensitizes

melanoma cells to cisplatin and temozolomide. J Invest Dermatol 2009;129(6):1500–15.

42. Ribas A, Hauschild A, Kefford R, et al. Phase III, open-label, randomized, comparative study of tremelimumab (CP-675,206) and chemotherapy (temozolomide [TMZ] or dacarbazine [DTIC]) in patients with advanced melanoma. J Clin Oncol 2008; 26(15S [May 20 Suppl]):abstract 9011.

43. Hodi FS, O'Day SJ, McDermott DF, et al. Improved survival with ipilimumab in patients with metastatic melanoma. N Engl J Med 2010;363(8):711–23.

44. Hamid O, Urba WJ, Yellin M, et al. Kinteics of response to ipilimumab (MDX-010) in patients with stage III/IV melanoma. J Clin Oncol 2007;25(June 20 Supplement):abstract 8525.

45. Wolchok JD, Hoos A, O'Day S, et al. Guidelines for the evaluation of immune therapy activity in solid tumors: immune-related response criteria. Clin Cancer Res 2009;15(23):7412–20.

46. Wolchok JD, Neyns B, Linette G, et al. Ipilimumab monotherapy in patients with pretreated advanced melanoma: a randomised, double-blind, multicentre, phase 2, dose-ranging study. Lancet Oncol 2010; 11(2):155–64.

47. Di Giacomo AM, Biagioli M, Maio M. The emerging toxicity profiles of anti-CTLA-4 antibodies across clinical indications. Semin Oncol 2010;37(5):499–507.

48. Fourcade J, Kudela P, Sun Z, et al. PD-1 is a regulator of NY-ESO-1-specific CD8+ T cell expansion in melanoma patients. J Immunol 2009;182(9):5240–9.

49. Parry RV, Chemnitz JM, Frauwirth KA, et al. CTLA-4 and PD-1 receptors inhibit T-cell activation by distinct mechanisms. Mol Cell Biol 2005;25(21): 9543–53.

50. Iwai Y, Ishida M, Tanaka Y, et al. Involvement of PD-L1 on tumor cells in the escape from host immune system and tumor immunotherapy by PD-L1 blockade. Proc Natl Acad Sci U S A 2002;99(19):12293–7.

51. Brahmer JR, Drake CG, Wollner I, et al. Phase I study of single-agent anti-programmed death-1 (MDX-1106) in refractory solid tumors: safety, clinical activity, pharmacodynamics, and immunologic correlates. J Clin Oncol 2010;28(19):3167–75.

52. Sznol M, Powderly JD, Smith DC, et al. Safety and antitumor activity of biweekly MDX-1106 (Anti-PD-1, BMS-936558/ONO-4538) in patients with advanced refractory malignancies. J Clin Oncol 2010;28(15s): (suppl; abstr 2506).

Radiation Therapy for Cutaneous Melanoma

Christopher A. Barker, MD*, Nancy Y. Lee, MD

KEYWORDS

- Cutaneous melanoma • Radiation therapy • Lentigo maligna • Desmoplastic melanoma • Adjuvant
- High-risk • Nodal recurrence • Palliation

KEY POINTS

- Radiation therapy is infrequently used in the care of patients with cutaneous melanoma, despite research suggesting a benefit in certain clinical scenarios.
- Definitive radiation therapy may be a viable treatment option for lentigo maligna and lentigo maligna melanoma.
- Adjuvant radiation therapy to the site of a resected neurotropic melanoma may improve local control of the tumor.
- Adjuvant radiation therapy to the site of resected lymph node metastases from melanoma at high risk for recurrence may improve regional control of lymphatic metastases.
- Palliative radiation therapy is likely to yield a response in patients with distant metastases.

INTRODUCTION

In 2002, the Collaboration for Cancer Outcomes Research and Evaluation of Australia estimated that over the course of their disease approximately 23% of patients diagnosed with cutaneous melanoma (CM) would be appropriately treated with radiation therapy (RT) based on the best available evidence. Using population registry data, these investigators found that RT was part of the treatment of 13% of patients in New South Wales, Australia, and 1% to 6% of patients in the United States.[1] Others have noted the infrequent and dwindling use of RT for CM over time.[2,3] Awareness of the evidence supporting the use of RT for the treatment of CM is vital to delivering the optimal care of patients with this potentially lethal disease.

Several general aspects of RT for melanoma are not addressed in this review. The myth that melanoma is not responsive to RT has been adequately described and dispelled elsewhere.[3–5] The curative and organ-preserving potential of RT for uveal melanoma has been demonstrated by the Collaborative Ocular Melanoma Study[6] and is beyond the scope of this review. Likewise, the role of RT in the management of mucosal melanoma is beyond the scope of this article. Herein, data providing the highest levels of evidence supporting the use of RT for CM are presented and discussed, acknowledging a significant dearth of high-level evidence in many situations.

RADIATION THERAPY FOR THE PRIMARY TUMOR

Although the effective use of RT as definitive local therapy for primary CM has been described,[7–10] the therapeutic modality of choice for resectable CM in the medically operable patient is surgery. At present, pathologic staging by surgery provides the most valuable prognostic information available for early-stage CM. However, there are situations

The authors have no relevant conflicts of interest.
Department of Radiation Oncology, Memorial Sloan-Kettering Cancer Center, 1275 York Avenue, Box 22, New York, NY 10065, USA
* Corresponding author.
E-mail address: barkerc@mskcc.org

in which surgery might preclude acceptable functional or cosmetic outcomes to some patients.

Definitive Radiation Therapy for Lentigo Maligna and Lentigo Maligna Melanoma

Most frequently, RT for the primary tumor is considered for lentigo maligna (LM) and lentigo maligna melanoma (LMM). Because patients with LM and LMM are often elderly and present with large, superficial lesions on the face, alternatives to surgery are often considered to optimize cosmetic and functional outcome. Table 1 summarizes the outcome of RT for LM and LMM from the largest updated retrospective series from around the world.[11–17] Although follow-up has been limited, the pooled results demonstrate that the efficacy of RT compares favorably with other treatment modalities. Of note, relatively high rates of local recurrence have been noted in several series from North America, and may be related to RT technique. Although toxicity generally depends on the technique used, the outcome of skin RT is generally acceptable to elderly patients,[18] in whom LM and LMM are most common.

A recent retrospective comparative study of clinical outcomes in the management of CM in situ revealed no statistically significant difference in outcome between surgical excision and RT.[19] In this study, 15 patients were given RT to primary CM in situ in the head and neck region with a 10-kV superficial unit, to a total dose of 120 Gy in 6 fractions, with a security margin of 5 mm. Patients treated with RT were older than patients treated with surgical excision (mean 79 vs 59 years). The majority of patients undergoing excision had non–head and neck primary lesions. Among all patients, statistically significant higher rates of local recurrence were noted in patients older than 62 years or with head and neck lesions. Five-year rates of local recurrence were higher in patients treated with RT when compared with surgery (13.2% vs 6.8%), but this difference was not statistically significant. Statistically significant higher rates of 5-year of local recurrence were noted in patients treated with cryotherapy (34.3%, n = 22) and laser therapy (42.9%, n = 8) in comparison with surgery (6.8%, n = 1041).[19]

Use of RT for LM or LMM varies widely. As noted in Table 1, higher rates of recurrence have been observed in North American centers and may be part of the reason for geographic variations. Even within a single geographic region, there is evidence of disparate opinions about the appropriateness of RT of LM and LMM. For example, guidelines from the United Kingdom suggest that RT may be an appropriate treatment method,[20] but a survey of dermatologists in the United Kingdom found that few (18%) ever recommended RT for LM or LMM while only 13% considered it the treatment of choice for patients older than 70 years.[21]

Adjuvant Radiation Therapy After Resection of Primary Cutaneous Melanoma

Although adjuvant RT to the site of a resected primary tumor at high risk for local recurrence has been advocated, a single phase II study has assessed this prospectively. From 1983 to 1992, 174 patients were enrolled on a single-center study at the M.D. Anderson Cancer Center (MDACC). Patients with CM of the head or neck were eligible if they fulfilled criteria for 1 of 3 groups of patients (Table 2) thought to be at high risk for local (at the site of the excised primary tumor) or regional (in dermal or nodal lymphatics) recurrence. All patients in this study received adjuvant RT (before or after surgery) to the site of the excised primary, unless the primary tumor had been excised more than 1 year before nodal recurrence. A dose of 24 to 30 Gy in 4 to 5 fractions over 2.5 to 3 weeks was delivered, using mostly high-energy (9–12 MeV) electrons.

Overall, dermal recurrence was noted in 10 patients (5.7%). Among patients in group 1, a large proportion of patients harbored advanced tumors (61% with $\geq$T2, 27% with T4, by current American Joint Committee on Cancer staging criteria), and 2 (2.5%) experienced any dermal recurrence. Whether dermal recurrence represented tumor recurrence at the site of primary tumor excision site or in-transit dermal lymphatics was not specified by the report. Nevertheless, these favorable local control rates in high-risk patients suggest a benefit of adjuvant RT to the site of the primary tumor. Because of this study, a phase III trial (9302) of adjuvant RT for high-risk CM of the head and neck was initiated by the Radiation Therapy Oncology Group (RTOG) and the Eastern Cooperative Oncology Group (ECOG) in 1994, but this was subsequently closed because of poor accrual.

Adjuvant Radiation Therapy After Resection of Neurotropic Cutaneous Melanoma

Desmoplastic melanoma is an unusual subtype of CM that frequently occurs in the head and neck where adequate surgical margins can be difficult to obtain. Moreover, desmoplastic melanoma frequently exhibits neurotropism, which may increase the likelihood of local recurrence. For these reasons, many have used RT to the site of tumor (before, after, or in lieu of resection). The retrospective research presented in Table 3 suggests a benefit of adjuvant RT in patients with neurotropic CM with adverse features (ie, recurrent

Table 1
Outcomes of superficial radiotherapy (RT) for lentigo maligna (LM) and lentigo maligna melanoma (LMM)

Origin of Study[Ref.]	Disease	Patients n	Local Recurrence n	Local Recurrence %	Lymphatic Recurrence n	Lymphatic Recurrence %	Distant Recurrence n	Distant Recurrence %	Follow-Up
Netherlands[11]	LM	21	1	5	0	0	0	0	Median 3 y
Switzerland[12]	LM	93	5	5	0	0	0	0	Not reported (101 patients followed for at least 2 y)
	LMM	54	0	0	2	4	0	0	
Germany[13]	LM	42	0	0	0	0	0	0	Median 1.3 y
	LMM	22	2	9	0	0	1	5	
USA[14]	LM	15	4	27	1	7	3	20	Median 2.7 y
	LMM	1	0	0	0	0	1	100	
Canada[15]	LM	36	4	11	0	0	0	0	Median 6 y
Canada[16]	LM	31	9	29					Median 3.9 y
Australia[17]	LM	7	0	0	0	0	0	0	Median 1.3 y
Pooled estimates	LM	245	23	9	1	0	3	1	
	LMM	77	2	3	2	3	2	3	

Table 2
Treatment groups in phase II adjuvant radiotherapy (RT) study of high-risk cutaneous melanoma of the head and neck

Group	Patients (N)	Presentation	Tumor Criteria	Nodal Criteria	Treatment Rendered
1	79	Previously untreated	≥1.5 mm Thick or Clark level ≥4	None palpable	Wide local excision of primary tumor (margins 2–4 cm) and RT to tumor bed and ≥2 echelons of draining lymphatics
2	32	Previously untreated	Any thickness	Palpable	Wide local excision with limited neck dissection and RT to the tumor bed and ipsilateral neck to the supraclavicular fossa
3	63	Previously excised primary tumors with relapse in nodes only	Absent	Recurrent, palpable	Limited node dissection and RT to the tumor bed and ipsilateral neck

tumors, thick tumors, and tumors excised with narrow margins).[22–24] This topic is controversial, as some suggest that RT may not be necessary to achieve high rates of local tumor control.[25]

Two recent analyses of the Surveillance, Epidemiology, and End Result (SEER) program of the National Cancer Institute found that approximately 8% of patients in the United States with desmoplastic melanoma receive RT. The studies arrived at different conclusions, with one suggesting no survival effect of RT[26] and the other finding an association between RT and inferior survival.[27]

The investigators attributed the findings to the selection bias of treating physicians, although finding an association of survival and adjuvant RT would seem unlikely a priori. SEER data do not permit assessment of the local tumor control, the proposed benefit of adjuvant RT.

To further assess the effect of adjuvant RT for desmoplastic neurotropic CM, a phase II study (NCT00060333) was initiated by the North Central Cancer Treatment Group in 2003, the results of which are pending. The Australia and New Zealand Melanoma Trials Group (ANZMTG)

Table 3
Outcomes of adjuvant radiotherapy (RT) for desmoplastic melanoma with or without neurotropism

Origin of Study[Ref.]	Histology	Treatment	Patients n	Neurotropic n	Neurotropic %	Local Recurrence n	Local Recurrence %	Comments
USA[22]	Desmoplastic melanoma	Surgery + RT	15	21 of 44	50	0	0	All patients treated
	Desmoplastic melanoma	Surgery alone	29			4	14	with RT had locally recurrent tumors
Australia[23]	Desmoplastic melanoma	Surgery + RT	24	18	75	2	8	
Australia[24]	Desmoplastic neurotropic melanoma	Surgery + RT	27	27	100	2	7	Patients treated with RT had significantly more adverse features (thick tumors, narrow margins)
		Surgery alone	101	100	100	6	6	

and the Trans-Tasman Radiation Oncology Group (TROG) are currently conducting a phase III trial (NCT00975520) of adjuvant RT in patients with neurotropic CM of the head and neck, which will provide the high-level evidence that is currently lacking.

RADIATION THERAPY FOR REGIONAL LYMPH NODES

Regional RT has been studied extensively in retrospective series and has been well summarized by Guadagnolo and Zagars.[28] The topic is controversial, as evidenced by the inability to accrue patients to an intergroup trial of adjuvant RT initiated by the RTOG and ECOG (9302), or in another trial activated by ECOG alone (3697). However, 2 prospective, randomized controlled trials have been performed, and form the highest level of evidence available on this topic.

The first trial was conducted at the Mayo Clinic (Rochester, Minnesota).[29] Eighty-two patients were enrolled between 1972 and 1977, and 56 were ultimately included in the analysis. Patients with clinically involved and biopsy-confirmed nodal metastases from the primary CM of the extremities, trunk, or unknown site were eligible after undergoing staging (history, physical examination, liver and bone scan, hematologic and chemical assessment) and lymphadenectomy. Patients were randomly assigned to adjuvant RT or observation. RT was delivered with supervoltage therapy units using parallel-opposed fields, treating one field per day to a dose of 5000 rad (equivalent to cGy) at the midplane over 7 to 8 weeks, including a 3- to 4-week break during treatment.

The investigators found a doubling of disease-free survival, from 9 months to 20 months in patients who received RT, a marginally statistically significant finding ($P = .07$). Median duration of overall survival was extended by 50% in patients who received RT, also marginally statistically significant (median survival 33 months, vs 22 months in those undergoing observation; $P = .09$). Imbalances in

the treatment groups, suboptimal RT technique, and small power of the study limited the interpretation, which nevertheless suggested improved regional control of melanoma in lymph nodes with RT.[29]

The ANZMTG and TROG recently published the results of a practice-changing phase III trial (TROG 02.01/ANZMTG 01.02) evaluating the effect of adjuvant RT in patients with CM.[30] Based on phase II data,[31] the group evaluated patients with palpable metastatic melanoma in regional lymph nodes, and were thought to be at significant risk for future lymph node relapse. Risk factors constituting eligibility for the trial are listed in **Table 4**. Between 2002 and 2007, 250 patients were randomized to adjuvant RT or observation. RT was delivered using standardized fields,[31] to a dose of 48 Gy in 20 fractions over 4 weeks.

After a median potential follow-up of 40 months, the group of patients randomized to receive radiotherapy were found to have a significantly lower rate of lymph node field relapse than the group of patients initially observed ($P = .041$). RT was associated with a lower risk of nodal relapse in all of the lymph node regions studied. Three years after randomization, the cumulative risk of lymph node field relapse was 19% if patients that received RT, and 31% in patients who were initially observed. No significant difference in relapse-free or overall survival was noted. Radiation dermatitis was the most common acute grade 3 toxicity and present in 16% of patients 2 weeks after completing RT. The frequency of seroma, wound infection, nerve damage, wound necrosis, and pain did not appear to be more common in patients that received RT. Quality of life assessments are still being conducted and were not included as part of this report.[30]

RT-associated late toxicity was well characterized by the multicenter phase II study conducted by the TROG.[31] Two hundred thirty patients completed RT to a dose of 45 to 50 Gy in 20 to 21 fractions. Median follow-up was 58.4 months (range 21.2–158 months). Acute toxicity was not reported.

Table 4
Criteria for enrollment on the TROG 02.01/ANZMTG 01.02 trial of adjuvant radiotherapy after lymphadenectomy

Lymph Node Region	Criteria for Inclusion in Trial (Eligible if Any of These were Met)		
	Extracapsular Extension	Involved Lymph Nodes (n)	Size of Lymph Node (cm)
Parotid	Yes	≥ 1	≥ 3
Neck	Yes	≥ 2	≥ 3
Axilla	Yes	≥ 2	≥ 3
Groin	Yes	≥ 3	≥ 4

Lymphedema (moderate symptoms requiring treatment) was the most frequently observed moderately severe (grade 3) toxicity, observed in 9% of patients receiving treatment of the axilla and 19% of patients receiving treatment of the ilioinguinal region; grade 4 lymphedema (incapacitating or causing ulceration in skin creases) was not observed. Grade 1 and 2 skin effects (atrophy, hair loss, telangiectasias) were noted in 46% of patients, with grade 3 and 4 effects in 11%. Grade 1 and 2 subcutaneous effects (induration/fibrosis and loss of subcutaneous fat) were noted in 36% of patients, with grade 3 and 4 effects in 2%. These results indicate that adjuvant RT of regional lymphatics is well tolerated, with few severe side effects observed. While intensity modulation has improved the side-effect profile of RT in several randomized trials, confirmation of this benefit in CM is still lacking.[32]

The phase II study of adjuvant RT for CM of the head and neck conducted by Ang and colleagues[33] at MDACC described earlier also assessed the effect of adjuvant RT in the cervical lymphatics. Cervical lymph node recurrence occurred in 6%, 0%, and 2% of patients in groups 1, 2, and 3, respectively (see **Table 2** for description of groups). Of note, 2 of the 3 cervical lymph node recurrences occurred outside the RT field, indicating the importance of accurate target delineation and the low rate of cervical lymph node recurrence with appropriate field design. Treatment was well tolerated, with acute and transient parotitis being the most common side effect. In fewer than 5% of patients, moist desquamation and confluent mucositis of short duration were observed. One patient experienced each of the following side effects after RT: surgical-site infection, moderate neck fibrosis, mild ipsilateral hearing loss, transient exposure of external auditory canal cartilage.[33] These data indicate a low rate of nodal recurrence after RT for head and neck CM with high-risk features, using a safe and convenient RT regimen that differed from that used in studies conducted by the TROG.

RADIATION THERAPY FOR DISTANT METASTASES

RT is most commonly used for palliative purposes in patients with metastatic melanoma.[1] There is a wide variety of situations in which RT may be helpful. However, many of the research studies investigating the efficacy and toxicity of palliative RT have not focused specifically on metastatic melanoma. In many situations, extrapolating findings from other metastatic cancers is necessary. In this section, attention is paid to studies

specifically studying the role of palliative RT in metastatic melanoma.

Radiation Therapy for Brain Metastasis

The most common situation whereby palliative RT is used in the care of patients with metastatic melanoma is for the treatment of brain metastasis. In general, the prognosis of patients with brain metastasis from CM is poor. RT strategies typically consist of focal RT (by stereotactic radiosurgery [SRS][34] or other related techniques), whole-brain RT (WBRT), or both. The treatment modalities selected depend on several factors.

For patients with a single brain metastasis, focal palliative therapy (surgical resection,[35] SRS, or both) is typically used. A randomized comparison of surgery and SRS has never been performed adequately; a recent study attempted this, but was discontinued because of poor accrual.[36] Surgery generally has the advantage of providing tissue for diagnostic and prognostic purposes, relieving mass effect, and being safer for tumors larger than 4 cm. SRS is generally less morbid, with almost no risk of death as a result of the procedure. Retrospective data generally suggest that the oncologic outcomes are comparable. After focal therapy for a single brain metastasis, randomized trials have suggested that WBRT may be used to decrease the risk of recurrence of brain metastasis in regions harboring radiographically inapparent disease.[37,38] However, WBRT is associated with acute fatigue and hair loss, and may cause neurocognitive impairment or delay systemic therapy.[39] The role of WBRT in melanoma specifically is controversial, and a randomized controlled trial is currently under way to help define the effects.[40]

When few (variably defined, but typically <4) brain metastases are found, SRS is typically recommended. The ECOG conducted a phase II study (6397) of SRS in 31 eligible patients with 1 to 3 "radioresistant" brain metastases, including 14 patients with melanoma. After a median follow-up of 32.7 months, median survival was 8.3 months; neurologic cause of death was observed in 38% of patients. About half of the patients developed intracranial recurrence, with about 32.2% of these being outside the SRS treatment area and 32.2% being inside the SRS treatment area. Three grade 3 toxic events were recorded: cytopenia, fatigue, and seizure.[41]

When many (variably defined, but typically more than 3) brain metastases are found, WBRT is typically used. Alternative strategies including chemotherapy and immunotherapy have been also been used, but no single modality or combination has been proved to be clearly superior to others. A randomized multicenter trial conducted in France showed that patients with at least one unresectable brain metastasis from melanoma treated with WBRT and fotemustine demonstrated a statistically significantly longer time to cerebral progression than patients treated with fotemustine alone (49 vs 56 days), although the clinical significance of this is unclear.[42] In general, patients with brain metastases from melanoma respond to WBRT in a manner similar to patients with multiple brain metastases from other causes.[43]

Radiation Therapy for Bone Metastasis

RT is generally effective at alleviating pain in patients with metastatic cancer in the bone, with complete pain relief seen in 25% of patients, and at least 50% pain relief in 41% of patients (overall response rate of 66%).[44] A single-arm prospective study has assessed the effect of palliative RT for painful metastases in melanoma. The investigators found that pain was relieved in 67% of patients with metastatic melanoma, with responders experiencing pain relief for a median of 2.4 months, or 57% of their remaining lifetime.[45] Retrospective studies have suggested that appendicular metastases are more likely than axial metastases to respond.[46,47] Some retrospective studies have suggested higher response rates with higher doses per RT fraction, or higher total doses, although these are likely biased by patient selection. A randomized trial by the RTOG found no difference in non–bone metastatic tumor response rates using different fractionation regimens.[48]

Radiation Therapy for Dermal Metastasis

RT has been used in the palliative treatment of skin and subcutaneous metastases. Early reports suggested response rates of greater than 90% for patients with skin metastases treated with fractions of 6 Gy and higher, with no responses noted in patients treated with fractions less than 6 Gy.[49] A subsequent prospective, randomized controlled trial found no difference in response rate in patients with skin metastases treated with a high total dose of RT in different RT fraction sizes, with a complete response rate of 66% and partial response rate or 33% (overall response rate of 100%) noted.[50] Acute toxicity consisted of grade 2 and 3 erythema and was noted in 47% and 53% of patients, respectively. Late toxicity consisted of moderate fibrosis, although estimates of frequency were not given. A later randomized study of patients with metastatic melanoma in the skin found that complete response

rates were doubled when adjuvant hyperthermia was used with palliative high-dose RT.[51]

ADVANCED TECHNIQUES IN RADIATION THERAPY FOR TREATMENT OF METASTASES

Advanced techniques in RT have allowed for the delivery of a single or a few high doses to several sites of metastatic melanoma. Gerszten and colleagues[52] reported on the experience at the University of Pittsburgh, and found that 96% of patients reported long-term improvement in spine pain, with mean improvement of 7 points on a 10-point pain scale. Treatment with doses of 17.5 to 25 Gy was found to be safe, with no clinical or radiographic evidence of radiation-associated neurologic toxicity. Multicenter phase I/II trials of high-dose RT for lung[53] and liver[54] metastases (including, but not exclusively from, melanoma) have demonstrated safety and 2-year metastatic tumor control rates of 96% and 92%, respectively. Tumor-control probability modeling has suggested that a minimum dose of 48 Gy in 3 fractions is necessary to obtain metastatic tumor-control rates of greater than 90% in melanoma.[55]

SUMMARY

RT has a role in the management of patients with CM. As new data emerge on the relative efficacy and toxicity of RT, a change in practice patterns may be observed. Further carefully planned studies of RT in CM are necessary to optimize the outcomes of patients with this potentially lethal disease.

REFERENCES

1. Delaney G, Barton M, Jacob S. Estimation of an optimal radiotherapy utilization rate for melanoma: a review of the evidence. Cancer 2004;100(6):1293–301.
2. French J, McGahan C, Duncan G, et al. How gender, age, and geography influence the utilization of radiation therapy in the management of malignant melanoma. Int J Radiat Oncol Biol Phys 2006;66(4): 1056–63.
3. Williams MV, Drinkwater KJ. Radiotherapy in England in 2007: modelled demand and audited activity. Clin Oncol (R Coll Radiol) 2009;21(8):575–90.
4. Harwood AR, Cummings BJ. Radiotherapy for malignant melanoma: a re-appraisal. Cancer Treat Rev 1981;8(4):271–82.
5. Stevens G, McKay MJ. Dispelling the myths surrounding radiotherapy for treatment of cutaneous melanoma. Lancet Oncol 2006;7(7):575–83.
6. Hawkins BS. Collaborative Ocular Melanoma Study randomized trial of I-125 brachytherapy. Clin Trials 2011;8(5):661–73.

7. Papadopoulos T, Rasiah K, Thompson JF, et al. Melanoma of the nose. Br J Surg 1997;84(7):986–9.

8. Hellriegel W. Radiation therapy of primary and metastatic melanoma. Ann N Y Acad Sci 1963;100: 131–41.

9. Mortier L, Mirabel X, Modiano P, et al. Interstitial brachytherapy in management of primary cutaneous melanoma: 4 cases. Ann Dermatol Venereol 2006; 133(2):153–6 [in French].

10. Harwood AR. Radiotherapy of acral lentiginous melanoma of the foot. J La State Med Soc 1999; 151(7):373–6.

11. De Groot WP. Provisional results of treatment of the mélanose précancéreuse circonscrite Dubreuilh by Bucky-rays. Dermatologica 1968;136(5):429–31.

12. Farshad A, Burg G, Panizzon R, et al. A retrospective study of 150 patients with lentigo maligna and lentigo maligna melanoma and the efficacy of radiotherapy using Grenz or soft X-rays. Br J Dermatol 2002; 146(6):1042–6.

13. Schmid-Wendtner MH, Brunner B, Konz B, et al. Fractionated radiotherapy of lentigo maligna and lentigo maligna melanoma in 64 patients. J Am Acad Dermatol 2000;43(3):477–82.

14. Kopf AW, Bart RS, Gladstein AH. Treatment of melanotic freckle with x-rays. Arch Dermatol 1976;112(6): 801–7.

15. Tsang RW, Liu FF, Wells W, et al. Lentigo maligna of the head and neck. Results of treatment by radiotherapy. Arch Dermatol 1994;130(8): 1008–12.

16. Lee H, Sowerby LJ, Temple CL, et al. Carbon dioxide laser treatment for lentigo maligna: a retrospective review comparing 3 different treatment modalities. Arch Facial Plast Surg 2011;13(6):398–403.

17. Christie DR, Tiver KW. Radiotherapy for melanotic freckles. Australas Radiol 1996;40(3):331–3.

18. Cooper JS. Patients' perceptions of their cosmetic appearance more than ten years after radiotherapy for basal cell carcinoma. Radiat Med 1988;6(6): 285–8.

19. Zalaudek I, Horn M, Richtig E, et al. Local recurrence in melanoma in situ: influence of sex, age, site of involvement and therapeutic modalities. Br J Dermatol 2003;148(4):703–8.

20. Marsden JR, Newton-Bishop JA, Burrows L, et al. Revised UK guidelines for the management of cutaneous melanoma 2010. J Plast Reconstr Aesthet Surg 2010;63(9):1401–19.

21. Mahendran RM, Newton-Bishop JA. Survey of U.K. current practice in the treatment of lentigo maligna. Br J Dermatol 2001;144(1):71–6.

22. Vongtama R, Safa A, Gallardo D, et al. Efficacy of radiation therapy in the local control of desmoplastic malignant melanoma. Head Neck 2003;25(6):423–8.

23. Foote MC, Burmeister B, Burmeister E, et al. Desmoplastic melanoma: the role of radiotherapy in improving local control. ANZ J Surg 2008;78(4): 273–6.

24. Chen JY, Hruby G, Scolyer RA, et al. Desmoplastic neurotropic melanoma: a clinicopathologic analysis of 128 cases. Cancer 2008;113(10):2770–8.

25. Arora A, Lowe L, Su L, et al. Wide excision without radiation for desmoplastic melanoma. Cancer 2005;104(7):1462–7.

26. Feng Z, Wu XC, Chen V, et al. Incidence and survival of desmoplastic melanoma in the United States, 1992-2007. J Cutan Pathol 2011;38(8):616–24.

27. Wasif N, Gray RJ, Pockaj BA. Desmoplastic melanoma—the step-child in the melanoma family? J Surg Oncol 2011;103(2):158–62.

28. Guadagnolo BA, Zagars GK. Adjuvant radiation therapy for high-risk nodal metastases from cutaneous melanoma. Lancet Oncol 2009;10(4):409–16.

29. Creagan ET, Cupps RE, Ivins JC, et al. Adjuvant radiation therapy for regional nodal metastases from malignant melanoma: a randomized, prospective study. Cancer 1978;42(5):2206–10.

30. Burmeister BH, Henderson MA, Ainslie J, et al. Adjuvant radiotherapy versus observation alone for patients at risk of lymph-node field relpase after therapeutic lymphadectomy for melanoma: a randomised trial. Lancet oncology 2012. DOI:10.1016/ S1470-2045(12)70138-9.

31. Burmeister BH, Mark Smithers B, Burmeister E, et al. A prospective phase II study of adjuvant postoperative radiation therapy following nodal surgery in malignant melanoma-Trans Tasman Radiation Oncology Group (TROG) Study 96.06. Radiother Oncol 2006;81(2):136–42.

32. Staffurth J. A review of the clinical evidence for intensity-modulated radiotherapy. Clin Oncol (R Coll Radiol) 2010;22(8):643–57.

33. Ang KK, Peters LJ, Weber RS, et al. Postoperative radiotherapy for cutaneous melanoma of the head and neck region. Int J Radiat Oncol Biol Phys 1994;30(4):795–8.

34. Suh JH. Stereotactic radiosurgery for the management of brain metastases. N Engl J Med 2010; 362(12):1119–27.

35. Vogelbaum MA, Suh JH. Resectable brain metastases. J Clin Oncol 2006;24(8):1289–94.

36. Roos DE, Smith JG, Stephens SW. Radiosurgery versus surgery, both with adjuvant whole brain radiotherapy, for solitary brain metastases: a randomised controlled trial. Clin Oncol (R Coll Radiol) 2011;23(9):646–51.

37. Patchell RA, Tibbs PA, Regine WF, et al. Postoperative radiotherapy in the treatment of single metastases to the brain: a randomized trial. JAMA 1998; 280(17):1485–9.

38. Aoyama H, Shirato H, Tago M, et al. Stereotactic radiosurgery plus whole-brain radiation therapy vs stereotactic radiosurgery alone for treatment of brain

metastases: a randomized controlled trial. JAMA 2006;295(21):2483–91.

39. Chang EL, Wefel JS, Hess KR, et al. Neurocognition in patients with brain metastases treated with radiosurgery or radiosurgery plus whole-brain irradiation: a randomised controlled trial. Lancet Oncol 2009; 10(11):1037–44.

40. Fogarty G, Morton RL, Vardy J, et al. Whole brain radiotherapy after local treatment of brain metastases in melanoma patients—a randomised phase III trial. BMC Cancer 2011;11:142.

41. Manon R, O'Neill A, Knisely J, et al. Phase II trial of radiosurgery for one to three newly diagnosed brain metastases from renal cell carcinoma, melanoma, and sarcoma: an Eastern Cooperative Oncology Group study (E 6397). J Clin Oncol 2005;23(34): 8870–6.

42. Mornex F, Thomas L, Mohr P, et al. A prospective randomized multicentre phase III trial of fotemustine plus whole brain irradiation versus fotemustine alone in cerebral metastases of malignant melanoma. Melanoma Res 2003;13(1):97–103.

43. Carella RJ, Gelber R, Hendrickson F, et al. Value of radiation therapy in the management of patients with cerebral metastases from malignant melanoma: Radiation Therapy Oncology Group Brain Metastases Study I and II. Cancer 1980;45(4): 679–83.

44. McQuay HJ, Collins SL, Carroll D, et al. Radiotherapy for the palliation of painful bone metastases. Cochrane Database Syst Rev 2000;(2):CD001793.

45. Huguenin PU, Kieser S, Glanzmann C, et al. Radiotherapy for metastatic carcinomas of the kidney or melanomas: an analysis using palliative end points. Int J Radiat Oncol Biol Phys 1998;41(2):401–5.

46. Seegenschmiedt MH, Keilholz L, Altendorf-Hofmann A, et al. Palliative radiotherapy for recurrent and metastatic malignant melanoma: prognostic factors for tumor response and long-term outcome:

a 20-year experience. Int J Radiat Oncol Biol Phys 1999;44(3):607–18.

47. Konefal JB, Emami B, Pilepich MV. Analysis of dose fractionation in the palliation of metastases from malignant melanoma. Cancer 1988;61(2):243–6.

48. Sause WT, Cooper JS, Rush S, et al. Fraction size in external beam radiation therapy in the treatment of melanoma. Int J Radiat Oncol Biol Phys 1991; 20(3):429–32.

49. Habermalz HJ, Fischer JJ. Radiation therapy of malignant melanoma: experience with high individual treatment doses. Cancer 1976;38(6):2258–62.

50. Overgaard J, von der Maase H, Overgaard M. A randomized study comparing two high-dose per fraction radiation schedules in recurrent or metastatic malignant melanoma. Int J Radiat Oncol Biol Phys 1985;11(10):1837–9.

51. Overgaard J, Gonzalez Gonzalez D, Hulshof MC, et al. Randomised trial of hyperthermia as adjuvant to radiotherapy for recurrent or metastatic malignant melanoma. European Society for Hyperthermic Oncology. Lancet 1995;345(8949):540–3.

52. Gerszten PC, Burton SA, Quinn AE, et al. Radiosurgery for the treatment of spinal melanoma metastases. Stereotact Funct Neurosurg 2005;83(5–6): 213–21.

53. Rusthoven KE, Kavanagh BD, Burri SH, et al. Multi-institutional phase I/II trial of stereotactic body radiation therapy for lung metastases. J Clin Oncol 2009;27(10):1579–84.

54. Rusthoven KE, Kavanagh BD, Cardenes H, et al. Multi-institutional phase I/II trial of stereotactic body radiation therapy for liver metastases. J Clin Oncol 2009;27(10):1572–8.

55. Stinauer MA, Kavanagh BD, Schefter TE, et al. Stereotactic body radiation therapy for melanoma and renal cell carcinoma: impact of single fraction equivalent dose on local control. Radiat Oncol 2011;6:34.

New Diagnostic Aids for Melanoma

Laura Korb Ferris, MD, PhD*, Ryan J. Harris, MD

KEYWORDS

- Melanoma detection • Technology • Imaging • Biopsy • Automated diagnosis

KEY POINTS

- The incidence of melanoma is continuing to increase.
- Current methods commonly fail to diagnose melanoma at an early stage.
- Use of dermatoscopy has improved our diagnostic capabilities, but is highly user dependent and commonly misses the diagnosis.
- Recent advances have lead to new diagnostic technologies such as confocal scanning laser microscopy, MelaFind, SIAscopy, noninvasive genomic detection, and many others.
- Systems such as MelaFind are being created to provide an automated diagnosis to improve diagnostic accuracy and decrease the need for biopsy of benign lesions.
- Several barriers to implementation exist, including cost, time needed to become competent in use of new technologies, and lack of insurance reimbursement for use of new modalities.
- Proper implementation of new technologies will, it is hoped, lead to earlier diagnosis of melanoma, decreased mortality and morbidity, fewer biopsies of benign lesions, and decreased cost to the health care system.

INTRODUCTION

According to estimates, there will be approximately 70,000 new cases of melanoma and 8800 subsequent deaths in 2011. For 2012 the estimates are 76,250 cases and 9180 deaths.[1] The incidence of melanoma has been steadily increasing and has doubled in recent decades.[2] For lesions with a depth of less than 1 mm, surgical excision is usually curative and 5-year survival rate is 93% to 97%.[3] By contrast, distant metastatic melanoma has an extremely poor prognosis and 5-year survival ranges from 10% to 20%, depending on location of the metastasis.[3] Detection of melanoma at an early stage is critical for improving the survival rate. In addition to decreased survival of late-stage versus early-stage melanoma, the cost of treating a late-stage melanoma is dramatically higher.

Recent estimates show the total costs of in situ tumors to be around $4700, whereas a stage IV melanoma has a total cost of approximately $160,000.[4] The cost of treating late-stage melanoma is likely to increase with the implementation of newly approved treatments such as ipilimumab, which costs about $120,000 for a full treatment.

Despite advances in diagnostic aids such as dermatoscopy, detection has remained a significant challenge, and improved methods of accurately diagnosing melanoma are needed. Studies have shown that even for expert dermoscopists, accurately diagnosing melanoma, particularly in small-diameter lesions, is very challenging, with one study showing a biopsy sensitivity of 71% for melanomas of size less than 6 mm.[5] To measure specificity, numerous studies have looked at biopsy ratios (ie,

Funding Sources: Dr Ferris: NIH/NCRR grant number 5 UL1 RR024153-04. Dr Harris: None.
Conflicts of Interest: Dr Ferris: Served as an investigator and consultant for MELA Sciences and as an investigator for DermTech International. Dr Harris: No conflicts of interest to declare.
Department of Dermatology, University of Pittsburgh Medical Center, 3601 Fifth Avenue, Fifth Floor, Pittsburgh, PA 15213, USA
* Corresponding author.
E-mail address: ferrislk@upmc.edu

Dermatol Clin 30 (2012) 535–545
doi:10.1016/j.det.2012.04.012
0733-8635/12/$ – see front matter © 2012 Elsevier Inc. All rights reserved.

the number of biopsies of benign lesions performed to make the diagnosis of one skin cancer), and numbers vary widely. On the low end, a study from a specialized pigmented lesion clinic showed a biopsy ratio of approximately 5:1 (5 benign lesions per melanoma biopsied).[6] A recent retrospective study involving 8 practitioners at a single institution had a biopsy ratio of 15:1.[7] On the high end, a study involving a single physician over a 14-year period showed a biopsy ratio of more than 500:1 in patients with no history of melanoma.[8] Given these challenges, new diagnostic aids that could help increase both sensitivity and specificity of biopsies would be of great benefit to patients and physicians. Such improvements (**Table 1**) have the potential to lead to increased diagnosis of early lesions, which would improve survival and lower the overall cost of treating melanoma. In addition, improved diagnostic techniques would lead to fewer biopsies and decreased morbidity to patients.

ESTABLISHED METHODS
Physician and Patient Detection of Malignant Melanoma

Multiple studies have tried to assess who initially detects melanomas, with most finding that the majority of melanomas are detected by the patient.[9–11] Patient education, including the ABCDEs (Asymmetry, Border irregularity, Color variegation, Diameter of >6 mm, and Evolution) of melanoma will always be an important part of helping patients to diagnose melanoma.[12,13] In addition, regular self-examinations of the skin should be encouraged, as they have been associated with detection of thinner melanomas and may reduce mortality.[14–16] Self detection seems to be most successful in younger patients, as increased age has been associated with increased Breslow thickness in patients who have discovered melanoma by self examination.[17] Physician-detected melanomas, particularly melanomas detected by dermatologists, tend to be thinner.[9–11,15,18]

Dermatoscopy

Dermatoscopy, covered in depth by Rao and Ahn elsewhere in this issue, has been widely used by dermatologists to improve their abilities to accurately diagnose melanoma, and has been shown to improve early detection of melanoma[19] while reducing unnecessary biopsies.[20,21] A major drawback to dermatoscopy is that it is highly user dependent and varies with experience.[22] Despite the advantages of using dermatoscopy, only about 60% of dermatologists in the United States are trained in its use, and fewer than half report using dermatoscopy daily (**Fig. 1**).[23]

Temporal Analysis of the Skin

In addition to dermatoscopy alone, temporal analysis of the skin is commonly used. Individual lesions can be followed serially with dermatoscopy and/or photography. Total-body photography can be used to monitor for new or changing lesions, particularly in high-risk patients or patients with a large number of nevi. Temporal analysis has been shown to increase the sensitivity of melanoma detection when compared with dermatoscopy alone.[24] A perceived benefit of total-body photography would be to decrease the biopsy rate, and indeed this has been demonstrated in some studies,[25] although others have failed to show any noticeable change in number of biopsies performed.[26] Total-body photography seems to be most useful in older patients, as one study showed that in patients younger than 50 years fewer than 1% of new lesions identified by photography turned out to be melanoma, whereas in patients older than 50 years 30% of new lesions were melanomas on biopsy.[27]

Total-body photography has the limitation of being time consuming and laborious. Also, costs can run as high as $500 per person and are not typically covered by insurance. Imaging technologies including MoleMax (Derma Medical Systems, Vienna, Austria) and FotoFinder (FotoFinder Systems, Inc, Columbia, MD, USA) are computerized systems used to help the clinician to more rapidly and efficiently perform total-body cutaneous photography and dermatoscopy of individual lesions. MoleMax has software that analyzes pigmented lesions and provides a scoring system based on established criteria to aid clinicians in evaluating concerning lesions. The FotoFinder system also has software that aids in the detection of new nevi by comparing baseline photos with those taken at a follow-up visit, as well as software that rates the likelihood that a pigmented lesion is a melanoma. However, no large peer-reviewed studies have validated the accuracy of these systems.

RECENT ADVANCES
Confocal Scanning Laser Microscopy

Confocal scanning laser microscopy (CSLM) is a noninvasive imaging technology that provides in-vivo images of the epidermis and papillary dermis in real time. There are currently 2 forms of CSLM in use: reflectance mode, which is primarily used in clinical practice, and fluorescence mode, used primarily in research. Reflectance confocal microscopy (RCM) relies on the inherent reflective properties of tissue structures, whereas fluorescence CSLM relies on fluorescent dyes to provide contrast for images.[28] The contrast seen in RCM

Table 1
Comparison of technologies in melanoma diagnosis

Technology	Sensitivity (%)	Specificity (%)	Advantages	Disadvantages
Confocal scanning laser microscopy	88–98[32–34]	83–98[32–34]	Provides a "virtual biopsy" of concerning lesions. Low incremental cost per lesion after initial investment	Accuracy is user dependent; imaging depth only 300 μm; imaging system is expensive
MelaFind	98[42]	10[42,a]	Provides automated diagnosis, minimizing user dependence	Cost of imaging is $150, which must be covered by the patient
SIAscope	83–91[38]	80–91[38,39]	Provides high-resolution images of melanin, hemoglobin, and collagen content in the epidermis and papillary dermis	Accuracy is user dependent; diagnostic features may classify many benign lesions as malignant
Epidermal genetic information retrieval	100[48]	88[48]	Minimal special equipment or investment required up front	Samples must be sent to distant laboratory, delaying diagnosis
Electrical impedance spectroscopy	91–95[52,53]	49–64[52,53]	Provides automated diagnosis	Can be technically challenging; can take up to 5 minutes per lesion for evaluation

[a] Lesions evaluated in this study were enriched by preselection from a general population. Lesions were already scheduled for a biopsy because of high concern for melanoma, resulting in a lower specificity in comparison with other studies performed in lesions that were not preselected.

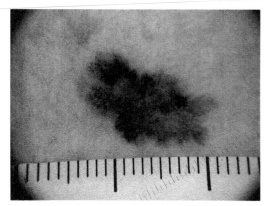

Fig. 1. Dermatoscopic image of an invasive melanoma.

images is due to the naturally occurring variations in refractive index of organelles and other structures within the skin. Melanin granules have a high refractive index, which causes more light to be reflected back to the confocal microscope. Thus areas of higher melanin concentration will appear as bright areas on a confocal image (**Fig. 2**). When used by those properly trained in confocal use, lesions can be evaluated based on characteristics such as cellular atypia, uniformity of pigment distribution, loss of keratinocyte borders, and rate of blood flow to help distinguish malignant from benign lesions. One of the unique features of CSLM is its ability to detect amelanotic melanoma because of the presence of melanosomes and rare melanin granules.[29]

CSLM works by intensely focusing a low-power laser beam on a specific point in the skin. Light from that point is then reflected from structures within the skin, and passes through a pinhole-sized aperture to a detection apparatus. The reflected light is transformed into an electrical signal to create a 3-dimensional image from the scanned horizontal sections.[30] Imaging depth is related to the

wavelength of light used, with longer wavelengths allowing deeper imaging. RCM uses a near-infrared 830-nm laser that provides an imaging depth of 250 to 300 μm in normal skin, allowing visualization to the level of the superficial dermis.[28] The images provide 1 to 2 μm of lateral resolution and 3 to 5 μm of axial resolution.[31] This resolution is comparable with that of standard pathology, which is typically based on 5-μm thin sections. CSLM has potential to provide a "virtual biopsy" of concerning skin lesions. Advantages of CSLM are that, like dermatoscopy, it is noninvasive and allows rapid imaging of multiple lesions, and can be used to follow lesions over time. CSLM is also similar to dermatoscopy in that it requires the reader's interpretation and is thus user dependent. Training required to accurately use CSLM has been reported to be less than that required for dermatoscopy, with subjects showing ability to correctly diagnose images of lesions from a test set after only 30 minutes of instruction in one study.[32]

CSLM has demonstrated high sensitivity and specificity in diagnosing melanoma from benign pigmented lesions. One study involving a test set of 27 melanomas and 90 benign nevi with images evaluated by 5 independent observers showed sensitivity of 88.15% and specificity of 97.6%.[32] A retrospective study of 3709 unselected CSLM melanocytic tumor images coming from 50 benign nevi and 20 melanomas showed sensitivity and specificity of 97.5% and 99%, respectively.[33] In comparison with standard dermatoscopy, another prospective study showed sensitivity and specificity of CSLM to be 97.3% and 83%, respectively, compared with sensitivity and specificity of 89.2% and 84.1% for dermatoscopy.[34] This study, however, involved only a single observer and evaluated 37 melanomas and 88 nevi.

CSLM has been tested with diagnostic imaging analysis for fully automated diagnosis,

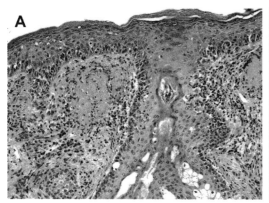

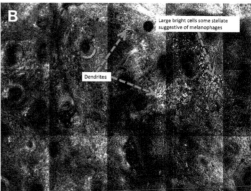

Fig. 2. Histopathology (*A*; H&E stain, original magnification ×10) and confocal microscopy (*B*; original magnification ×100) of an in situ melanoma. (*Courtesy of* Harold Rabinovitz, MD.)

and in the future such a system could possibly improve diagnostic accuracy and decrease user dependence.[35–37] CSLM is also limited by its cost. A commercially available unit costs approximately $50,000. Although the upfront cost of the device is high, the supplies to image individual lesions cost only about $1 per lesion, allowing imaging of multiple lesions with minimal increased cost to the patient per lesion.

Advances in CSLM technology continue to make it a more useful diagnostic tool. Newer devices use a single optical fiber to both illuminate and detect the laser light in place of the pinhole aperture detector found in earlier CSLM devices. This improvement has led to miniaturization of the confocal scanner into a flexible and more user-friendly handheld device. Multiple CSLM units are available and have Food and Drug Administration (FDA) 510(k) clearance, including the VivaScope 1500 and the handheld VivaScope 3000 (Lucid, Inc, Rochester, NY, USA).

Multispectral Imaging

The SIAscope (Spectrophotometric Intracutaneous Analysis, made by Biocompatibles, Farnham, Surrey, UK) emits radiation ranging from 400 to 1000 nm, and provides the user with 8 narrow-band spectrally filtered images that demonstrate the vascular composition and pigment network of a lesion. This multispectral imaging technology has FDA 510(k) clearance and uses a handheld imager to provide microarchitectural information for concerning lesions. The SIAscope measures levels of 3 chromophores (melanin, blood, and collagen) contained in the epidermis and papillary dermis. It is also able to show if melanin is confined to the epidermis, or whether it has penetrated into the deeper dermis. The clinician then interprets these images to determine whether a biopsy is necessary. In a study of 384 lesions, SIAscopy was found to have a sensitivity of 82.7% and specificity of 80.1%.[38] However, a larger study showed that SIAscopy had similar sensitivity and specificity to dermatoscopy performed by experienced dermatologists, and thus did not provide sufficient benefit in diagnosing melanoma to warrant its use.[39] One of the major criticisms of SIAscopy is that it uses features in its diagnostic classification that are common to benign lesions, such as seborrheic keratoses and hemangiomas, which causes many benign lesions to be classified as suspicious.[40] A recent study sought to develop a scoring system to correctly classify lesions and allow use of SIAscopy in a primary care setting.[40] The scoring system is still early in its development and needs further improvement and validation, but

such a system could provide primary care physicians with a useful tool to screen a larger population of patients, with referral to a dermatologist for suspicious lesions.

As most imaging modalities require user interpretation and are thus prone to varying levels of accuracy based on user experience, attempts have been made to create automated imaging systems to improve diagnostic accuracy. MelaFind (MELA Sciences, Inc, Irvington, NY, USA) is a handheld imager that evaluates lesions with multispectral images in 10 different spectral bands, from blue (430 nm) to near infrared (950 nm). The images are processed with proprietary software, which generates a 10 digital image sequences in less than 3 seconds. The software determines the border of the lesion and analyzes the lesion for asymmetry, color variation, perimeter changes, texture changes, and wavelet maxima (Fig. 3).[41] The Mela-Find device then provides the user with a recommendation of whether or not to perform a biopsy based on this analysis. The algorithm for determining biopsy recommendation comes from a database of over 9000 biopsied lesions from 7000 patients, consisting of in vivo skin lesion images and corresponding histopathologic results.

A recent large multicenter study evaluated the diagnostic accuracy of MelaFind, and found it to have a sensitivity of 98.4% and a specificity superior to that of expert dermatologists using dermatoscopy.[42] In the study, MelaFind had a biopsy ratio of 10.8:1 for melanomas, and a ratio of 7.6:1 if borderline lesions (high-grade dysplastic nevus, atypical melanocytic hyperplasia, and atypical melanocyte proliferation) were also included.[42] Such a biopsy ratio is better than most ratios from reported literature. An earlier study evaluated the ability of MelaFind to diagnose melanoma in small pigmented lesions (smaller than 6 mm) and showed sensitivity of 98% for melanoma.[5] This study also showed sensitivity superior to expert dermatologists with similar levels of specificity.

MelaFind was approved for use in Europe in September 2011, and in the United States in November of 2011. In contrast to other devices that have only FDA 510(k) clearance, MelaFind has FDA premarket approval. MelaFind differs from other diagnostic modalities in that it provides the user with a recommendation as to whether or not to biopsy, whereas many other technologies completely rely on user interpretation for the decision to biopsy. As such, MELA Sciences has strict quality controls in place, and would need to maintain ownership of the device to assure that devices are properly updated and maintained. MelaFind is expected to be made available to dermatologists, with doctors paying a one-time fee to lease the

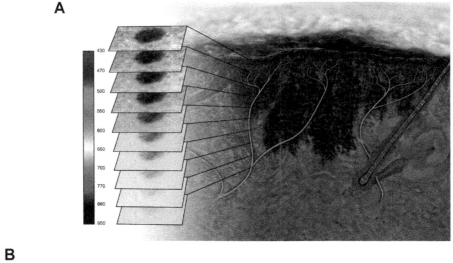

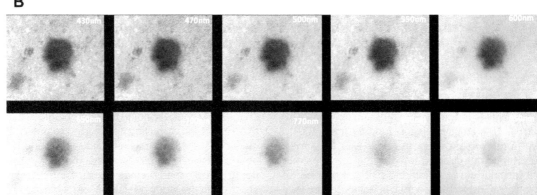

Fig. 3. (*A*) A representative multispectral image analysis of a pigmented lesion showing 10 images from multiple depths within the skin. (*B*) Actual images from multispectral image analysis showing a digitally detected margin from most superficial (430 nm) to deepest (950 nm). (*Image courtesy of* MELAScience, Inc.)

device and receive training. At the time of publication, insurance coverage was not available for use of the device, so this fee will be an out-of-pocket expense to the patient. Given that the price per use is targeted to be less than the cost of biopsy and histopathology, MelaFind could provide a cost-effective means of reducing numbers of biopsies while improving diagnostic accuracy.

OTHER IMAGING TECHNOLOGIES

Optical coherence tomography (OCT) is a well-established tool in ophthalmology. OCT is commonly used as a diagnostic aid for uveal melanoma[43] and has shown usefulness in dermatology as well. OCT is analogous to ultrasound imaging, except that it uses light rather than sound waves. OCT uses a low-coherence-length light source to evaluate lesion architecture up to 1 mm in depth.[44] One study showed that OCT allows for in vivo correlation between dermatoscopic parameters and histopathologic analysis in melanocytic lesions.[45]

Resolution in OCT is insufficient to show morphology of single cells, but does allow for evaluation of architectural changes.[46] OCT is further limited, as it has shown inability to properly image lesions that are raised or hyperkeratotic. The resolution in OCT lies between that of ultrasonography and CSLM, and at this point is best suited for measuring depth of invasion rather than diagnosing melanoma.

Reflex transmission imaging (RTI) is a form of high-resolution ultrasonography that can be combined with white-light digital photography to classify pigmented lesions. In one study, RTI was found to discriminate between melanoma, seborrheic keratoses, and nevi based on quantitative methods involving various sonographic parameters.[47] When parameters were set to yield 100% sensitivity for distinguishing melanoma from seborrheic keratoses and benign pigmented lesions, RTI provided 79% specificity for differentiation of seborrheic keratoses from melanoma, and specificity of 55% for differentiating benign pigmented lesions from melanoma.[47] RTI has yet to be validated in prospective studies, but results from initial studies warrant further investigation into its clinical applications.

UPCOMING TECHNOLOGIES
Noninvasive Genomic Detection

Epidermal genetic information retrieval (EGIR; DermTech International, La Jolla, CA, USA) uses an adhesive tape placed on suspicious lesions to sample cells from the stratum corneum noninvasively. RNA isolated from cells is amplified using real-time polymerase chain reaction and then hybridized with Affymetrix human genome U133 plus 2.0 GeneChip. Gene expression is then analyzed. Using this technology, 312 genes that are differentially expressed between melanoma, nevi, and normal skin were identified.[48] Subsequent analysis has reduced the number or genes needed to be analyzed to differentiate melanoma from nevi to 17.[48] The 17 genes used in the analysis are known to be involved in functions such as melanocyte development, pigmentation signaling, hair and skin development, melanoma progression, cell death, cellular development, and cancer. Using this 17-gene classifier, EGIR was able to accurately differentiate between in situ and invasive melanomas from nevi with 100% sensitivity and 88% specificity.[48]

EGIR has many potential advantages. It is noninvasive, and samples can be easily obtained in the office setting. Multiple lesions can be quickly sampled, preventing initial need for biopsies, and in studies to date EGIR has shown high sensitivity and specificity. The major disadvantage is that it requires the tape sample to be sent to a distant laboratory, so results would not be available on the same day as they would be with other imaging technologies. Patients would be required to return at a later date for a biopsy if indicated by the test results, which could raise the possibility of patients being lost to follow-up.

As the RNA analyzed with EGIR is isolated from cells found in the stratum corneum, it is interesting that diagnosis of melanoma can be made by tape stripping, considering the fact that melanocytes generally reside deeper, at the dermal-epidermal junction. It is unclear whether the RNA sampled comes directly from the melanocytes, is due to the effect of melanocytes on surrounding keratinocytes through cell-cell cross-talk, or is a result of pagetoid spread of melanocytes into the epidermis. Regardless of the mechanism, EGIR has great potential and represents a novel technique in diagnosing melanoma, although initial studies are limited by sample size.

Electrical Impedance Spectroscopy

Electrical impedance spectroscopy (EIS) is an investigational technology that has shown promise in its ability to assist in diagnosing melanoma. EIS uses an impedance spectrometer probe to measure opposition to flow of alternating currents from one pole to another across a lesion at various frequencies. The probe consists of many microscopic pins designed to penetrate the stratum corneum and pass a low-voltage current to allow measurement of electrical impedance of the tissue. EIS works on the premise that cancer cells have electrochemical properties that are distinct from those of healthy cells.[49] EIS has demonstrated the ability to distinguish different stages of breast cancer cell lines.[50] In vitro studies using cultured mouse melanoma cells show reduced membrane capacitance typical of other types of cancer cells, supporting the possibility the EIS could be useful in melanoma detection.[51]

Two recent in vivo studies evaluated EIS using an automated algorithm to distinguish between melanoma and benign lesions. One study evaluated 62 malignant melanomas and 148 various benign lesions, and showed sensitivity to melanoma of 95% and specificity of 49%.[52] These numbers were similar to results of a previous study that showed sensitivity of 91% and specificity of 64%.[53] While EIS is a promising new technology, it does have limitations and improvements still need to be made. Despite the fact that EIS uses an automated algorithm, it is still somewhat user dependent in accurately providing a diagnosis. The procedure for evaluating a lesion involves soaking the skin in saline solution for 60 seconds before impedance measurement to facilitate better contact between the skin and electrode system. One EIS measurement takes approximately 20 seconds, and measuring an entire lesion typically takes less than 5 minutes. It is also necessary to measure EIS in perilesional skin for calibration to compensate for intersubject variation due to factors such as age, gender, body location, and seasonal variation.[52] In most cases, EIS is more time consuming than a skin biopsy and other diagnostic modalities, and is also more technically challenging. Despite these limitations, its ability to noninvasively analyze a lesion and accurately recommend the need for biopsy make it an intriguing technology for further study.

Fiber Diffraction

The α keratins in hair and nail proteins produce a characteristic x-ray fiber diffraction pattern in all mammals, regardless of age or species.[54] Recent studies have shown that some cancers, including melanoma, cause detectable alterations in the molecular patterns of macromolecules in hair, nails, and skin. A recent blinded retrospective study looking at multiple forms of cancer was able to detect changes in x-ray fiber diffraction from skin samples in all 28 patients diagnosed with melanoma.[55] The diffraction pattern for all melanoma patients had a single additional ring in the same location, which was not appreciated in any of the other 238 patients consisting of controls as well as patients with other cancers or systemic diseases.[55] There is currently no biological mechanism to explain the changes in diffraction patterns, but results have been consistent and specific to the type of malignancy, and have not resulted in any false negatives. Large prospective studies are still needed to clarify sensitivity and specificity, and this technique would only indicate the presence of melanoma somewhere in the patient but would not identify specific lesions of concern. However, fiber diffraction is certainly an intriguing possibility for melanoma detection or screening, particularly in high-risk patients.

Tissue Elastography

Real-time tissue elastography is a technology under very early investigation, which is based on the principle that softer, normal tissue deforms more easily than harder, malignant tissue.[56] Lesions are evaluated by manually applying light pressure with an ultrasound transducer with simultaneous imaging by ultrasonography. A recent report showed that tissue elastography was able to correctly identify cutaneous melanoma in 2 patients.[57] Similar to other evaluative methods, tissue elastography is highly operator dependent. It has been shown to be a useful diagnostic tool in the detection of breast cancer and prostate cancer.[58] With further refinement, tissue elastography could someday be an affordable, noninvasive diagnostic tool for diagnosing melanoma.

Thermal Imaging

Like many other cancers, melanoma lesions have higher metabolic activity than normal healthy tissue. This property could be exploited using dynamic thermal imaging to examine lesions with infrared imaging. Early results show that there are detectable temperature differences between melanoma and healthy tissue. This technique is currently technically challenging, as the skin must be cooled to accentuate temperature differences and sophisticated motion tracking is needed to compensate for movement of the patient while acquiring thermal images.[59]

Melanoma-Sniffing Dogs

A recent study in detection of lung cancer has shown promise in the ability of dogs to detect cancer in patients. In this study, dogs examined 220 exhalation samples from a combination of patients with and without lung cancer. The dogs were able to correctly identify 71% of the samples coming from those with lung cancer, and correctly identified 93% of the samples that were cancer free.[60] A similar study also showed promise with detection of breast cancer from exhalation samples.[61] There have been isolated case reports of dogs identifying skin cancers in patients. In one case, a dog continually showed interest in a mole belonging to its owner, and even tried to bite off the mole, which eventually led the owner to seek medical advice. The mole was excised and found to be invasive melanoma.[62] A similar case was reported in a patient with a lesion later found to be a basal cell carcinoma.[63] The experiences in lung and breast cancer suggest that trained canines may hold promise as aides in the dermatology office for the detection of melanoma, although clinical trials will be needed to see whether the evidence goes beyond anecdotal.

SUMMARY

Despite recent advances in the diagnosis and treatment of malignant melanoma, it still remains a potentially devastating disease if not diagnosed early and treated properly. With incidence continuing to increase, advances in diagnostic techniques are necessary because diagnosing melanoma is difficult and current methods still miss too many cases, especially in small-diameter lesions. Moreover, biopsying benign lesions can lead to increased morbidity to patients and increased cost to the health care system. Many available technologies are underutilized, with more promising technologies on the way.

There are significant barriers to implementation that must be overcome, including the time, training, and experience needed to properly use many of these technologies, and costs associated with developing and adopting new technologies. Also, none of these modalities currently are reimbursed by insurance carriers. Ideally new technologies would: (1) have increased sensitivity and specificity in comparison with current methods; (2) be able to be used in a time-efficient manner, such that the time needed to use the diagnostic aid is equivalent to or less than the time it takes to perform a biopsy; (3) have some reimbursement through insurance if proved to decrease the number of benign biopsies performed, to encourage their widespread use; and (4) be accessible to a wide range of patients and physicians, including nondermatologists, as a significant proportion of melanomas are diagnosed by primary care providers and other physicians.

With proper implementation of these technologies, it is hoped that the ultimate goal of reducing the morbidity and mortality associated with melanoma can be reached.

REFERENCES

1. Siegel R, Naishadham D, Jemal A. Cancer statistics, 2012. CA Cancer J Clin 2012;6(1):10–29.

2. Siegel R, Ward E, Brawley O, et al. Cancer statistics, 2011: the impact of eliminating socioeconomic and racial disparities on premature cancer deaths. CA Cancer J Clin 2011;61:212–36.

3. Balch CM, Gershenwald JE, Soong SJ, et al. Final version of 2009 AJCC melanoma staging and classification. J Clin Oncol 2009;27:6199–206.

4. Alexandrescu DT. Melanoma costs: a dynamic model comparing estimated overall costs of various clinical stages. Dermatol Online J 2009;15:1.

5. Friedman RJ, Gutkowicz-Krusin D, Farber MJ, et al. The diagnostic performance of expert dermoscopists vs a computer-vision system on small-diameter melanomas. Arch Dermatol 2008;144:476–82.

6. Carli P, Nardini P, Crocetti E, et al. Frequency and characteristics of melanomas missed at a pigmented lesion clinic: a registry-based study. Melanoma Res 2004;14:403–7.

7. Wilson RL, Yentzer BA, Isom SP, et al. How good are US dermatologists at discriminating skin cancers? A number-needed-to-treat analysis. J Dermatolog Treat 2012;23(1):65–9.

8. Cohen MH, Cohen BJ, Shotkin JD, et al. Surgical prophylaxis of malignant melanoma. Ann Surg 1991;213:308–14.

9. Brady MS, Oliveria SA, Christos PJ, et al. Patterns of detection in patients with cutaneous melanoma. Cancer 2000;89:342–7.

10. Epstein DS, Lange JR, Gruber SB, et al. Is physician detection associated with thinner melanomas? JAMA 1999;281:640–3.

11. Kantor J, Kantor DE. Routine dermatologist-performed full-body skin examination and early melanoma detection. Arch Dermatol 2009;145:873–6.

12. Abbasi NR, Shaw HM, Rigel DS, et al. Early diagnosis of cutaneous melanoma: revisiting the ABCD criteria. JAMA 2004;292:2771–6.

13. Rigel DS, Friedman RJ, Kopf AW, et al. ABCDE—an evolving concept in the early detection of melanoma. Arch Dermatol 2005;141:1032–4.

14. Berwick M, Begg CB, Fine JA, et al. Screening for cutaneous melanoma by skin self-examination. J Natl Cancer Inst 1996;88:17–23.

15. Carli P, De Giorgi V, Palli D, et al. Dermatologist detection and skin self-examination are associated with thinner melanomas: results from a survey of the Italian Multidisciplinary Group on Melanoma. Arch Dermatol 2003;139:607–12.

16. Pollitt RA, Geller AC, Brooks DR, et al. Efficacy of skin self-examination practices for early melanoma detection. Cancer Epidemiol Biomarkers Prev 2009;18:3018–23.

17. Trolle L, Henrik-Nielsen R, Gniadecki R. Ability to self-detect malignant melanoma decreases with age. Clin Exp Dermatol 2011;36:499–501.

18. Fisher NM, Schaffer JV, Berwick M, et al. Breslow depth of cutaneous melanoma: impact of factors related to surveillance of the skin, including prior skin biopsies and family history of melanoma. J Am Acad Dermatol 2005;53:393–406.

19. de Troya-Martin M, Blazquez-Sanchez N, Fernandez-Canedo I, et al. Dermoscopic study of cutaneous malignant melanoma: descriptive analysis of 45 cases. Actas Dermosifiliogr 2008;99:44–53 [in Spanish].

20. Carli P, de Giorgi V, Chiarugi A, et al. Addition of dermoscopy to conventional naked-eye examination in melanoma screening: a randomized study. J Am Acad Dermatol 2004;50:683–9.

21. Carli P, De Giorgi V, Crocetti E, et al. Improvement of malignant/benign ratio in excised melanocytic lesions in the 'dermoscopy era': a retrospective study 1997-2001. Br J Dermatol 2004;150:687–92.

22. Piccolo D, Ferrari A, Peris K, et al. Dermoscopic diagnosis by a trained clinician vs. a clinician with minimal dermoscopy training vs. computer-aided diagnosis of 341 pigmented skin lesions: a comparative study. Br J Dermatol 2002;147:481–6.

23. Noor O 2nd, Nanda A, Rao BK. A dermoscopy survey to assess who is using it and why it is or is not being used. Int J Dermatol 2009;48:951–2.

24. Haenssle HA, Krueger U, Vente C, et al. Results from an observational trial: digital epiluminescence microscopy follow-up of atypical nevi increases the sensitivity and the chance of success of conventional dermoscopy in detecting melanoma. J Invest Dermatol 2006;126:980–5.

25. Menzies SW, Emery J, Staples M, et al. Impact of dermoscopy and short-term sequential digital dermoscopy imaging for the management of pigmented lesions in primary care: a sequential intervention trial. Br J Dermatol 2009;161:1270–7.

26. Risser J, Pressley Z, Veledar E, et al. The impact of total body photography on biopsy rate in patients from a pigmented lesion clinic. J Am Acad Dermatol 2007;57:428–34.

27. Banky JP, Kelly JW, English DR, et al. Incidence of new and changed nevi and melanomas detected using baseline images and dermoscopy in patients at high risk for melanoma. Arch Dermatol 2005;141:998–1006.

28. Meyer LE, Otberg N, Sterry W, et al. In vivo confocal scanning laser microscopy: comparison of the reflectance and fluorescence mode by imaging human skin. J Biomed Opt 2006;11:044012.

29. Busam KJ, Hester K, Charles C, et al. Detection of clinically amelanotic malignant melanoma and

assessment of its margins by in vivo confocal scanning laser microscopy. Arch Dermatol 2001;137:923–9.

30. Ono I, Sakemoto A, Ogino J, et al. The real-time, three-dimensional analyses of benign and malignant skin tumors by confocal laser scanning microscopy. J Dermatol Sci 2006;43:135–41.

31. Rajadhyaksha M, Gonzalez S, Zavislan JM, et al. In vivo confocal scanning laser microscopy of human skin II: advances in instrumentation and comparison with histology. J Invest Dermatol 1999;113:293–303.

32. Gerger A, Koller S, Kern T, et al. Diagnostic applicability of in vivo confocal laser scanning microscopy in melanocytic skin tumors. J Invest Dermatol 2005;124:493–8.

33. Gerger A, Hofmann-Wellenhof R, Langsenlehner U, et al. In vivo confocal laser scanning microscopy of melanocytic skin tumours: diagnostic applicability using unselected tumour images. Br J Dermatol 2008;158:329–33.

34. Langley RG, Walsh N, Sutherland AE, et al. The diagnostic accuracy of in vivo confocal scanning laser microscopy compared to dermoscopy of benign and malignant melanocytic lesions: a prospective study. Dermatology 2007;215:365–72.

35. Gerger A, Wiltgen M, Langsenlehner U, et al. Diagnostic image analysis of malignant melanoma in in vivo confocal laser-scanning microscopy: a preliminary study. Skin Res Technol 2008;14:359–63.

36. Koller S, Wiltgen M, Ahlgrimm-Siess V, et al. In vivo reflectance confocal microscopy: automated diagnostic image analysis of melanocytic skin tumours. J Eur Acad Dermatol Venereol 2011;25:554–8.

37. Wiltgen M, Bloice M, Koller S, et al. Computer-aided diagnosis of melanocytic skin tumors by use of confocal laser scanning microscopy images. Anal Quant Cytol Histol 2011;33:85–100.

38. Moncrieff M, Cotton S, Claridge E, et al. Spectrophotometric intracutaneous analysis: a new technique for imaging pigmented skin lesions. Br J Dermatol 2002;146:448–57.

39. Haniffa MA, Lloyd JJ, Lawrence CM. The use of a spectrophotometric intracutaneous analysis device in the real-time diagnosis of melanoma in the setting of a melanoma screening clinic. Br J Dermatol 2007;156:1350–2.

40. Emery JD, Hunter J, Hall PN, et al. Accuracy of SIAscopy for pigmented skin lesions encountered in primary care: development and validation of a new diagnostic algorithm. BMC Dermatol 2010;10:9.

41. Gutkowicz-Krusin D, Elbaum M, Jacobs A, et al. Precision of automatic measurements of pigmented skin lesion parameters with a MelaFind(TM) multispectral digital dermoscope. Melanoma Res 2000;10:563–70.

42. Monheit G, Cognetta AB, Ferris L, et al. The performance of MelaFind: a prospective multicenter study. Arch Dermatol 2011;147:188–94.

43. Kivela T. Diagnosis of uveal melanoma. Dev Ophthalmol 2012;49:1–15.

44. Vogt M, Knuttel A, Hoffmann K, et al. Comparison of high frequency ultrasound and optical coherence tomography as modalities for high resolution and non invasive skin imaging. Biomed Tech 2003;48:116–21.

45. de Giorgi V, Stante M, Massi D, et al. Possible histopathologic correlates of dermoscopic features in pigmented melanocytic lesions identified by means of optical coherence tomography. Exp Dermatol 2005;14:56–9.

46. Welzel J. Optical coherence tomography in dermatology: a review. Skin Res Technol 2001;7:1–9.

47. Rallan D, Bush NL, Bamber JC, et al. Quantitative discrimination of pigmented lesions using three-dimensional high-resolution ultrasound reflex transmission imaging. J Invest Dermatol 2007;127:189–95.

48. Wachsman W, Morhenn V, Palmer T, et al. Noninvasive genomic detection of melanoma. Br J Dermatol 2011;164:797–806.

49. Cone CD Jr. The role of the surface electrical transmembrane potential in normal and malignant mitogenesis. Ann N Y Acad Sci 1974;238:420–35.

50. Han A, Yang L, Frazier AB. Quantification of the heterogeneity in breast cancer cell lines using whole-cell impedance spectroscopy. Clin Cancer Res 2007;13:139–43.

51. Alqabandi JA, Abdel-Motal UM, Youcef-Toumi K. Extracting cancer cell line electrochemical parameters at the single cell level using a microfabricated device. Biotechnol J 2009;4:216–23.

52. Aberg P, Birgersson U, Elsner P, et al. Electrical impedance spectroscopy and the diagnostic accuracy for malignant melanoma. Exp Dermatol 2011;20:648–52.

53. Har-Shai Y, Glickman YA, Siller G, et al. Electrical impedance scanning for melanoma diagnosis: a validation study. Plast Reconstr Surg 2005;116:782–90.

54. Astbury WT, Street A. X-ray studies of the structure of hair, wool, and related fibres. I. General. Trans R Soc Lond 1931;230:75–101.

55. James VJ. Fiber diffraction of skin and nails provides an accurate diagnosis of malignancies. Int J Cancer 2009;125:133–8.

56. Ophir J, Cespedes I, Ponnekanti H, et al. Elastography: a quantitative method for imaging the elasticity of biological tissues. Ultrason Imaging 1991;13:111–34.

57. Hinz T, Wenzel J, Schmid-Wendtner MH. Real-time tissue elastography: a helpful tool in the diagnosis of cutaneous melanoma? J Am Acad Dermatol 2011;65:424–6.

58. Ginat DT, Destounis SV, Barr RG, et al. US elastography of breast and prostate lesions. Radiographics 2009;29:2007–16.

59. Herman C, Cetingul MP. Quantitative visualization and detection of skin cancer using dynamic thermal imaging. J Vis Exp 2011;(51). pii: 2679.

60. Ehmann R, Boedeker E, Friedrich U, et al. Canine scent detection in the diagnosis of lung cancer: revisiting a puzzling phenomenon. Eur Respir J 2012;39(3):669–76.

61. McCulloch M, Jezierski T, Broffman M, et al. Diagnostic accuracy of canine scent detection in early- and late-stage lung and breast cancers. Integr Cancer Ther 2006;5:30–9.

62. Williams H, Pembroke A. Sniffer dogs in the melanoma clinic? Lancet 1989;1:734.

63. Church J, Williams H. Another sniffer dog for the clinic? Lancet 2001;358:930.

Index

Note: Page numbers of article titles are in **boldface** type.

A

ABCD rule
  in dermatoscopy for melanoma and pigmented
    lesions, 416–417
Acrolentiginous melanoma
  pathologic features of, 450
Age
  in melanoma prognosis, 477–478
AJCC. *See* American Joint Committee on Cancer
  (AJCC)
American Joint Committee on Cancer (AJCC)
  melanoma classification by, 469–477. *See also*
    Melanoma, classification of, by AJCC
  melanoma database of
    electronic prediction tool based on, 477–479
      age as factor in, 477–478
      exclusion of mitotic rate in, 477
  melanoma staging guidelines of, 457–458,
    469–477
Anesthesia/anesthetics
  in biopsy of pigmented lesions, 436–437
Animal melanoma
  pathologic features of, 451
Anti–cytotoxic T-lymphocyte antigen-4 monoclonal
  antibodies
  in metastatic melanoma, 520–521
Anti–programmed death 1 monoclonal antibodies
  in metastatic melanoma, 522
Array comparative genomic hybridization
  in histopathologic diagnosis of melanoma, 456
Artifact(s)
  from Monsel solution
    vs. cutaneous melanoma, 454
Artificial UV tanning
  melanoma related to, 364–365
ASAP algorithm
  in dermatoscopy for melanoma and pigmented
    lesions, 423–427
Atypical melanocytic cutaneous lesions of uncertain
  diagnosis
  surgical treatment of, 496
Avobenzone
  in sunscreens, 372

B

B-K mole syndrome, 389
Balloon cell melanoma
  pathologic features of, 451–452

Benzophenones
  in sunscreens, 372
Biomarker(s)
  genetic
    melanoma, 482–483
Biopsy. *See also specific types and indications*
  of pigmented lesions, **435–443**. *See also*
    Pigmented lesions, biopsy of
Bone metastasis
  radiation therapy for, 531
Brain metastasis
  radiation therapy for, 530–531
Breslow depth
  in melanoma prognosis, 458

C

C-kit inhibitors
  for metastatic melanoma, 520
CASH algorithm
  in dermatoscopy for melanoma and pigmented
    lesions, 420–423
Central nervous system (CNS)
  CMN effects on, 380–381
Children
  cutaneous melanoma in
    pathologic features of, 452–453
  scalp nevi in
    biopsy in evaluation of, 441
Cinnamates
  in sunscreens, 371
Clark levels
  in melanoma prognosis, 460
Clear cell sarcoma
  pathologic features of, 452
CMN. *See* Congenital melanocytic nevi (CMN)
CNS. *See* Central nervous system (CNS)
Confocal microscopy
  for melanoma, 511
Confocal scanning laser microscopy (CSLM)
  in melanoma, 536–539
Congenital melanoblastic proliferation
  vs. cutaneous melanoma, 454
Congenital melanocytic nevi (CMN)
  CNS involvement
    risk of, 380–381
  malignancy related to
    risk of, 381–383
  management of

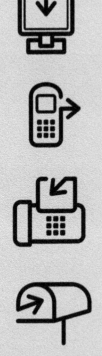

Printed and bound by CPI Group (UK) Ltd, Croydon, CR0 4YY
03/10/2024
01040354-0019